AF352353

Migraine

Migraine

Pharmacology and genetics

Edited by

Merton Sandler
Department of Chemical Pathology, Queen Charlotte's and Chelsea Hospital, UK

Michel Ferrari
Department of Neurology, University Hospital, Leiden, The Netherlands

and

Sara Harnett
UK

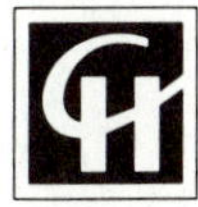

Altman
An imprint of Chapman & Hall

London • Glasgow • Weinheim • New York • Tokyo • Melbourne • Madras

Published by Altman, an imprint of Chapman & Hall, 2–6 Boundary Row, London SE1 8HN, UK

Chapman & Hall, 2–6 Boundary Row, London SE1 8HN, UK

Blackie Academic & Professional, Wester Cleddens Road, Bishopbriggs, Glasgow G64 2NZ, UK

Chapman & Hall GmbH, Pappelallee 3, 69469 Weinheim, Germany

Chapman & Hall USA, 115 Fifth Avenue, New York, NY 10003, USA

Chapman & Hall Japan, 1TP-Japan, Kyowa Building, 3F, 2–2–1 Hirakawacho, Chiyoda-ku, Tokyo 102, Japan

Chapman & Hall Australia, 102 Dodds Street, South Melbourne, Victoria 3205, Australia

Chapman & Hall India, R. Seshadri, 32 Second Main Road, CIT East, Madras 600 035, India

First edition 1996

© 1996 Chapman & Hall

Typeset in Palatino 10/12pt by Photoprint, Torquay, Devon
Printed in Great Britain by Cambridge University Press

ISBN 1 86036 006 8

A catalogue record for this book is available from the British Library

Library of Congress Catalog Card Number: 96–83041

∞ Printed on permanent acid-free text paper, manufactured in accordance with ANSI/NISO Z39.48–1992 and ANSI/NISO Z39.48–1984 (Permanence of Paper).

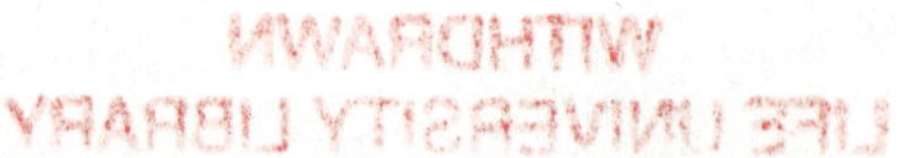

Contents

Contents

List of contributors

F. Ahmed
Department of Neurology
Charing Cross Hospital
London
UK

J.A. Bard
Synaptic Pharmaceutical Corporation
215 College Road
Paramus
New Jersey 07652
USA

W.A. Bax*
Department of Pharmacology
Erasmus University
Rotterdam
The Netherlands

D.T. Beattie
Systems Biology
Glaxo Wellcome Research
Stevenage
Herts
SG1 2NY
UK

I. Bouchelet
Montreal Neurological Institute
3801 University Street
Montréal
Québec
Canada
H3A 2B4

T.A. Branchek*
Synaptic Pharmaceutical Corporation
215 College Road
Paramus
New Jersey 07652
USA

G.W. Bruyn*
Department of Neurology
University Hospital
Leiden
The Netherlands

Z. Cohen
Montreal Neurological Institute
3801 University Street
Montréal
Québec
Canada
H3A 2B4

H.E. Connor*
Receptor Pharmacology
Glaxo Wellcome Research
Stevenage
Herts
SG1 2NY
UK

P. de Vries
Department of Pharmacology
Erasmus University
Rotterdam
The Netherlands

H.C. Diener*
Department of Neurology
University of Essen
45122 Essen
Germany

L. Edvinsson*
Department of Internal Medicine
Lund University Hospital
S-221 85 Lund
Sweden

M.D. Ferrari*
Department of Neurology
University Hospital
2300 RC Leiden
The Netherlands

J.R. Fozard*
Sandoz Pharma Ltd
CH-4002 Basel
Switzerland

R.R. Frants*
MGC Department of Human Genetics
Leiden University
Leiden
The Netherlands

P.J. Goadsby*
Institute of Neurology
Queen Square
London
WC1N 3BG
UK

V. Glover*
Department of Paediatrics
Queen Charlotte's and Chelsea Hospital
Goldhawk Road
London
W6 0XG
UK

J. Haan*
Department of Neurology
University Hospital
Leiden
The Netherlands

E. Hamel*
Montreal Neurological Institute
3801 University Street
Montréal
Québec
Canada
H3A 2B4

P.P.A. Humphrey*
Glaxo Institute of Applied Pharmacology
University of Cambridge
Tennis Court Road
Cambridge
CB2 1QJ
UK

N. Hussein
Kingston University
Kingston upon Thames
UK

J. Jarman
Kingston University
Kingston upon Thames
UK

N. Jarrett
Department of Paediatrics
Queen Charlotte's and Chelsea Hospital
Goldhawk Road
London
W6 0XG
UK

S.A. Kucharewicz
Synaptic Pharmaceutical Corporation
215 College Road
Paramus
New Jersey 07652
USA

J.W. Lance*
Suite 5A
66 High Street
Randwick
New South Wales 2031
Australia

D. Lindhout
Department of Clinical Genetics
Erasmus University
Rotterdam
The Netherlands

A. Maassen van den Brink
Department of Pharmacology
Erasmus University
Rotterdam
The Netherlands

G.R. Martin*
Receptor Pharmacology Group
Wellcome Research Laboratories
Langley Court
Beckenham
Kent
BR3 3BS
UK

R.S. Martin
Receptor Pharmacology Group
Wellcome Research Laboratories
Langley Court
Beckenham
Kent
BR3 3BS
UK

A. May
Department of Neurology
University of Essen
45122 Essen
Germany

K.R. Merikangas*
Genetic Epidemiology Research Unit
Yale University School of Medicine
40 Temple Street
New Haven
Connecticut 06510
USA

M.A. Moskowitz*
Stroke and Neurovascular Regulation
Neurology and Neurosurgery
Massachusetts General Hospital
Harvard Medical School
Boston
Massachusetts 02114
USA

J. Olesen
Department of Neurology
Glostrup Hospital
University of Copenhagen
DK-2600 Glostrup
Denmark

R.A. Ophoff
MGC Department of Human Genetics
Leiden University
Leiden
The Netherlands

R.C. Peatfield*
The Princess Margaret Migraine Clinic
Charing Cross Hospital
Fulham Palace Road
London
W6 8RF
UK

A. Pilgrim*
Glaxo Research and Development
Greenford
Middlesex
UB6 0HE
UK

K.A. Sandkuijl
MGC Department of Human Genetics
Leiden University
Leiden
The Netherlands

M. Sandler*
Department of Chemical Pathology
Queen Charlotte's and Chelsea Hospital
Goldhawk Road
London
W6 0XG
UK

P.R. Saxena
Department of Pharmacology
Erasmus University
Rotterdam
The Netherlands

J. Schoenen*
Department of Neurology
University of Liège
CHR Citadelle
Boulevard du 12eme de Ligne 1
B-400 Liège
Belgium

P. Séguéla
Montreal Neurological Institute
3801 University Street
Montréal
Québec
Canada H3A 2B4

G.M. Terwindt
Department of Neurology
University Hospital
Leiden
The Netherlands

L.L. Thomsen*
Department of Neurology
Glostrup Hospital
University of Copenhagen
DK-2600 Glostrup
Denmark

E. Tournier-Lasserve*
INSERM U 25
Faculte de Medecine Necker Enfants-Malades
156 rue de Vaugirard
75730 Paris
Cedex 15
France

C. Urban
Department of Neurology
Essen University
Essen
Germany

R. van Eijk
MGC Department of Human Genetics
Leiden University
Leiden
The Netherlands

W.H. Visser
Department of Neurology
University Hospital
2300 RC Leiden
The Netherlands

R.L. Weinshank
Synaptic Pharmaceutical Corporation
215 College Road
Paramus
New Jersey 07652
USA

* Participant in Migraine Research Symposium (Malaga, Spain, 18–20 May 1995).

Preface

The nature of migraine continues to elude us. Even so, there has been massive progress in this field in recent years, largely based on the therapeutic benefit resulting from the interaction of drugs, such as sumatriptan, with certain 5-hydroxytryptamine receptors.

Taken together with the arrival of new and sophisticated imaging techniques and the insights provided by the latter-day genetic revolution, many key researchers in the field believe that the old kaleidoscopic image bequeathed by Wolff is broken and that a new picture has begun to emerge. They decided to take stock and this book is the result.

Many of these reinterpretations and, indeed, a substantial proportion of the new findings presented within, are startling. What is the role of the neurotrophins and does nerve growth factor form the basis of migraine pain? How do we interpret the PET scan changes revealed in the medulla during a migraine attack? How close are we to cracking the genetic basis of migraine? The contents of this book cannot fail to be of crucial interest to pharmacologists, geneticists, neurologists and, indeed, to all with an interest in this fascinating topic.

1

Whither migraine research?

G.W. Bruyn

The purpose of this compilation is to reflect on migraine research in the next millennium, a subject perhaps more seductive and appropriate for ambitious futurologists than for clinical and basic researchers. Inasmuch as today is the parent of an uncertain tomorrow, this introductory chapter might serve our objective best by critically cataloguing what we know and understand of such a complex, endemic and intriguing disorder as migraine.

SEMANTIC PROBLEMS

As insufficient distinction is made between a migrainous attack and migraine as a disorder, the annual yield of more than 600 papers on migraine tends to create a Babel-like confusion. Introduction of the International Headache Society (IHS) diagnostic criteria (Headache Classification Committee 1988) ought to have prevented, or at least reduced, such a state of affairs. However, the attack criteria include 3–5 variables, each comprising 1–4 subvariables, an ensemble inviting misdiagnosis: if, according to these criteria, a patient develops a 76-hour continuous headache which limits day-to-day activities, worsens on routine physical exertion and is associated with photophobia, the diagnosis of migraine without aura may be applied. The patient might just as easily, however, have meningitis, dural sinus thrombosis, or a subarachnoid bleed.

Migraine: Pharmacology and genetics
Edited by Merton Sandler, Michel Ferrari and Sara Harnett
Published in 1996 by Chapman & Hall
ISBN 1 86036 006 8

The IHS criteria for migraine as a disease remain silent about such discriminant factors as: 1) attacks over a sufficiently extended minimum period of time; 2) the stereotypy of migraine's sequence of stages and of symptom pattern; 3) the side-alternation of features; 4) the absence of post-ictal sequelae; 5) the diagnostic weight of such factors as age at onset and sex; and 6) the relevance of the course of the disorder. This is made clear by the numerous reported instances of symptomatic 'migraine' with intracranial tumours, arteriovenous malformation, mitochondrial encephalopathy with lactic acidosis and strokes (MELAS), polycythaemia and even C_2-root neurinoma (Bruyn 1984a, Shimizu *et al*. 1993, Goldhammer 1993).

How can one expect a physician to make a correct diagnosis, when the IHS criteria permit the absence of components, as in 'migraine without aura', 'migraine sine hemicrania', 'incomplete migraine' (which themselves vary in frequency, duration and intensity)?

Refinement and revision of these 1988 IHS criteria should not be impossible during the coming decade. A multi-centre, statistically planned analysis of accurately recorded clinical features and their duration, sequence and intensity in, say, 3000 well-diagnosed migraine patients may well be practicable with present-day information technology.

CLASSIFICATION

Taxonomies of the past, as devised, for example, by Aristotle, Linnaeus (a dysphrenic migraineur with Doppelgänger auras), Buffon, or de Sauvages, were idiosyncratic and, inevitably, based on phenomenology. The present-day revolution in neurological classification brought about by molecular biology has underscored the importance of fundamental knowledge. Such knowledge is lacking in the field of migraine and we still have to classify its complex manifestations at the lowest, i.e. descriptive, level of sophistication. As a solace, the virtue of any accepted classification lies in its power to have everyone make identical mistakes.

The 1988 IHS classification needs a critical reevaluation. Deletion of such varieties as 'abdominal', 'retinal', 'ophthalmoplegic', 'facioplegic', 'hemiplegic' and 'familial hemiplegic' migraine, as well as 'benign paroxysmal vertigo' and 'alternating juvenile hemiplegia' should be considered. The first five, like MELAS, appear to be different disorders, occasionally or regularly associated with symptomatic migrainous attacks, and the last two may not even be associated with headache. Familial hemiplegic migraine, like hereditary episodic ataxia, is most likely to be an allelic heterogenic variant of the chromosome 19-associated vascular disorder CADASIL. 'Familial hemiplegic migraine with nystagmus and/or retinal degeneration and/or deafness' (Codina *et al*.

1971a, b, Zifkin *et al.* 1980) is another variety that needs reclassification. On the contrary, the revised classification should include 'dysphrenic migraine' and consider inclusion or, rather, the definition of 'migraine with CSF pleocytosis with or without ataxia and/or spastic paraparesis' (Bruyn *et al.* 1984, Marti Massi *et al.* 1984, Stamboulis *et al.* 1987, Goldstein *et al.* 1990), and 'dystonic/choreatic migraine' (Bruyn and Ferrari 1984).

Finally, the prevalent IHS distinction between migraine with and without aura constitutes a challenging cognitive exercise for a future IHS committee. The study by Sanin *et al.* (1994) on 400 patients showed that 96% of migraine patients with aura attacks also had non-aura attacks, a perfect example of a Popperian 'invalidation' study.

EPIDEMIOLOGY

One area which future migraine research can safely do without is epidemiology. Epidemiological studies, consuming considerable energy, time and money, vary so widely in their results as to be scientifically meaningless. Ziegler (1990) found the reported prevalence to range between 1 and 85%, and Stewart *et al.* (1994) between 1.7 and 48%, confirming the wide prevalence gap of between 0 and 38% recorded by Bruyn (1985) in a review of prevalence figures reported between 1930 and 1984. In this context, an interesting study was reported by Mitsikostas *et al.* (1994) concerning migraine prevalence among the 1500 monks of Athos, a monastery on a peninsula where no woman is allowed to set foot. These monks fast for six months per year, avoid milk and fats, and have religious services from 2 a.m. until 8 a.m. Migraine prevalence in this rigidly religious community amounted to a mere 1.7%, which may show that celibacy and lack of sleep or food are not risk factors!

Apart from prevalence, severity is an issue that must be taken into account. Blau (1994), for instance, found that the annual migraine-induced absence from work among 50 migrainous colleagues amounted to less than half a day.

PATHOGENESIS

The absence of neuropathological as well as of unequivocally specific biochemical data in a disorder which manifests with episodic transient dysfunction without sequelae (like paroxysmal tachycardia, intestinal colic or muscle cramp) makes for a degree of pathogenetic uncertainty that provides fertile soil for speculation. Thus, three major hypotheses of migraine pathogenesis hold sway, humoral, vascular and neurogenic, depending on the surmised primacy of the attack-provoking factor or mechanism and the importance of the constitution underlying the disease. Their boundaries are blurred and tend to merge.

Humoral hypothesis

This theory holds that one or more biochemical compounds, present or circulating in body fluids and normally playing an unobtrusive part in metabolism, suddenly appear (or disappear) beyond normal limits and initiate the attack. Since Harold G. Wolff's neurokinin, attention has focused successively on histamine, tyramine, prostaglandins and calcium overload, and only serotonin (5-hydroxytryptamine, 5-HT) has survived as a possible humoral factor. The origins of its putative role lay with Sicuteri (1959) who noted the prophylactic effect of methysergide, and observed increased urinary 5-hydroxyindoleacetic acid (5-HIAA) excretion during attacks (Sicuteri *et al.* 1961), a finding soon corroborated by Curran *et al.* (1965). Kimball *et al.* (1960) treated reserpine-induced attacks by intravenous (iv) 5-HT injection whilst Anthony *et al.* (1967) observed a drop in plasma 5-HT during spontaneous episodes.

Although Ferrari *et al.* (1989) were unable to confirm the existence of Anthony's (1986) platelet serotonin-releasing factor (PSRF) in serum of migraine patients, the phenomenon, particularly in the prodromal stage might well repay further study.

The focus of interest on 5-HT as a humoral factor has now shifted to one of its receptors, the 5-HT_{1D} subtype. That such a receptor subclass rather suddenly becomes hypoactive, only to resume its normal state of activity after the attack, seems unlikely. The migraine-alleviating effects of 5-HT_{1D} agonists such as sumatriptan may well owe their success to some pharmacological action of these drugs rather than by entering into some physiological sequence.

In the past few years, two new humoral factors or, rather, humoral-endothelial factors, have entered the scene. One is the potent local vasodilator, nitric oxide (NO), synthesized in the endothelium, macrophages and certain (NADH-diaphorase-positive) neurons in the cortex, olfactory bulbs, cerebellum, neostriatum and two hypothalamic nuclei. The substrate is arginine, the enzyme acting on it is NO synthase (NOS; diaphorase), using Ca^{2+}, calmodulin and tetrahydrobiopterin as cofactors. The endproducts are citrulline and NO. Its half-life is about six seconds and its relaxant effect on vascular myocytes is mediated by cGMP. Although NOS-positive fibres are present in the meningeal arteries (Berger *et al.* 1994) and glutamate-induced activation of *N*-methyl-D-aspartate (NMDA) receptors leads to NO formation, its role in migraine pathogenesis has remained uncertain despite a huge literature on NO and expectations that spreading oligaemia would show unequivocal concomitant NO changes.

The potent local (venous) vasoconstrictors known as endothelins 1, 2 and 3 are also synthesized in the endothelium, by endopeptidases from the 203–213 aminoacid-containing preproendothelin via the 38 amino acid peptide, proendothelin 1, and act on two receptor classes, ET-A and ET-B. Again, despite a prolific literature, the endothelins have not yet proved their significance in migraine pathogenesis. Like NO, their effects on glia and venous (more than arterial) microvasculature did not fulfil their promise.

Vascular hypothesis

The vascular hypothesis of migraine pathogenesis boasts a venerable pedigree, dating from the days of Liveing, Dubois-Reymond and Möllendorf. Following the 150-year span between the old distinction between 'white' and 'red' migraines and Harold G. Wolff's proposition of penury perfusion in the cerebral followed by luxury perfusion in the dural arterial systems (exerting its spell to the mid-seventies), realization has dawned that migrainous vascular phenomena are an epiphenomenon rather than a primary, causative factor. The observations and arguments militating against a vascular pathogenetic theory include the following: migraine attacks usually appear about (pre-)puberty when the vascular tree is healthy, and disappear in the age-groups prone to vascular accidents; the clinical symptomatology of transient ischaemic attacks, cerebral infarctions, etc. are quite unlike those of classical migraine attacks; migraine preferentially involves the posterior cerebral circulation, autonomically innervated by the vertebrobasilar plexus, while the posterior fossa's dural innervation is vagal and hypoglossal rather than trigeminal; the duration of premonitory symptoms (6–48 h) appears incompatible with vasospasm (Isler 1986); no incontrovertible angiographic evidence of spasm during an attack has been presented; vasospasm is incapable of explaining the caudorostral spread of the scintillating scotoma (Bruyn 1982) and also fails to explain the occurrence of hemi/monoparesis, cheiro-oral auras (the postcentral and precentral convolutions being supplied by the same branches of the middle cerebral artery); the unilaterality of the presumed vasospasm, which induced Lance and coworkers (Goadsby *et al.* 1982, 1985, Lance *et al.* 1983, 1990, Lambert *et al.* 1984) to perform their exemplary experiments on the monkey's coeruleus, raphe and trigeminal nuclei; the rare but direct observations of cerebral bulging (brain oedema) through cranial burr holes or developmental foramina parietalia permagna during a migraine attack (Goltman 1935–36, Olsen *et al.* 1984, Blau and Solomon 1985, Meyer 1985, Goldstein *et al.* 1990); the absence of migraine symptoms in (generalized) temporal arteritis, whereas headache, nausea and vomiting are cardinal features of leptomeningeal irritation, as occurs, for example, in meningitis, subarachnoid haemorrhage and dural sinus thrombosis (Blau 1978, Blau and Dexter 1981).

The moribund vascular theory, ready to receive the coup de grâce by the humoral 5-HT receptor hypothesis, was granted a stay of execution by the Scandinavian observation of oligaemia, spreading at a rate of approximately 2 mm/min in an occipitofrontal direction in aura attacks provoked by carotid puncture, whilst not manifesting, or rarely so, in non-aura attacks (Olesen *et al.* 1981, 1982, Lauritzen *et al.* 1983, Lauritzen and Olesen 1984). In a recent review, Lauritzen (1994) drew attention to disparity between provoked and spontaneous spreading oligaemia.

The discovery of cortical spreading hypoperfusion ignited an explosion of enthusiasm throughout the migraine community because of its potential connection with Leão's neurogenic spreading depression, despite the fact that Stirling Meyer's group, using a somewhat comparable technique, had consistently found a 30% hyperaemia in well over 400 cases (Kobari *et al.* 1990).

What seemed a rejuvenating paradigm for the vascular theory in agonal state, soon proved to be a false lead. Was the spreading hypoperfusion equivalent to cerebral ischaemia? Original figures yielded a 20–30% reduction in regional cerebral blood flow (rCBF) following intracarotid ^{133}Xe-injection, distinctly above the level of neuronal ischaemia (Olesen *et al.* 1981, Lauritzen *et al.* 1983). In spontaneously occurring attacks, using the ^{133}Xe inhalation method, single photon emission computed tomography (SPECT) data yielded an average reduction of 17 ± 7% about two hours after attack onset (Lauritzen and Olesen 1984). Subsequent reports ranged from 12% (Friberg *et al.* 1994a) and 20–25% (Lauritzen 1994) to 60% (Olsen 1990 1993), giving rise to rather fruitless discussion on the Compton scatter effect. The cerebral tolerance limit for hypoperfusion is 18 ml/min/100g (Heiss 1983), i.e. a rCBF reduction of 65%. The spreading hypoperfusion respected anatomical, but disregarded arterial supply boundaries, which rather disposed of an arteriospastic pathogenesis. This finding appeared more in line with Leão's phenomenon.

Disquieting conflicting findings by the Scandinavian group were pointed out earlier (Bruyn 1984b): in some attacks hypoperfusion was not observed; in some it manifested bilaterally although the aura was unilateral (Lauritzen 1987), thus ending Compton-scatter and ischaemia discussions; it occurred also in some common migraine attacks, dispelling the notion (never entertained by clinicians; Wilkinson and Blau 1985) that common and classical migraine are different entities; in one of the original cases, there was spreading oligaemia but no migraine attack; in most patients, the oligaemia preceded or lasted well beyond the aura stage, a disjunction between rCBF and symptoms that cast doubt on the causal significance of oligaemia (Andersen *et al.* 1988). The

[133]Xe method measures CBF particularly in cerebral convexity surfaces. It does not convincingly visualize cuneate and lingual gyri (Brodmann area 17) bordering the calcarine sulcus on the mesial, deeply-hidden surface of the brain, where the scintillating scotoma is generated. Also, theoretically, spreading oligaemia proceeding on the brain's convexity from the tip of the occipital lobe (the extremity of area 17) towards postcentral areas 3, 1, 2 and 5, thereby passing through areas 18, 19, 39 and 40, should produce clinically a limited central scotoma, followed by visual hallucinations, receptive aphasia, terminating with cheiro-oral paraesthesias, a sequence of aura symptoms I have never seen and doubt whether anyone else has.

The hypoperfusion, also mentioned in a neglected positron emission tomography (PET) study by Herold *et al.* (1985), received anecdotal confirmation by PET findings made in a 28-year old migraineuse who had bilateral spreading hypoperfusion during a spontaneous common migraine attack (Woods *et al.* 1994). Clearly, then, the vascular theory is left without its trump card, a caudorostral ripple of hypoperfusion that may (usually) occur during a classical (but also a common) migraine attack; (rarely) without an attack; not during such an attack; bilaterally in a unilateral attack; and, finally, not being a primary vasospastic event. For all we know, cortical spreading depression (SD) might occur in cluster headache, trigeminal neuralgia, or even in healthy persons, as a sort of 'self-purgation' function of the brain to rid itself of 1/F noise and re-set cortical networks.

Even if the relationship between clinical symptoms and rCBF data appears tenuous, the agenda for future research on the significance of occipito-rostral spreading oligaemia should focus on: the effect of prolonged eye-closure, or loud phono- or bright photostimulation, or raised intracranial pressure through impeded venous return (Valsalva-manoeuvre, straining) on the generation or progress of spreading oligaemia; identification of oligaemia in patients with (exclusive) cheiro-oral, dysphrenic, aphasic or dysosmic auras; refinement of PET techniques to study calcarine phenomena (if any) more closely; and structural and ultrastructural study of possible differences between corticopial capillary and venular systems of occipital and frontal lobes that may account for the predominant frequency of visual auras and the rarity of frontal or temporal auras cf. spreading oligaemias.

Neurogenic hypothesis

Clinical evidence, as well as experimental work, persuasively argues in favour of a primary neural cause of migraine, with vascular epi-phenomena, rather than *vice versa* (Blau 1984). Several hypothetical approaches to the neural pathophysiology of migraine have been suggested.

Sicuteri's (1976) central dysnociception theory is based on a series of pharmacological findings, from which he argued that central 5-HT deficiency would produce a denervation supersensitivity, inhibiting the endogenous pontomesencephalic opioid receptor system which, in turn, inhibits spinotrigeminothalamic nociceptor afferents. This was an original concept, supported by the strong resemblance of the symptoms of migraine to those of the morphine withdrawal syndrome, as well as by reportedly low CSF endorphin values and modern anatomical data (Basbaum and Fields 1978, Baskin *et al.* 1986, Raskin *et al.* 1987). Sicuteri's can be epitomized as the first of the brainstem theories.

Lance began a series of experiments in monkeys to explain migraine's lateralization and trigeminocervical territory of symptoms. Electro-stimulation of the serotonergic dorsal raphe nucleus produced vaso-dilatation in extra- and intracranial arterial trees, and stimulation of the noradrenergic locus coeruleus gave rise to vasoconstriction of cerebral and dilatation of extracranial vasculature. Presumed concomitant activation of the spinal descending trigeminal nucleus would, by antidromic pulse flow, produce increased permeability of dural vessels (so-called neurogenic inflammation) and pain in one side of the head, as well as parasympathetic effects via the greater superficial petrosal nerve, the orthodromic arm of a trigeminovascular reflex. Coerulean nor-adrenaline (NA) release would induce platelet 5-HT release and inhibit the central nociceptive control system of trigeminothalamic afferents. This articulate and intelligent construct, Lance's 'coeruleo-raphe con-cept' can be regarded as the second brainstem theory.

The crucial questions remain, however, as to what the pathophysio-logical equivalent of animal electrostimulation is in man, and how the alleged coeruleo-raphe discharge is generated. How do we explain that the adjacent salivary and ambiguus nuclei (autonomic symptoms!) escape immediate involvement or that the alleged activation of the spinal descending Vth nerve nucleus remains limited to its most caudal part (corresponding to its ophthalmic branch) which is farthest away from the raphe and coerulean nuclei and close to ambiguus, dorsal vagal, cuneate and gracile nuclei? The neuroanatomical obstacles to the model proposed by Lance (and Moskowitz, see below) are simple, notwithstanding the recent breakthrough discovery by Diener of contralateral pontomesencephalic hyperaemia (Diener and May, this volume): a presumed coeruleo-raphe discharge, triggering a spinal descending Vth nerve nucleus (caudal part) discharge, would in itself not only be an extraordinary event, but would also activate coerulean efferents, i.e. Probst's bundle to the Xth nerve nucleus dorsalis, Schütz's dorsal longitudinal fasciculus and the lateral tegmentoreticular tract. At best, this might produce pain according to the central representation pattern of facial sensation known as van Sölden's lines (and not a peripheral Vth nerve ophthalmic pattern). Secondly, coeruleo-raphe activation would primarily affect intraparenchymal cortical micro-vasculature, and the antidromic trigeminal discharge cannot remain restricted to the dura and its vessels, but must also affect the pial network because the leptomeningeal rami are branches of the dural nerves. The question of 5-HT and NA innervation of either large or small arteries in cortex, dura or pia mater was essentially clarified by Reinhard *et al.* (1979), Edvinsson *et al.* (1983), Bonvento *et al.* (1991) and, definitively, by Mathiau *et al.* (1993).

Finally, an ipsilateral superior cervical ganglion-derived rich neuro-peptide Y/tyrosine hydroxylase (NPY/TH) and poor substance P/calcitonin gene-related peptide/vasoactive intestinal peptide (SP/CGRP/VIP) innerva-tion of anterior/middle cerebral arteries, arterioles and veins, as opposed to a sparse innervation of the posterior circulation which seems predominantly involved in migraine (Edvinsson *et al.* 1994), is neglected in both Lance's and Moskowitz's models, as is the role of the sphenopalatine relay ganglion. The attack abortive effect of intranasal 4% lidocaine spray points to the significance of this circuit (Kudrow *et al.* 1995).

The model known as the 'trigeminovascular theory', originally suggested (Moskowitz *et al.* 1979) and championed by Moskowitz on the basis of a long, cohesive series of experiments, is essentially another brainstem theory. Its roots go back a century to the observations that either local application of mustard oil, xylene, or capsaicin (8-methylnonene-6-oxyvanillylamide, the active ingredient of red peppers) or antidromic electrostimulation of nociceptive C-fibres produce: a) hyperaemia due to vasodilatation; and b) oedema stemming from increased vasopermeability, with plasma protein exudate, a reaction known as neurogenic inflammation. This is caused by calcium-dependent release of SP and CGRP from C-fibre axon terminals, causing vasodilation. Substance P (like neurokinin A) also provokes oedema. Neurogenic inflammation can be abolished by SP antagonists, somatostatin (Lembeck *et al.* 1982, Foreman and Jordan 1984), ergotamine, indo-methacin, lofentanil, sumatriptan, methysergide, and a number of 5-HT$_1$ receptor agents (Krootila *et al.* 1992, Moskowitz 1992, Goadsby and Edvinsson 1993, Moussaoui *et al.* 1993).

The model proposes that an antidromic Vth nerve discharge produces dural neurogenic inflammation which, in its turn, orthodromically causes head pain as well as activation of the spinal descending Vth nerve nucleus with a parasympathetic VIP-mediated reflex through the greater superficial petrosal nerve. By methodical animal experimentation, SP was shown to be present in the walls of the middle cerebral artery and its proximal branches. Horseradish peroxidase, applied to the middle segment of the middle cerebral artery and to the middle meningeal artery, retrogradely stained approximately 0.05% of ipsilateral Gasserian ganglion cells, mainly in its ophthalmic branch portion. When it was applied to the superior sagittal sinus, these neurons stained bilaterally. Conspicuously, in all experiments, superior cervical ganglion cells stained, and when the peroxidase was applied to distal middle cerebral artery branches, Gasserian ganglion cells failed to take up stain, while superior cervical ganglion cells did so. The next step necessary to make the middle cerebral artery/dura/forehead pain relationship likely was made by O'Connor and van der Kooy (1986), whose experiments indicated that the Gasserian ganglion cells, innervating middle cerebral artery, middle meningeal artery and forehead, tended to cluster, although big Gasserian ganglion cells rather than small SP-containing cells stained. They hypothesized that these cell clusters might converge centripetally in the descending Vth nerve tract. Indeed, Strassman *et al.* (1986) during electrostimulation of the mesencephalic periaqueductal grey (Sicuteri's and Lance's central nociception inhibiting system), suppressed the response of spinal Vth nerve nucleus neurons to electrostimulation of the infraorbital nerve and the dura overlying the middle meningeal artery and superior sagittal sinus.

In addition, c-*fos* immunostaining was expressed in caudal Vth nerve nucleus neurons (Rexed laminae I and II equivalents) on noxious stimulation of the middle meningeal artery (Hunt *et al.* 1987) and Moskowitz *et al.* (1993) showed that cortical SD also causes c-*fos* expression in these neurons (as well as in the cortex; Herrera *et al.* 1993), which is blocked by sumatriptan, morphine and dihydroergotamine. In this way, the SD aura stage was linked to the pain stage, and a connection between cortical SD and trigeminovascular models (neuroanatomically improbable) experimentally established.

This, in brief, is a description of Moskowitz's trigeminovascular model, as shaped by a long series of methodical and intelligent animal experiments (Goadsby and Edvinsson 1993, Moskowitz and Macfarlane 1993). In spite of its appealing elegance, a number of considerations remain that question its clinical applicability, even apart from Diener's work showing that something happens in the brainstem during an attack (Diener and May, this volume): neurogenic inflammation can be elicited in the dura (external carotid supply!) but not in the brain and pia, despite rich pial vessel innervation (but the endothelial tight junctions there, constituting the blood–brain barrier, might prevent it); neurogenic inflammation occurs in 80% of ipsilateral postcapillary venules (Majno and Palade 1961, McDonald 1987, Dimitriadou *et al.* 1992) about which little is known concerning their trigeminal innervation; dural neurogenic inflammation has not been observed in man. The basic question (as with Lance's model) remains how the primary Vth nerve discharge is triggered and generated, because cortical SD certainly does not qualify as a cause, despite the animal c-*fos* data. One cannot equate 5 Hz, 5 min, 1 mA, 10 msec trains of square electrostimuli with physiological neuronal firing and the five per 10 000 Gasserian ganglion cells that stain with horseradish peroxidase appear to be well below the numerical threshold for physiological effects such as neurogenic inflammation and pain. If occipital spreading depression produces spinal Vth nerve tract c-*fos* expression, the neuroanatomist will wish to know which (antidromic) occipito-trigeminal tract mediates this event. The model does not account for the fact that an estimated 50% of migraine patients initially experience their pain in the occipito-nuchal area, which is devoid of Vth nerve innervation. Also a consequence of the model is that aura and head pain should invariably be experienced in opposite body-halves (which is usually but not always the case) (Peatfield *et al.* 1982, Jensen *et al.* 1986). SP and CGRP release in jugular venous blood during migraine attacks and on animal Vth nerve stimulation (Goadsby *et al.* 1988, 1990) could not be confirmed in man (Friberg *et al.* 1994b). The model fails to explain why such an unequivocal discharge as in trigeminal neuralgia does not bear any of the features on which the 'trigeminovascular' model rests: trigeminal neuralgia attacks last less than three minutes, manifest predominantly in the second and third divisions of the nerve and are not associated with autonomic disturbances. Cluster headache attacks, with their neurogenic inflammatory features of vasodilatation (conjunctival redness) and oedema (blocked, running nose) fit the model better. The intriguing neurogenic inflammatory changes in the venules are ignored.

The 'cerebral hyperexcitability state theory' (Welch *et al.* 1990, 1993) rests upon findings obtained with ^{31}P NMR spectroscopy in 17 migraine patients (14 with aura). The patients showed large-amplitude waves, long-lasting amplitude decrements and large-amplitude DC shifts during and between attacks. Taken together with known electrophysiological abnormalities of migraine patients, such as Golla's photic driving response at 22 Hz and increased contingent negative variation (CNV) amplitudes, as well as reduced intracellular cortical Mg^{2+} during attacks, a latent state of cortical hyperexcitability can be inferred.

The 'cortical spreading depression theory' is a derivative of the spreading oligaemia findings. Despite the fact that SD has not been observed in man (as countless neurosurgeons testify), it is well established in the experimental animal (for reviews, see Do Carmo 1992, Lauritzen 1987, 1994). SD is mechanically, electronically or chemically initiated (pin-prick, electrostimulation or application of cysteic acid or K^+) or receptor-mediated by glutamate/aspartate release, activating NMDA receptors. Pin-pricks elicit single SDs and cysteic acid or K^+

recurrent ones. Receptor-mediated SD spreads faster than K^+-induced SD, but is blocked by Mg^{2+}, which the latter is not.

An SD episode consists of a brief period of intense spiking, followed by a 15–60 mV negative deviation of the cerebral steady potential (due to synchronous depolarization of many apical dendrites of adjacent pyramidal cells and of glia), followed by a positive wave lasting 3–6 min, spreading tangentially over the cortex at 2–3 mm/min and 1–2 mm down into it. Electroencephalogram activity stops, sensory evoked responses show diminished amplitudes, cortical impedance increases by 17%, and massive ion shifts (Cl^-, Na^+ and Ca^{2+} influx, K^+ efflux) underlie the depolarization. The impedance increase is caused by cellular H_2O influx, so that the cells swell by 25–50% with a commensurate decrease of the interstitial space. Astrocytes can swell to five times their original volume without bursting (Tomita *et al.* 1994). The glial cell population is overtaxed with K^+ redistribution, there is massive though brief release of amino acids, and a decease of interstitial pH. Briefly, intracortical and pial vessels constrict, followed by opening of arteriovenous (AV) shunts and dilatation. SD spreads via the external granular and molecular layers and not via pyramidal axons, the pia-arachnoid or an electric field. The cortex returns to its normal state within 5–10 min after the spreading wave has passed.

It is doubtful whether cortical SD can explain the aura symptoms (as indicated above in the section on vascular pathogenesis), or is sufficient to explain migraine as a disease in its rich variety and complexity. The only direct, but partial, evidence we have of cortical SD is the spreading oligaemia, possibly caused by shunting away of superficial cortical blood through AV shunts. There might be another explanation for the spreading oligaemia. As indicated earlier (Bruyn 1984b), there is an interface in the brain where all (humoral, vascular, neurogenic) models meet, i.e. the astrocytes, whose myriads of 'little feet' form the liaison between vascular and neuronal domains. Astrocytes induce the formation of capillary and venular endothelial tight junctions (Arthur *et al.* 1987), thus creating the blood–brain barrier; they convert neuronally released glutamate and cysteine to glutamine and cystine for re-use; they are the sole K^+ redistributors, as proved by the SD-blocking effect of $BaCl_2$ which inhibits the glial Na-K-pump; an enzyme they contain, carbonic anhydrase, converts CO_2 and H_2O into HCO_3^- and H^+, thus regulating cellular pH (Sykova and Chvatal 1993); they produce NO and endothelin 3, 2, and 1. If, by any chance, cortical SD were the primary or causative event in a migraine attack, the oligaemia could readily be explained by cell swelling, narrowing the intercellular space (already small in the brain at 15%) and increasing its pressure to exceed the intravenular pressure (14 mm H_2O) to squeeze blood out of the superficial cortical venous bed.

The experiments necessary to test the SD theory would require interventions either during (occipital) craniotomy or implantation of microelectrodes/pipettes through dentist-drill burr holes, with prolonged signal recording on portable-recorders in ambulant patients. Such a programme is, for obvious ethical reasons, as unlikely as it would be enlightening. Be this as it may, both venous endothelium and glia appear promising fields for future research. Before this century comes to a close and the next millennium commences, we may expect a decisive leap forward in finding a solution to the enigma of migraine.

REFERENCES

Andersen, A.R., Friberg, L. and Olsen, T.S. (1988) Delayed hyperemia following hypoperfusion in classic migraine. *Archives of Neurology*, **45**, 154–159.

Anthony, M. (1986) The biochemistry of migraine. In: *Handbook of Clinical Neurology*, vol. 48, (eds P.J. Vinken, G.W. Bruyn and F. Clifford Rose), pp. 85–105. Elsevier, Amsterdam.

Antony, M., Hinterberger. H. and Lance, J.W. (1967) Plasma serotonin in migraine and stress. *Archives of Neurology*, **16**, 544–552.

Arthur, F.E., Shivers, R.R. and Bowman, P.D. (1987) Astrocyte-mediated tight junctions in brain capillary endothelium. *Developmental Brain Research*, **36**, 155–159.

Basbaum, A.I. and Fields, H.L. (1987) Endogenous pain control mechanism. *Annals of Neurology*, **4**, 451–462.

Baskin, D.S., Mehler, W.R. and Hosobuchi, Y. (1986) Autopsy analysis of the safety, efficacy and cartography of electrostimulation of the central gray. *Brain Research*, **371**, 231–236.

Berger, R.J., Zuccarello, M. and Keller, J.T. (1994) NOS-immunoreactivity in rat dura mater. *NeuroReport*, **5**, 519–521.

Blau, J.N. (1978) Migraine: vasomotor instability of the meningeal circulation. *Lancet*, **ii**, 1136–1139.

Blau, J.N. (1984) Migraine pathogenesis: the neural hypothesis. *Journal of Neurology, Neurosurgery and Psychiatry*, **47**, 437–442.

Blau, J.N. (1994) Migraine in doctors: work loss and consumption of medication. *Lancet*, **344**, 1623–1624.

Blau, J.N. and Dexter S.L. (1981) The site of pain origin during migraine attacks. *Cephalalgia*, **1**, 143–147.

Blau, J.N. and Solomon, F.(1985) Migraine and intracranial swelling. *Lancet*, **ii**, 718.

Bonvento, R., Lacombe, P. and MacKenzie, E.T. (1991) Differing origins of 5HT innervation of major arteries and small pial vessels in the rat. *Journal of Neurochemistry*, **56**, 681–689.

Bruyn, G.W. (1982) Cerebral cortex and migraine. In: *Advances in Neurology. Headache: Physiopathological and Clinical Concepts*, (eds M. Critchley, A.P. Friedman, S. Gorini and F. Sicuteri), Vol 33, pp. 151–161. Raven Press, New York.

Bruyn, G.W. (1984a) Intracranial AVM and migraine. *Cephalalgia*, **4**, 191–207.

Bruyn, G.W. (1984b) The pathomechanism of migraine as a basis for pharmacotherapy. In: *The Pharmacological Basis of Brain Therapy*, (eds W.K. Amery, J.M. van Nueten and A. Wauquier), pp. 267–278. Pitman Press, London.

Bruyn, G.W. (1985) Prevalence and incidence of migraine: a critical review. In: *Migraine and Beta-Blockade*, (eds J.D. Carroll, V. Pfaffenrath and O. Sjaastad), pp. 99–109. A.B. Hässle, Mölndal, Sweden.

Bruyn, G.W. and Ferrari, M.D. (1984) Chorea and migraine: 'Hemicrania choreatica'?. *Cephalalgia*, **4**. 119–124.

Bruyn, G.W., Ferrari, M.D. and De Beer, F.C. (1984) Migraine, Tolosa-Hunt syndrome and pleocytosis. *Clinical Neurology and Neurosurgery*, **86**, 33–41.

Codina, A., Acarin, P.N. and Miguel, F. (1971a) Migrana hemiplejica familiar asociada a nistigmo. *Medicina Clinica (Barcelona)*, **57**, 841–846.

Codina, A., Acarin, P.N. and Miguel, F. (1971b) *Revue Neurologique (Paris)*, **124**, 526–530.

Curran, D.A., Hinterberger, H. and Lance, J.W. (1965) Total plasma serotonin, 5HIAA and p-hydroxy-m-methoxy mandelic acid excretion in normal and migrainous subjects. *Brain*, **88**, 997–1010.

Diener, H.C. and May, A. (1996) Positron emission tomography studies in acute migraine attacks. In: *Migraine: Pharmacology and Genetics*, (eds M. Sandler, M.D. Ferrari and S. Harnett) pp. 109–115. Chapman & Hall, London.

Dimitriadou, V., Buzzi, M.G., Theoharides, T.C. and Moskowitz, M.A. (1992) Ultrastructural evidence for neurogenically mediated changes in blood vessels. *Neuroscience*, **48**, 187–203.

Do Carmo, R.J. (1992) *Spreading Depression*. Springer Verlag, Berlin.

Edvinsson, L., Degueurce, A. and Duverger, D. (1983) Central serotonergic nerves project to the pial vessels. *Nature*, **306**, 55–57.

Edvinsson, L., Jansen, I., Cunha e Sa, M. and Gulbenkian, S. (1994) Neuropeptide containing nerves and vasomotor responses in human cerebral arteries. *Cephalalgia*, **14**, 88–96.

Ferrari, M.D., Odink, J., Frolich, M., Tapparelli, C. and Portielje, J.E.A. (1989) Release of platelet Met-enkephalin, but not serotonin, in migraine. A platelet response unique to migraine patients? *Journal of the Neurological Sciences*, **93**, 51–60.

Foreman, J.C. and Jordan, C.C. (1984) Neurogenic inflammation. *Trends in Pharmaceutical Science*, **5**, 116–119.

Friberg, L., Olesen, J. and Lassen, N.A. (1994a) Cerebral oxygen extraction, consumption and rCBF during the aura phase of migraine. *Stroke*, **25**, 974–979.

Friberg, L., Olesen J. and Olsen, T.S. (1994b) Absence of vasoactive peptide release from brain to circulation during migraine with aura. *Cephalalgia*, **14**, 47–54.

Goadsby, P.J. and Edvinsson, L. (1993) The trigeminovascular system and migraine. *Annals of Neurology*, **33**, 48–56.

Goadsby, P.J., Lambert, G.A and Lance, J.W. (1982) Differential effects on the carotid circulation of the monkey evoked by locus coeruleus stimulation. *Brain Research*, **249**, 247–254.

Goadsby, P.J., Rjor, R.D., Lambert, S.A. and Lance, J.W. (1985) Effects of nucleus raphe dorsalis stimulation on carotid blood flow. *American Journal of Physiology*, **428**, 257–262.

Goadsby, P.J., Edvinsson, L. and Ekman, R. (1988) Release of vasoactive peptides in extracerebral circulation of man and cat during activation of the trigeminovascular system. *Annals of Neurology*, **26**, 193–196.

Goadsby, P.J., Edvinsson, L. and Ekman, R. (1990) Vasoactive peptide release in human extracerebral circulation during migraine headache. *Annals of Neurology*, **28**, 183–187.

Goldhammer, L. (1993) Second cervical root neurofibroma and ipsilateral migraine headache. *Cephalalgia*, **13**, 132–134.

Goldstein, J.M., Shaywitz, B.A. and Sze, G. (1990) Migraine with focal cerebral edema, CSF pleocytosis and progressive cerebellar ataxia. *Neurology*, **40**, 1284–1287.

Goltman, A.M. (1935–36) The mechanism of the brain. *Journal of Allergy*, **7**, 351–355.

Headache Classification Committee of the International Headache Society (J. Olesen *et al.*) (1988) Classification and diagnostic criteria for headache disorders, cranial neuralgias and facial pain. *Cephalalgia*, **8** (Suppl. 7), 1–97.

Heiss, W.D. (1983) Flow thresholds of functional and morphological damage of brain tissue. *Stroke*, **14**, 329–331.

Herrera, D.G., Maysinger, D. and Gadient, R. (1993) Spreading depression induces C-fos-like immunoreactivity and NGF mRNA in rat cerebral cortex. *Brain Research*, **602**, 99–103.

Herold, S., Gibbs, J.M. and Jones, A.K.P. (1985) Oxygen metabolism in migraine. *Journal of Cerebral Blood Flow and Metabolism*, **5**, S445–446.

Hunt, S.P., Pini, A. and Evan, G. (1987) Induction of C-fos-like protein in spinal cord neurons following sensory stimulation. *Nature*, **328**, 632–634.

Isler, M. (1986) Frequency and time course of premonitory phenomena. In: *The Prelude to the Migraine Attack*, (eds W.K. Amery and A. Wauquier), pp. 44–53. Bailliere Tindall, Eastbourne.

Jensen, K., Tfelt-Hansen, P., Lauritzen, M. and Olesen, J. (1986) Classic migraine: a prospective recording of symptoms. *Acta Neurologica Scandinavica*, **73**, 359–362.

Kimball, R.W., Friedman, A.P. and Vallejo, E. (1960) Effect of serotonin in migraine. *Neurology*, **10**, 107–111.

Kobari, M., Meyer, J.S. and Ichijo, M. (1990) Cortical and subcortical hyperfusion during migraine. *Neuroradiology*, **32**, 4–11.

Krootila, K., Oksala, O. and Zschauer, A. (1992) Inhibitory effect of methysergide on CGRP-induced vasodilation. *British Journal of Pharmacology*, **106**, 404–408.

Kudrow L., Kudrow, D.B. and Sandweiss, J.H. (1995) Effect of intranasal lidocaine on migraine-attacks. *Headache*, **35**, 79–82.

Lambert, S.A., Bogduk, N., Goadsby, P.J., Duchworth, J.W. and Lance, J.W. (1984) Decreased carotid arterial resistance in cat in response to trigeminal stimulation. *Journal of Neurosurgery*, **61**, 307–315.

Lance, J.W., Lambert, G.A. and Goadsby, P.J. (1983) Brainstem influences on the cephalic circulation. *Headache*, **23**, 258–265.

Lance, J.W., Lambert, G.A. and Goadsby, P.J. (1990) Contribution of experimental studies to the pathophysiology of migraine. In: *Migraine: A Spectrum of Ideas*, (eds M. Sandler and G. Collins), pp. 21–36. Oxford University Press.

Lauritzen, M. (1987) Cerebral blood flow in migraine and cortical SD. *Acta Neurologica Scandinavica*, **76** (Suppl. 113), 9–34.

Lauritzen, M. (1994) Pathophysiology of the migraine aura. The spreading depression theory. *Brain*, **117**, 199–210.

Lauritzen, M. and Olesen, J. (1984) rCBF during migraine attacks by 133 Xe-inhalation and SPECT. *Brain*, **107**, 447–461.

Lauritzen, M., Olsen, T.S. and Lassen, N.A. (1983) Changes in rCBF during the course of classical migraine attacks. *Annals of Neurology*, **13**, 633–641.

Lembeck, F., Donnerer, J. and Barthu, L. (1982) Inhibition of neurogenic inflammation by SP antagonists, somatostatin and enkephalin. *European Journal of Pharmacology*, **85**, 171–176.

Majno, G. and Palade, G.E. (1961) Studies of inflammation. *Journal of Biophysical and Biochemical Cytology*, **11**, 571–626.

Marti Massi, J.F., Obeso, J.A. and Carrera, N. (1984) Seudomigrana con liquido cefalorraquideo inflamato. Un sindromo benigno. *Medicina Clinica (Barcelona)*, **83**, 665–667.

Mathiau P., Escurat, M. and Aubineau, P. (1993) Absence of central neuron projection to pial blood vessels and dura mater. *Neuroscience*, **52**, 667–676.

McDonald, D.M. (1987) Neurogenic inflammation in the respiratory tract. *American Review of Respiratory Disease*, **136**, 65–72.

Meyer, J.S. (1985) Migraine and intracranial swelling. *Lancet*, **ii**, 1308–1309.

Mitsikostas, D.D., Thomas, A. and Gatzonis, S. (1994) An epidemiological study of headache among the monks of Athos. *Headache*, **34**, 539–541.

Moskowitz, M.A. (1992) Neurogenic vs. vascular mechanisms of sumatriptan and ergot alkaloids in migraine. *Trends in Pharmaceutical Science*, **13**, 307–311.

Moskowitz, M.A. and Macfarlane, R. (1993) Neurovascular and molecular mechanisms in migraine headaches. *Cerebrovascular Brain Metabolism Review*, **5**, 159–177.

Moskowitz M.A., Nozaki, K. and Kraig, R.D. (1993) Cortical spreading depression provokes C-fos proteinlike immunoreactivity within V nucleus caudalis. *Journal of Neuroscience*, **13**, 1167–1177.

Moskowitz, M.A., Reinhard, J.F. and Romero, J. (1979) Neurotransmitters and the fifth cranial nerve. Relation to the headache phase of migraine? *Lancet*, **ii**, 883–885.

Moussaoui, S.M., Philippe, L. and Le Prado, N. (1993) Inhibition of neurogenic inflammation in the meninges by a non-peptide NK_1 receptor antagonist. *European Journal of Pharmacology*, **238**, 421–424.

O'Connor, T.P. and Van Der Koor, D. (1986) Intra- and extracranial projections of trigeminal ganglion cells. *Journal of Neuroscience*, **6**, 2200–2207.

Olesen, J., Larsen, B. and Lauritzen, M. (1981) Focal hyperemia followed by spreading oligemia and impaired rCBF activation in classic migraine. *Annals of Neurology*, **9**, 344–352.

Olesen, J., Lauritzen, M. and Tfelt-Hansen, P. (1982) Spreading cerebral oligaemia in classical and normal blood flow in common migraine. *Headache*, **42**, 242–248.

Olsen, A., Jensen, I.W. and Olano, F.J. (1984) Kortikalt oden ved hemiplegisk migraene. *Ugeskrift for laeger*, **146**, 1861–1863.

Olsen, T.S. (1990) Migraine with and without aura: the same disease due to cerebral vasospasm of different intensity. *Headache*, **30**, 269–272.

Olsen, T.S. (1993) Spreading oligemia in the migraine aura. *Cephalalgia*, **13**, 86–88.

Peatfield, R.C., Gawel, M.J. and Clifford Rose, F. (1982) Asymmetry of aura and pain in migraine. *Journal of Neurology Neurosurgery and Psychiatry*, **44**, 846–848.

Raskin, N.Y., Hosobuchi, Y. and Lamb, S. (1987) Headache may arise from perturbation of the brain. *Headache*, **27**, 416–420.

Reinhard, J.F., Liebma, J,F., Schlosba, A.J. and Moskowitz, M.A. (1979) Serotonin neurons project to small blood vessels in the brain. *Science*, **206**, 85–86.

Sanin, L.C., Mathew, T.N. and Bellmeyer, L.R. (1994) The IHS headache classification as applied to a headache clinic population. *Cephalalgia*, **14**, 442–446.

Shimizu, Y., Yamana, K. and Tsutsuni, Y. (1993) Migraine due to meningioma. *Rinsho Shinkeigaku*, **33**, 396–399.

Sicuteri, F. (1959) Prophylactic properties of UML-491 in migraine. *International Archives of Allergy and Applied Immunology*, **15**, 300–307.

Sicuteri, F. (1976) Migraine: a central biochemical dysnociception. *Headache*, **16**, 145–159.

Sicuteri F., Testi, A. and Anselmi, B. (1961) Increase in 5HIAA excretion during migraine attacks. *International Archives of Allergy and Applied Immunology*, **19**, 55–58.

Stamboulis, E., Spengos, M., Rombos, M. and Haidemenos, A. (1987) Aseptic inflammatory meningeal reaction manifesting as a migrainous syndrome. *Headache*, **27**, 439–441.

Stewart, W.K., Schechter, A. and Rasmussen, B.K. (1994) Migraine prevalence. *Neurology*, **44** (Suppl. 4), S17–S23.

Strassman, A., Mason, P. and Moskowitz, M.A. (1986) Response of brain stem trigeminal neurons to electrostimulation of dura. *Brain Research*, **379**, 242–252.

Sykova, E. and Chvatal, A. (1993) Extracellular ionic and volume changes: the glia–neuron interaction. *Journal of Chemical Neuroanatomy*, **6**, 247–260.

Tomita, M., Fukuuchi, Y. and Terakawa, S. (1994) Differential behavior of glia and neurons exposed to hypotonic solutions. *Acta Neurochirurgica*, Suppl.60, 31–33.

Welch, K.M.A., D'Andrea, G. and Tepley, N. (1990) The concept of migraine as a state of central neuronal hyperexcitability. *Neurology Clinic*, **8**, 817–828.

Welch, K.M.A., Barkely, G.L. and Tepley, N. (1993) Central neurogenic mechanisms of migraine. *Neurology*, **43** (Suppl. 3), S21–S25.

Wilkinson, M. and Blau, J.N. (1985) Are classic and common migraine different entities? *Headache*, **25**, 211–212.

Woods, R.P., Jacobine, M. and Mazziotta, J.C. (1994) Bilateral spreading cerebral hypoperfusion during spontaneous migraine headache. *New England Journal of Medicine*, **331**, 1689–1692.

Ziegler, D. (1990) Headache public health problem. *Neurology Clinic*, **8**, 781–791.

Zifkin, B., Andermann, E. and Andermann, F. (1980) An autosomal dominant syndrome of hemiplegic migraine, nystagmus and tremor. *Annals of Neurology*, **8**, 329–332.

2
5-Hydroxytryptamine receptor subtypes and migraine

Helen E. Connor and David T. Beattie

INTRODUCTION

In the last few years, a number of novel 5-hydroxytryptamine (5-HT, serotonin) receptor subtypes have been identified, largely through the use of molecular cloning techniques. Hence, seven different 5-HT receptor families (5-HT_1–5-HT_7) are now thought to exist, some of which are heterogeneous and contain several subtypes. For example, the 5-HT_1 receptor family contains at least five subtypes. Our current understanding of 5-HT receptor subtypes and their classification using molecular, pharmacological and transduction criteria have been reviewed in detail by Hoyer *et al.* (1994).

This advance in our knowledge of 5-HT receptor heterogeneity has importance for the disease of migraine, particularly with respect to migraine treatment. The antimigraine drug sumatriptan was identified as a selective agonist for the 5-HT_1 receptor subtype mediating vascular contraction (Humphrey *et al.* 1989). However, it is now known that sumatriptan has affinity for a number of the recently described 5-HT_1 receptor subtypes (Table 2.1). Furthermore, other recently described drugs of this class (e.g. 311C90 (zolmitriptan), MK-462) now in clinical trials for migraine have a very similar 5-HT receptor profile (Table 2.1). This has raised interest as to which of these receptor subtypes is important for antimigraine efficacy in man. Indeed, there has been much debate about the specific mechanism of action of sumatriptan in

Migraine: Pharmacology and genetics
Edited by Merton Sandler, Michel Ferrari and Sara Harnett
Published in 1996 by Chapman & Hall
ISBN 1 86036 006 8

Table 2.1 Binding affinity (pK_i or pIC_{50}) values for sumatriptan, and related compounds, at 5-HT$_1$ receptor subtypes

	Sumatriptan	*311C90*	*MK-462*
5-HT$_{1A}$	6.0	6.5	6.3
5-HT$_{1D\alpha}$	8.5	8.5	7.7*
5-HT$_{1D\beta}$	8.1	8.1	7.3*
5-HT$_{1E}$	5.6	<5	6.5
5-HT$_{1F}$	7.6	7.1*	nd

Data from Adham *et al.* 1993b, Martin 1994, McAllister *et al.* 1992, Street *et al.* 1995, Weinshank *et al.* 1992.
* H. Giles and G.R. Martin, unpublished data; nd, no data.

migraine: is this attributable to cranial vasoconstriction, trigeminal neuronal inhibition, or a combination of both actions (Humphrey and Feniuk 1991, Moskowitz 1992, Humphrey and Goadsby 1994)? The molecular identity of the 5-HT receptor mediating these two actions of sumatriptan, and related drugs, can now be investigated to see whether different receptors may be involved. This review will focus on the 5-HT$_1$ receptor family and look at which of these novel 5-HT$_1$ subtypes may be a target for antimigraine drugs.

5-HT RECEPTOR SUBTYPE MEDIATING CRANIAL VASOCONSTRICTION

The ability of sumatriptan to constrict intracranial blood vessels is now well established. Related compounds of this class, such as 311C90 and MK-462, have the same profile of action. The 5-HT$_1$ receptor subtype mediating contraction of intracranial arteries shows close pharmacological similarity to, but not identity with the 5-HT$_{1D}$ receptor (Perren *et al.* 1991), as initially defined in brain tissue using radioligand binding. However, more recently, 5-HT$_{1D}$ receptors have been shown to be heterogeneous, with two closely related, but molecularly distinct, subtypes (termed 5-HT$_{1D\alpha}$ and 5-HT$_{1D\beta}$) being cloned and characterized (Weinshank *et al.* 1992). Differences across species have been found with this receptor group: for example, the 5-HT$_{1B}$ receptor is the rat homologue of the human 5-HT$_{1D\beta}$ receptor but has a different pharmacology (Adham *et al.* 1992), and the dog 5-HT$_{1D\alpha}$ receptor shows approximately 30-fold lower affinity for ketanserin than the human 5-HT$_{1D\alpha}$ receptor (Branchek 1995). However, human 5-HT$_{1D\alpha}$ and 5-HT$_{1D\beta}$ receptors appear to have a very similar pharmacological profile, with over 30 structurally distinct compounds showing similar affinity (Hartig

Table 2.2 Calculated correlation coefficients (r) for comparison of functional potency at the 5-HT$_1$ receptor mediating contraction of dog isolated basilar artery with binding affinity at human 5-HT$_{1D\alpha}$ and 5-HT$_{1D\beta}$ receptors for agonists ($n = 16$) and antagonists ($n = 8$)

	Binding affinity	
Functional potency	*Human 5-HT$_{1D\alpha}$* *(pK$_i$)*	*Human 5-HT$_{1D\beta}$* *(pK$_i$)*
Agonists (pEC$_{50}$)	r = 0.46	r = 0.83
Antagonists (pK_B)	r = −0.15	r = 0.80

pEC$_{50}$, potency of agonists to cause constriction; pK_B, potency of antagonists to block contractile effects of sumatriptan.

et al. 1992). Interestingly, ketanserin shows some difference, with approximately 70-fold higher affinity at human 5-HT$_{1D\alpha}$ compared to 5-HT$_{1D\beta}$ receptors (Kaumann *et al.* 1993).

Molecular studies by Hamel *et al.* (1993) described the presence of mRNA for the 5-HT$_{1D\beta}$ receptor in human cerebral arteries, whilst mRNA for the 5-HT$_{1D\alpha}$ receptor was not detected in this tissue. Control experiments showed that both subtypes could be detected in human brain. These data provide convincing evidence for the 5-HT$_{1D\beta}$ receptor being the molecular correlate of the pharmacologically defined vascular 5-HT$_1$ receptor. Pharmacological studies support this conclusion. Hence correlation analysis of the potency of nine relatively non-selective compounds (seven agonists and two antagonists) at the 5-HT$_1$ receptor mediating contraction of human cerebral artery showed a better correlation with binding affinities at the human 5-HT$_{1D\beta}$ (r = 0.94) compared to the 5-HT$_{1D\alpha}$ receptor (r = 0.75) (Hamel *et al.* 1993). Unpublished studies conducted at Glaxo, using 16 agonists and eight antagonists, correlating functional potency at the contractile 5-HT$_1$ receptor in dog isolated basilar artery with binding affinity at the human 5-HT$_{1D\alpha}$ and 5-HT$_{1D\beta}$ receptors, showed considerably better correlation for the 5-HT$_{1D\beta}$ compared to the 5-HT$_{1D\alpha}$ receptor (Table 2.2; H.E. Connor and D.T. Beattie, unpublished data).

GR127935 is the first selective 5-HT$_{1D}$ receptor antagonist to be described (Skingle *et al.* 1993, 1995). This novel compound dissociates slowly from the receptor, possibly due to high lipophilicity. Therefore, although it is a potent antagonist of the 5-HT$_1$ receptor subtype mediating vascular contraction, its unsurmountable antagonist profile (Skingle *et al.* 1995) limits its value as an *in vitro* drug tool. GR55562 (3-[3-(dimethylamino)propyl-4-hydroxy-N-[4-(4-pyridinyl)phenyl]benzamide)

Table 2.3 5-HT receptor profile of GR55562, a selective 5-HT$_{1D}$ receptor antagonist

5-HT receptor	Binding affinity/Functional potency (pK_i/pK_B)
5-HT$_{1A}$	5.3
5-HT$_{1D\alpha}$	6.2
5-HT$_{1D\beta}$	7.4
5-HT$_{1F}$	5.6
5-HT$_{2A}$	5.6
5-HT$_3$	5.0
5-HT$_4$	<5
5-HT$_{5A}$	<5

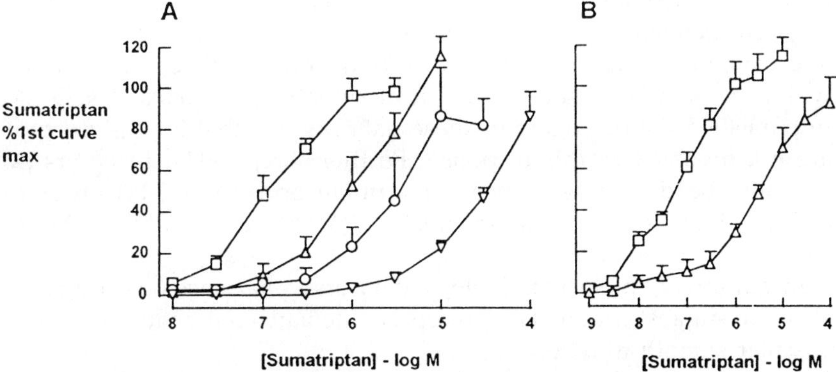

Figure 2.1 Effects of GR55562 against sumatriptan-induced contraction of dog (A) and monkey (B) isolated basilar artery. Control (□) and following pre-treatment with GR55562 0.1 (△), 0.3 (○) and 1 (▽) μM. Values are means ± SEM, n = 3–4.

is a structurally related, selective 5-HT$_{1D}$ receptor antagonist (Table 2.3), but with lower lipophilicity than GR127935, and a competitive profile of action (Glaxo R & D Ltd, unpublished data). GR55562 is a functional antagonist at the human cloned 5-HT$_{1D\beta}$ receptor with a pK_B value (vs sumatriptan-induced inhibition of cAMP) of 7.4 ± 0.2 SEM. This is approximately 16-fold higher than its functional potency at the human 5-HT$_{1D\alpha}$ receptor (pK_B = 6.2 ± 0.1 SEM). GR55562 competitively blocks sumatriptan-induced contractions of dog (pA_2 = 7.9 ± 0.2 SEM; Figure 2.1A) and monkey isolated basilar artery (pK_B = 7.7 ± 0.03 SEM; Figure 2.1B) with a potency very similar to its potency at human 5-HT$_{1D\beta}$ rather than at 5-HT$_{1D\alpha}$ receptors. These data using this novel, selective compound further suggest that the 5-HT_1 receptor mediating cerebral vasoconstriction is the $5\text{-HT}_{1D\beta}$ subtype.

In addition to its affinity for $5\text{-HT}_{1D\alpha}$ and $5\text{-HT}_{1D\beta}$ receptors, sumatriptan also has high binding affinity (pK_i = 7.6, Table 2.1) and functional agonist activity (inhibition of forskolin-stimulated cAMP accumulation; pEC_{50} = 7.5, Adham *et al.* 1993a,b) at human 5-HT_{1F} receptors. Other 5-HT_1 receptor agonists currently in clinical trials (e.g. 311C90) appear to have a similar receptor profile. Hence, could 5-HT_{1F} receptors play a role in the vasoconstrictor actions of these compounds, and thus confer antimigraine activity? Two pieces of evidence suggest that this is not the case. Firstly, 5-carboxamidotryptamine (5-CT) is approximately 30-fold weaker than sumatriptan as an agonist at human cloned 5-HT_{1F} receptors (pEC_{50} = 6.1; Adham *et al.* 1993b), whilst being about 10-fold more potent than sumatriptan at contracting human isolated basilar artery (Parsons *et al.* 1989). Secondly, a sumatriptan analogue which has low affinity at 5-HT_{1F} receptors (mouse clone; pK_i = 5.4), but retains high affinity at $5\text{-HT}_{1D\alpha}$ and $5\text{-HT}_{1D\beta}$ receptors (pK_i approximately 8) has been found to contract dog isolated basilar artery with a potency very similar to that of sumatriptan (Glaxo R & D Ltd, unpublished data). Together, these data suggest that 5-HT_{1F} receptors are not involved in this response. Furthermore, 5-HT_{1E} receptors can probably be discounted since sumatriptan and other 5-HT_1 receptor agonists have a low affinity at this site (McAllister *et al.* 1992, Martin 1994).

In summary, molecular biology data and pharmacological analysis strongly suggest that $5\text{-HT}_{1D\beta}$ receptors mediate contraction of cerebral vascular smooth muscle.

5-HT RECEPTOR SUBTYPE MEDIATING NEUROGENIC INHIBITION

Sumatriptan and related 5-HT_1 receptor agonists (e.g. 311C90) inhibit plasma protein extravasation in the dura mater evoked by electrical stimulation of the trigeminal ganglion in anaesthetised rats and guinea-pigs (Buzzi and Moskowitz 1990, Martin 1994). This animal model is suggested to mimic the neurogenic inflammatory events thought to occur during migraine headache. The action of sumatriptan has been ascribed to an effect at prejunctional inhibitory 5-HT_1 receptors on trigeminal nerve terminals innervating the dural vasculature, leading to inhibition of the release of the vasoactive neurotransmitter, substance P (Moskowitz 1992). Interestingly, this effect is specific for the dura: no inhibition of plasma protein extravasation is seen in extracranial tissues, which suggests that prejunctional 5-HT_1 receptors are specifically located on intracranial dural trigeminal nerve terminals (Buzzi and

Moskowitz 1990). Evidence for the ability of sumatriptan to inhibit trigeminal sensory nerves has also been obtained *in vitro*: in guinea-pig isolated basilar artery sumatriptan inhibits sensory nerve-mediated relaxations via a pre- rather than a postjunctional action (O'Shaughnessy and Connor 1994).

The identity of the 5-HT_1 receptor subtype mediating inhibition of trigeminal sensory nerve terminals is unclear. The selective 5-HT_{1D} receptor antagonist GR127935 (Skingle *et al.* 1995) blocks sumatriptan-induced inhibition of dural plasma protein extravasation in guinea-pigs (Yu *et al.* 1995), suggesting that $5\text{-HT}_{1D\alpha}$ and/or $5\text{-HT}_{1D\beta}$ receptors are involved. However, until compounds which show some selectivity between these receptor subtypes are tested in this model, it is impossible to draw any conclusions as to which subtype is involved. Ketanserin is the one compound reported to date to show some selectivity between these sites (see above) but there are no published data on whether, at doses likely to block only $5\text{-HT}_{1D\alpha}$ sites, it prevents sumatriptan-induced inhibition of dural plasma protein extravasation. An involvement of 5-HT_{1F} receptors in trigeminal nerve inhibition can be excluded since 5-CT, which is a relatively weak agonist at human (see above; Adham *et al.* 1993b) and mouse (Amlaiky *et al.* 1992) 5-HT_{1F} receptors, is a very potent agonist at inhibiting dural plasma protein extravasation (Buzzi *et al.* 1991). Similarly, a role for 5-HT_{1E} receptors can be discounted since both 5-CT and sumatriptan have low affinity at this site (McAllister *et al.* 1992).

Molecular studies have also been conducted to try and determine the 5-HT receptor subtype present on trigeminal nerve terminals. Hence, a number of research groups investigated the distribution of $5\text{-HT}_{1D\alpha}$ and $5\text{-HT}_{1D\beta}$ receptor mRNA in rat, guinea-pig and human trigeminal ganglion because mRNA for receptors present on the nerve terminals would be expressed and located in this region. Using *in situ* hybridization, 5-HT_{1B} (rat equivalent of the $5\text{-HT}_{1D\beta}$) receptor mRNA has been identified in rat trigeminal ganglia (Bruinvels *et al.* 1992). Using the polymerase chain reaction (PCR) a single mRNA, which could not be definitively identified, was detected in guinea-pig trigeminal ganglia: it was 85% and 71% identical to the human $5\text{-HT}_{1D\alpha}$ and $5\text{-HT}_{1D\beta}$ receptor DNA sequences respectively (Rebeck *et al.* 1994). In human trigeminal ganglia, using a similar PCR-based approach, $5\text{-HT}_{1D\alpha}$ but not $5\text{-HT}_{1D\beta}$ receptor message was found, but this was only in two of eight post-mortem samples. In the other six ganglia no message for either receptor was detected: the reasons for this difference were not clear, but it seems unlikely to be related to post-mortem delay (Rebeck *et al.* 1994). In studies at Glaxo, again using a PCR approach, mRNA for neither the $5\text{-HT}_{1D\alpha}$ nor the $5\text{-HT}_{1D\beta}$ receptor could be detected in two human trigeminal ganglia samples (G.H. Disney, unpublished data). Additionally, no mRNA for the 5-HT_{1F} receptor could be detected (G.H. Disney, unpublished data). Oligonucleotide probes used in this study showed good signals in cell lines transfected with the human cloned receptors. Hence, at present it is difficult to draw definitive conclusions about which receptor subtype is present on trigeminal nerves, and species differences may well occur. However, experiments in human tissue suggest a low expression of the $5\text{-HT}_{1D\alpha}$ subtype in some (approx. 25%) trigeminal ganglia.

CP-122,288: A NEURONALLY SELECTIVE COMPOUND

CP-122,288, a structural analogue of sumatriptan, inhibits dural plasma protein extravasation in anaesthetised guinea-pigs at extremely low doses (ID_{50} = 0.5 ng/kg iv), being about 2000-fold more potent than sumatriptan in this model (Lee and Moskowitz 1993). This effect appears to be attributable to inhibition of trigeminal neurotransmission, since CP-122,288, like sumatriptan, does not modify dural plasma protein extravasation evoked by substance P administration (Lee and Moskowitz 1993). The remarkable potency of CP-122,288 to block dural plasma protein extravasation has been confirmed in anaesthetised rats and, furthermore, its effects are specific for the dura since extravasation in extracranial tissues (e.g. eyelid, lip) is unaffected (Beattie and Connor 1995). Interestingly, at these low doses, CP-122,288 does not have vasoconstrictor effects (Lee and Moskowitz 1993, Beattie and Connor 1995). However, at higher doses CP-122,288 causes vasoconstriction *in vitro* and *in vivo* (isolated cerebral arteries, anaesthetised dog carotid vascular bed) with a very similar potency to sumatriptan (Beattie and Connor 1995). Hence, CP-122,288 is a compound which appears to have a novel profile of action: a selective inhibitory effect on trigeminal nerves at low doses.

These observations raise several questions. Firstly and importantly, would a compound with this profile of action have antimigraine activity in man? This, of course, will only be answered by clinical testing in migraine patients. The crucial question is whether antimigraine activity is seen at very low doses, equivalent to those which block dural plasma extravasation without causing vasoconstriction. At higher doses, where the compound has a cranial vasoconstrictor profile like that of sumatriptan, relief of migraine headache is likely to occur. Evaluation of this type of compound in the future will provide valuable insight into the importance of neurogenic inflammation to the migraine process. Secondly, what is the mechanism by which CP-122,288 inhibits dural plasma protein extravasation with such exquisite potency? Understanding this would enable the relevance of this effect (seen only in rat and guinea-pig to date) to be considered for, and extrapolated to, humans. The mechanism is unlikely to be attributable to activity at either $5\text{-HT}_{1D\alpha}$ or $5\text{-HT}_{1D\beta}$ receptors, since CP-122,288 has a very similar affinity to sumatriptan at these human subtypes (pK_i for CP-122,288 and sumatriptan, respectively at: $5\text{-HT}_{1D\alpha}$, 8.1 and 8.0; and $5\text{-HT}_{1D\beta}$, 7.3 and 7.1, Beattie and Connor 1995). In support of this Yu *et al.* (1995) reported that the selective 5-HT_{1D} antagonist GR127935, which blocks the inhibitory effects of sumatriptan in the dural extravasation model, did **not** block CP-122,288-induced dural inhibition. Furthermore, an action at other known 5-HT receptor subtypes seems unlikely, given the known potencies of sumatriptan and other compounds with activity in the dural extravasation model at these receptors. Therefore the most likely explanation at present is that CP-122,288 is activating some as yet unknown receptor to cause its effects. We continue to try to identify this target.

SUMMARY

The field of 5-HT receptor research has been very productive for identifying antimigraine drugs. Sumatriptan, the first of a new class of drugs for effective treatment of migraine, was originally developed as a selective agonist for the 5-HT_1 receptor mediating cranial vasoconstriction. However, following the identification and cloning of several novel 5-HT receptor subtypes, it is now apparent that sumatriptan has high affinity for $5\text{-HT}_{1D\alpha}$, $5\text{-HT}_{1D\beta}$ and 5-HT_{1F} receptors. This review has considered which of these novel receptors may be important targets for migraine treatment. The 5-HT_{1F} receptor can probably be discounted: there is no evidence to support an action at this receptor type being important in alleviating this disease. In contrast, convincing molecular and pharmacological evidence identifies the receptor mediating cranial vasoconstriction as the $5\text{-HT}_{1D\beta}$ receptor. The identity of the 5-HT_1 receptor subtype mediating inhibition of trigeminal nerves is still not clearly established: evidence in human tissue points to $5\text{-HT}_{1D\alpha}$, but functional demonstration of this, in animal or humans, has not yet been obtained. The importance of cranial vasoconstriction versus trigeminal neuronal inhibition in the alleviation of migraine headache by sumatriptan, and other 5-HT_1 receptor agonists currently in clinical trials, continues to be debated. The sumatriptan analogue, CP-122,288 has been identified in animal experiments as a compound with a selective inhibitory action on trigeminal nerves. The mechanism of this action is unknown, but is unlikely to be due to effects at either $5\text{-HT}_{1D\alpha}$ or $5\text{-HT}_{1D\beta}$ receptors. Compounds with this neuronal-selective profile will, in the future, provide the opportunity to determine the importance of trigeminal nerve inhibition for conferring antimigraine activity.

REFERENCES

Adham, N., Romanienko, P., Hartig, P.R., Weinshank, R.L. and Branchek, T. (1992) The rat 5-hydroxytryptamine$_{1B}$ receptor is the species homologue of the human 5-hydroxytryptamine$_{1D\beta}$ receptor. *Molecular Pharmacology*, **41**, 1–7.

Adham, N., Borden, L.A., Schechter L.E., Gustafson, E.L., Cochran, T.L., Vaysse, P. J-J., Weinshank, R.L. and Branchek, T. (1993a) Cell-specific coupling of the cloned human 5-HT$_{1F}$ receptor to multiple signal transduction pathways. *Naunyn-Schmiedeberg's Archives of Pharmacology*, **348**, 566–575.

Adham, N., Kao, H-T., Schechter, L.E., Bard, J., Olsen, M., Urquhart, D., Durkin, M., Hartig, P.R., Weinshank, R.L. and Branchek, T. (1993b) Cloning of a novel serotonin receptor (5-HT$_{1F}$): a fifth 5-HT$_1$ receptor subtype coupled to the inhibition of adenylate cyclase. *Proceedings National Academy Sciences USA*, **90**, 408–412.

Amlaiky N., Ramboz, S., Boschert U., Plassat, J-L. and Hen R. (1992) Isolation of a mouse '5-HT$_{1E}$-like' serotonin receptor expressed predominantly in hippocampus. *Journal of Biological Chemistry*, **267**, 19761–19764.

Beattie, D.T. and Connor, H.E. (1995) The pre- and postjunctional activity of CP-122, 288, a conformationally restricted analogue of sumatriptan. *European Journal of Pharmacology*, **276**, 271–276.

Branchek, T. Bard, J.A., Kucharewicz, S.A., Zgombick, J.M., Weinshank, R.L., Cohen, M.L (1995) Migraine: relationship to cloned canine and human 5-HT$_{1D}$ receptors. In: *Experimental Headache Models*, (eds J. Olesen and M.A. Moskowitz), pp. 125–134. Raven Press, New York.

Bruinvels, A.T., Landwehrmeyer, B., Moskowitz, M.A. and Hoyer, D. (1992) Evidence for the presence of 5-HT$_{1B}$ receptor messenger RNA in neurons of the rat trigeminal ganglia. *European Journal of Pharmacology (Molecular Section)*, **227**, 357–359.

Buzzi, M.G. and Moskowitz, M.A. (1990) The antimigraine drug, sumatriptan (GR43175), selectively blocks neurogenic plasma extravasation from blood vessels in dura mater. *British Journal of Pharmacology*, **99**, 202–206.

Buzzi, M.G., Moskowitz, M.A., Peroutka, S.J. and Byun, B. (1991) Further characterisation of the putative 5-HT receptor which mediates blockade of neurogenic plasma extravasation in rat dura mater. *British Journal of Pharmacology*, **103**, 1421–1428.

Hamel E., Fan, E., Linville, V., Ting, V., Villemure, J. and Chia, L. (1993) Expression of mRNA for the serotonin 5-hydroxytryptamine$_{1D\beta}$ receptor subtype in human and bovine cerebral arteries. *Molecular Pharmacology*, **44**, 242–246.

Hartig, P.R., Branchek, T.A. and Weinshank, R.L. (1992) A subfamily of 5-HT$_{1D}$ receptor genes. *Trends in Pharmacological Science*, **13**, 152–159.

Hoyer, D., Clarke, D.E., Fozard, J.R., Hartig, P.R., Martin, G.R., Mylecharlane, E.J., Saxena, P.R. and Humphrey P.P.A. (1994) International Union of Pharmacology classification of receptors for 5-hydroxytryptamine (serotonin). *Pharmacology Reviews*, **46**, 157–203.

Humphrey, P.P.A. and Feniuk, W. (1991) Mode of action of the anti-migraine drug sumatriptan. *Trends in Pharmacological Science*, **12**, 444–446.

Humphrey, P.P.A. and Goadsby, P.J. (1994) The mode of action of sumatriptan is vascular? A debate. *Cephalalgia*, **14**, 401–410.

Humphrey, P.P.A., Feniuk, W., Perren, M.J., Connor, H.E., and Oxford, A. (1989) The pharmacology of the novel 5-HT$_1$-like receptor agonist, GR43175. *Cephalalgia*, **9** (Suppl. 9), 21–33.

Kaumann A.J., Parsons, A.A. and Brown, A.M. (1993) Human arterial constrictor serotonin receptors. *Cardiovascular Research*, **27**, 2094–2103.

Lee, W.S. and Moskowitz, M.A. (1993) Conformationally restricted sumatriptan analogues, CP-122, 288 and CP-122, 638 exhibit enhanced potency against neurogenic inflammation in dura mater. *Brain Research*, **626**, 303–305.

Martin, G.R. (1994) Pre-clinical profile of the novel 5-HT$_{1D}$ receptor agonist 311C90. In: *New Advances in Headache Research*, Vol. 4, (ed. F. Clifford Rose), pp. 3–4. Smith Gordon Nishimura.

McAllister, G., Charlesworth, A., Snodin, C., Beer, M.S., Noble, A.J., Middlemiss, D.N., Iverson, L.L. and Whiting, P. (1992) Molecular cloning of a serotonin receptor from human brain (5-HT$_{1E}$): a fifth 5-HT$_1$-like subtype. *Proceedings National Academy of Science USA*, **89**, 5517–5521.

Moskowitz, M.A. (1992) Neurogenic versus vascular mechanisms of sumatriptan and ergot alkaloids in migraine. *Trends in Pharmacological Science*, **13**, 307–312.

O'Shaugnessy, C.T. and Connor, H.E. (1994) Activation of sensory nerves in guinea-pig isolated basilar artery by nicotine: evidence for inhibition of trigeminal sensory neurotransmission by sumatriptan. *European Journal of Pharmacology*, **259**, 37–42.

Parsons, A.A., Whalley, E.T., Feniuk, W., Connor, H.E. and Humphrey, P.P.A. (1989) 5-HT$_1$-like receptors mediate 5-hydroxytryptamine-induced contraction of human isolated basilar artery. *British Journal of Pharmacology*, **96**, 434–449.

Perren, M.J., Feniuk, W. and Humphrey, P.P.A. (1991) Vascular 5-HT$_1$-like receptors that mediate contraction of the dog isolated saphenous vein and carotid arterial vasoconstriction in anaesthetised dogs are not of the 5-HT$_{1A}$ or 5-HT$_{1D}$ subtype. *British Journal of Pharmacology*, **102**, 191–197.

Rebeck, G.W., Maynard K.I., Hyman, B.T. and Moskowitz, M.A. (1994) Selective 5-HT$_{1D\alpha}$ serotonin receptor gene expression in trigeminal ganglia: implications for antimigraine drug development. *Proceedings National Academy Science USA*, **91**, 3666–3669.

Skingle, M., Scopes, D.I.C., Feniuk, W., Connor, H.E., Carter, M.C., Clitherow, J.W. and Tyers, M.B. (1993) A potent and orally active 5-HT$_{1D}$ receptor antagonist. *British Journal of Pharmacology*, **110**, 9P.

Skingle, M., Beattie, D.T., Scopes, D.I.C., Starkey, S.J., Connor, H.E., Feniuk, W. and Tyers, M.B. (1996) GR127935: a potent and selective 5-HT$_{1D}$ receptor antagonist. *Behavioral Brain Research*, in press.

Street, L.J., Baker, R., Davey, W.B., Guiblin, A.R., Jelley, R.A., *et al.*, (1995) Synthesis and serotonergic activity of N,N-dimethyl-2-[5(1,2,4-triazol-1-ylmethyl)-1H-indol-3-yl]ethylamine and analogues: potent agonists for 5-HT$_{1D}$ receptors. *Journal of Medicinal Chemistry*, **38**, 1799–1810.

Weinshank R.L., Zgombick, J.M., Macchi, M., Branchek, T.A. and Hartig P.R. (1992) Human serotonin $_{1D}$ receptor is encoded by a subfamiliy of two distinct genes: 5-HT$_{1D\alpha}$ and 5-HT$_{1D\beta}$. *Proceedings National Academy of Science*, **89**, 3630–3634.

Yu, X.-J., Waeber, C. and Moskowitz, M.A. (1995) Additional 5-HT receptor subtypes inhibit (besides 5-HT$_{1D}$) neurogenic plasma extravasation within guinea-pig dura mater. *Cephalalgia*, **15** (Suppl. 14), 117.

DISCUSSION

Sandler: Dr Moskowitz, your data (Rebeck *et al.* 1994) indicated that a 5-$HT_{1D\alpha}$ receptor agonist might avoid damaging side-effects, such as coronary artery spasm. Do you still hold this view?

Moskowitz: Yes. I would urge those who can develop drugs which discriminate between the α and β receptor subtypes to develop a 5-$HT_{1D\alpha}$-selective agonist. There are other approaches as well. Our findings (Lee and Moskowitz 1993) that the sumatriptan analogue CP-122,288, at dosages which do not constrict, blocks plasma extravasation and the c-*fos* response (which is a more direct reflection of activity in a primary afferent system) suggest that it might be possible to treat a painful condition like migraine with less drug than required with sumatriptan and at dosages which do not cause vasoconstriction.

Secondly, in our experiments with knock-out mice that lack the 5-HT_{1B} receptor (Moskowitz, this volume), we tested three compounds: CP-93,129, which is very selective for the 5-HT_{1B} receptor in *in vitro* assays; sumatriptan, which does not discriminate; and CP-122,288. As expected, in the wild type mouse we saw inhibition of extravasation within dura mater by all three compounds. In the mutant mouse, however, we saw no inhibition with CP-93,129 or sumatriptan, but significant inhibition with CP-122,288. Hence, the mouse 5-HT_{1B} receptor mediates the effect of sumatriptan and CP-93,129, whereas CP-122,288 clearly has a different mechanism of action. I do not know if that mechanism is 5-HT receptor-mediated. Perhaps CP-122,288 is working on a second messenger system and not directly on a receptor. It is an open question.

Goadsby: Is anyone making a 5-$HT_{1D\alpha}$ knock-out mouse?

Moskowitz: We do not yet know if there is any expression of 5-$HT_{1D\alpha}$ receptors in mouse ganglion.

Connor: In terms of the 5-HT receptor subtype mediating trigeminal nerve inhibition, do you believe that there is a species difference between mouse and man?

Moskowitz: That puzzled us because in the rat CP-93,129 clearly works via a 5-HT_{1B} receptor mechanism and theoretically the homologue in man should be the 5-$HT_{1D\beta}$ receptor. There are a number of examples where the isoform of a receptor-mediated response switches between species, particularly in the alpha-adrenergic system in the liver.

Fozard: When you see something *in vivo* and do not see it *in vitro* there may be a metabolite involved. Could that be an explanation for the remarkable potency of CP-122,288 *in vivo*?

Moskowitz: *In vivo* the action is pretty quick, but I don't think we can rule out that possibility.

Fozard: In your experiments, is the CP-122,288 given systemically?

Moskowitz: It is given intravenously ten minutes before we stimulate the ganglion.

Connor: Similar profiles are seen with 5-carboxamidotryptamine and CP-122,288. It is not just specific to CP-122,288, so you would have to argue that metabolites were seen with each of these compounds.

Fozard: Your data suggest that the effect of CP-122,288 reflects an action on neurons in your model. Have you investigated whether CP-122,288 opens a potassium channel or in some way changes the membrane characteristics by a channel mechanism to make it less likely that those neurons fired?

Connor: CP-122,288 has been tested at two types of potassium channel and the activity at both was very low. However, there are now known to be many different potassium channels.

Ferrari: Does ketanserin block both α and β subtypes of the 5-HT$_{1D}$ receptor?

Connor: No, it blocks the 5-HT$_{1D\alpha}$ subtype but not the 5-HT$_{1D\beta}$ subtype, except at very high concentrations.

Ferrari: Sumatriptan is still effective in patients who are on ketanserin.

Branchek: In man, the dose may not be high enough to block the 5-HT$_{1D\alpha}$ receptor. The affinity is several orders of magnitude lower than at 5-HT$_2$ receptors. Ketanserin's only interesting feature is that it is one of the few compounds that discriminate at all between 5-HT$_{1D\alpha}$ and 5-HT$_{1D\beta}$ subtypes.

Connor: That is correct. One would have to use a higher dose in man to investigate that.

Branchek: Yes, but then ketanserin has other actions, such as at α_1-adrenoceptors.

Ferrari: What is the significance of the different results on 5-HT$_{1D\alpha}$ and 5-HT$_{1D\beta}$ expression in human trigeminal ganglia?

Branchek: In the literature on biogenic amine receptors, comparison of data from different laboratories or localization studies applying different types of techniques, such as Northern blot analyses, polymerase chain reaction (PCR), and *in situ* hybridization studies, shows good concordance for regions with a very high abundance signal. However, for medium to low expression of any gene the correspondence falls apart dramatically. It does appear that these 5-HT$_{1D}$ receptors, particularly the 5-HT$_{1D\alpha}$ subtype, are of low abundance. I think that explains the apparent inconsistencies in the limited amount of data available, particularly as these are very small tissues and it is not easy to get fresh human samples.

Hamel: Some of our results (Bouchelet *et al.*, this volume) might be explained by the differences in sensitivity that exist between PCR and Northern blots. As Dr Branchek said, the way these experiments are done can affect the answer, particularly when you look at low levels of gene expression.

Humphrey: We should avoid oversimplistic interpretation. We are talking about experiments where mRNA is measured. But we do not know how that is translated and how much receptor protein there is. Even if you looked at the protein, you might fail to find it but still get a very good functional response, as Dr Martin has found with the 5-HT$_{1B}$ receptor in CHO cells (Giles *et al.* 1994). You cannot ignore the possibility that you may need a very low receptor density to observe a profound effect.

Moskowitz: The bottom line is that we need to develop compounds selective for 5-HT$_{1D\alpha}$ or 5-HT$_{1D\beta}$ receptors and that will resolve the issue.

Edvinsson: Dr Connor, did you not look at the trigeminal ganglion cells and find that sumatriptan had no effect upon the membrane potential?

Connor: Yes, but that was looking at cell bodies where functional receptors may not be present. But another explanation might be that the abundance of receptors was so low that we could not see a response.

Moskowitz: The receptors are not expressed on the membrane of trigeminal ganglion cell bodies, but presumably are on the nerve terminals.

Edvinsson: Why is it important that the receptors are expressed in the ganglion cells?

Moskowitz: If the mRNA is not present, then the protein is not synthesized. The fact that we have identified expression of the 5-HT$_{1D\alpha}$ mRNA means that there is at least the possibility of receptor protein synthesis, and therefore the possibility for specific receptor binding.

Hamel: You would not expect to find a message in the terminal area; it has to be located within the cell body. Even if the protein does not have a final location in the cell soma, the message has to be there so the protein can be synthesized and transported to the terminal.

Branchek: As Dr Hamel says, you would not look for the message in the terminal. We must use a complementary study employing an antibody or a selective radioligand, or a functional assay. Such data can then be correlated based on the neuroanatomy of the system.

Sandler: I assume GR55562 has not been used in man yet. You suggest it might be clinically helpful in certain contexts, but would you not expect it, as it is an antagonist, to provoke migraine attacks, as sumatriptan is an agonist and helps migraine?

Connor: You would only expect GR55562, as an antagonist, to have such an effect if there was endogenous 5-HT tone in the system. GR127935, a compound with a similar profile of action, has been given to man and I am not aware of reports of headache.

REFERENCES

Bouchelet, I., Cohen, Z., Séguéla, P. and Hamel, E. (1996) Differential expression of sumatriptan-sensitive 5-HT$_1$ receptors in human neuronal and vascular tissues. In: *Migraine: Pharmacology and Genetics*, (eds M. Sandler, M.D. Ferrari and S. Harnett), pp. 55–66. Chapman & Hall, London.

Giles, H., Lansdell, S.J., Fox, P., Lockyer, M., Hall, V. and Martin, G.R. (1994) Characterisation of a 5-HT$_{1B}$ receptor on CHO cells: functional responses in the absence of radioligand binding. *British Journal of Pharmacology*, **112**, 317P.

Lee, W.S. and Moskowitz, M.A. (1993) Conformationally restricted sumatriptan analogues CP-122, 288 and CP-122, 638 exhibit enhanced potency against neurogenic inflammation in dura mater. *Brain Research*, **626**, 303–305.

Moskowitz, M.A. (1996) 5-HT$_{1D}$ and GABA$_A$ receptors in migraine. In: *Migraine: Pharmacology and Genetics*, (eds M. Sandler, M.D. Ferrari and S. Harnett), pp. 144–153. Chapman & Hall, London.

Rebeck, G.W., Maynard, K.I., Hyman, B.T. and Moskowitz, M.A. (1994) Selective 5-HT $_{1D\alpha}$ serotonin receptor gene expression in trigeminal ganglia: implications for anti-migraine drug development. *Proceedings of the National Academy of Sciences USA*, **91**, 3666–3669.

3

Molecular perspectives on 5-hydroxytryptamine receptor subtypes related to migraine models

Theresa A. Branchek, Stefan A. Kucharewicz, Jonathan A. Bard and Richard L. Weinshank

INTRODUCTION

The involvement of serotonergic systems in migraine is indicated by the therapeutic success of agents acting at various serotonin (5-hydroxytryptamine, 5-HT) receptors. Both acute and prophylactic treatments based on serotonin receptor activity have been found useful. Serotonin receptors suggested to play a role in this process include the 5-$HT_{1D\alpha}$ and 5-$HT_{1D\beta}$ subtypes, based on the action of the 5-HT agonist sumatriptan. In addition, correlations of the prophylactic effect of methysergide and other agents have been made to 5-HT_{2B} and 5-HT_{2C} receptors. The search for potent and efficacious drugs to treat acute migraine has produced a set of compounds related to sumatriptan (311C90, MK-462, naratriptan) which all appear to display activity at 5-HT_{1D} receptor subtypes (see Connor and Beattie, this volume). Various animal models have used many different species, including rat (Buzzi *et al.* 1991), guinea-pig (Lee and Moskowitz 1993), dog (Connor *et al.* 1989), pig (Den Boer *et al.* 1991), cat (Goadsby and Edvinsson 1993) and rabbit (Martin and MacLennan 1990). However, species differences in receptor

Migraine: Pharmacology and genetics
Edited by Merton Sandler, Michel Ferrari and Sara Harnett
Published in 1996 by Chapman & Hall
ISBN 1 86036 006 8

pharmacology have been a source of confusion in receptor identification throughout the history of pharmacology. The identification of serotonin receptors, in particular the 5-HT$_{1B/1D}$ receptor family, has also suffered from this (Hartig *et al.* 1992). Furthermore, a large collection of functional responses to 5-HT, particularly in vascular preparations, remain classified as '5-HT$_1$-like' (Hoyer *et al.* 1994). The definition of a 5-HT$_1$-like receptor is based on agonist responses to 5-carboxamidotryptamine (5-CT) and antagonism by methiothepin (Bradley *et al.* 1986). We now know that several distinct molecular entities satisfy these criteria and that revision according to structural, transductional and operational criteria using more selective pharmacological agents is required (Hoyer *et al.* 1994). New tools to evaluate the impact of species differences in receptor structure have been provided by molecular biological techniques. To explore the role of species differences in 5-HT$_{1D}$ receptor pharmacology, we have cloned the 5-HT$_{1D\alpha}$ and 5-HT$_{1D\beta}$ receptors from the rabbit and attempted to align the profiles of the agonist and antagonist binding affinities with functional responses from rabbit blood vessels producing 5-HT$_1$-like responses. The rabbit saphenous vein (RbSV, Martin and MacLennan 1990) was chosen for comparison as it has been used in the discovery of 5-HT$_{1D}$ agonists.

CLONING OF THE RABBIT 5-HT$_{1D\alpha}$ AND 5-HT$_{1D\beta}$ RECEPTOR GENES

The rabbit homologues of the human 5-HT$_{1D\alpha}$ and 5-HT$_{1D\beta}$ receptor genes were obtained by screening a rabbit genomic library, using probes to the third intracellular loops of the human 5-HT$_{1D\alpha}$ and 5-HT$_{1D\beta}$ genes. The rabbit 5-HT$_{1D\alpha}$ gene encodes a predicted receptor protein of 377 amino acids, the same size as its human homologue. The rabbit 5-HT$_{1D\alpha}$ receptor exhibited 91% amino acid identity to the human 5-HT$_{1D\alpha}$ receptor and 62% to the human 5-HT$_{1D\beta}$ receptor. The rabbit 5-HT$_{1D\beta}$ gene encodes a predicted receptor protein of 389 amino acids. The human 5-HT$_{1D\beta}$ receptor protein contains an additional amino acid in its amino tail and, therefore, has a coding region of 390 amino acids. The rabbit 5-HT$_{1D\beta}$ receptor gene was 93% identical to the human 5-HT$_{1D\beta}$ receptor and 62% to the rabbit 5-HT$_{1D\beta}$ receptor. Figure 3.1 shows the relationship of the deduced amino acid sequences of the rabbit and human 5-HT$_{1D\alpha}$ receptors. Fifty-five to sixty percent of the amino acid residues of the 5-HT$_{1D}$ receptors are identical between rabbit and human. However, there are 33 amino acids which differ between the rabbit and human 5-HT$_{1D\alpha}$ receptors, and nine of these (shaded amino acids in Figure 3.1) fall within transmembrane domains (Table 3.1). Figure 3.2 shows the relationship of the deduced amino acid sequences

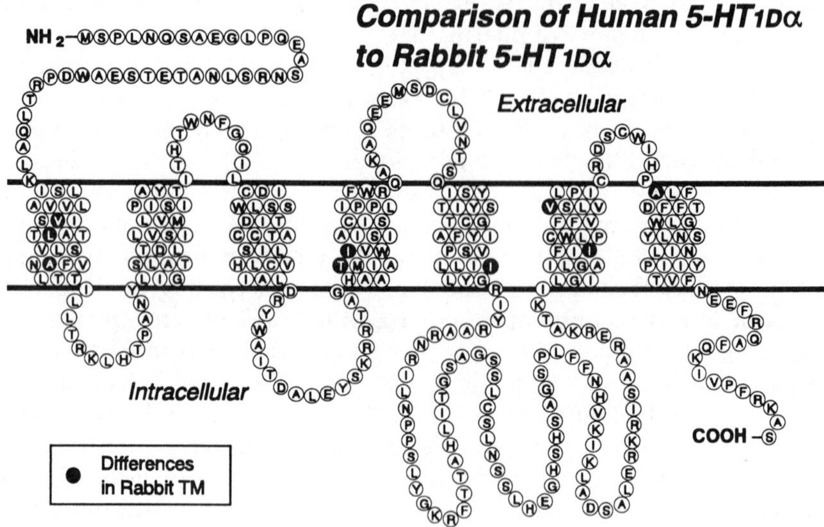

Figure 3.1 The deduced amino acid sequence of the human 5-HT$_{1D\alpha}$ receptor. Residues in the transmembrane region where the rabbit receptor is divergent are indicated in black.

Table 3.1 Comparison of structural properties of the 5-HT$_{1D\alpha}$ and 5-HT$_{1D\beta}$ receptor homologues in various species. Of particular note are the transmembrane (TM) regions

	Human	Rat	Dog	Rabbit
5-HT$_{1D\alpha}$				
Amino acids	377	374	377	377
% Overall identity vs human	100	91	88	91
% TM identity vs human	100	95	93	95
Differences in TM vs human	0	8	12	9
5-HT$_{1D\beta}$				
Amino acids	390	386	389	389
% Overall identity vs human	100	94	95	93
% TM identity vs human	100	96	99	94
Differences in TM vs human	0	6	2	11

of the rabbit and human 5-HT$_{1D\beta}$ receptors. Similarly, species differences for the 5-HT$_{1D\beta}$ receptor occur at 28 amino acids, with 11 residing within transmembrane domains (Table 3.1). Because the ligand-binding pocket for 5-HT is thought to reside in the outer third of the transmembrane

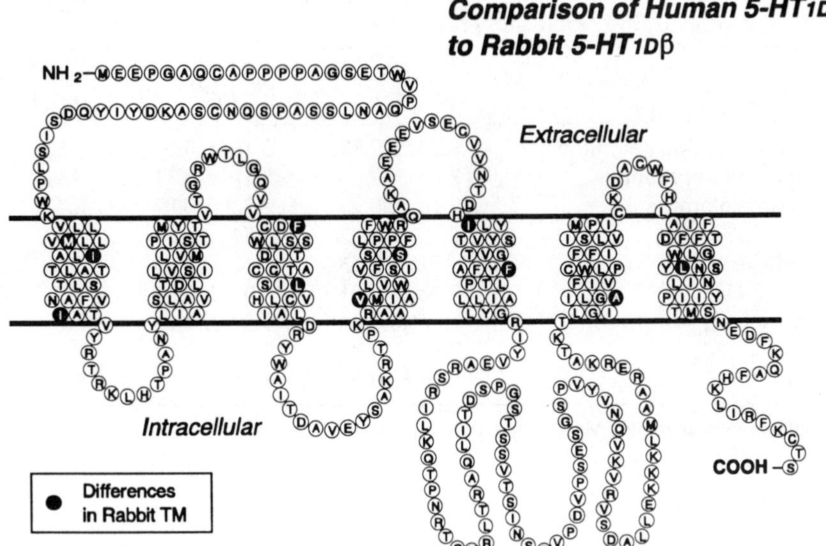

Figure 3.2 The deduced amino acid sequence of the human 5-HT$_{1D\beta}$ receptor. Residues in the transmembrane region where the rabbit receptor is divergent are indicated in black.

region, the number of residues for ligand interaction is limited, and species differences in pharmacology may be attributed to key amino acids.

PHARMACOLOGICAL CHARACTERIZATION OF CLONED RABBIT 5-HT$_{1D\alpha}$ OR 5-HT$_{1D\beta}$ RECEPTORS

Monkey kidney cells transiently expressing the gene encoding the rabbit 5-HT$_{1D\alpha}$ or 5-HT$_{1D\beta}$ receptor genes were used for pharmacological evaluation. The K_d values determined for cloned rabbit 5-HT$_{1D\beta}$ and 5-HT$_{1D\beta}$ receptors were 4.02 ± 0.16 nM and 6.46 ± 0.76 nM respectively using [^{3}H]5-HT as a radioligand. The B_{max} values were 235 ± 41.5 fmol/mg and 740 ± 72 fmol/mg protein respectively. The rank order of binding affinities for the cloned rabbit 5-HT$_{1D}$ receptors was as follows: for 5-HT$_{1D\alpha}$, 5-CT > 5-HT > sumatriptan > 2-CH$_3$-5-HT; and for 5-HT$_{1D\beta}$, 5-CT = 5-HT > sumatriptan > 2-CH$_3$-5-HT. When compared with each other, these subtypes are highly correlated (Table 3.2). However, ketanserin and methiothepin appear to discriminate modestly between rabbit 5-HT$_{1D\alpha}$ and 5-HT$_{1D\beta}$ receptors: the former has higher affinity for rabbit 5-HT$_{1D\alpha}$, whereas the latter has higher affinity for rabbit 5-HT$_{1D\beta}$. Several differences between rabbit and human homologues were also

Table 3.2 Comparison of binding affinities of cloned rabbit 5-HT$_{1D}$ receptors with potencies in the rabbit saphenous vein

Compound	5-HT$_{1D\alpha}$ (pK$_i$)	5-HT$_{1D\beta}$ (pK$_i$)	RbSV[a] (pK$_A$)
5-Carboxamidotryptamine	8.53 ± 0.12	8.16 ± 0.06	7.53
5-Hydroxytryptamine	7.88 ± 0.08	8.17 ± 0.11	7.12
5-CH$_3$-tryptamine	7.70 ± 0.23	7.32 ± 0.07	6.43
Sumatriptan	7.12 ± 0.08	6.84 ± 0.06	
α-CH$_3$-5-HT	6.52 ± 0.13	6.48 ± 0.03	5.68
2-CH$_3$-5-HT	5.38 ± 0.01	5.39 ± 0.11	4.7
Ketanserin	7.66 ± 0.08	6.30 ± 0.14	7.0*
Methysergide	7.05 ± 0.08	7.10 ± 0.03	
Methiothepin	6.64 ± 0.07	7.86 ± 0.08	9.45*

[a] Data from Martin and MacLennan 1990
* pK$_B$

observed. For example, 5-methyl tryptamine, ketanserin, methiothepin, 5-methoxytryptamine and methysergide all show significant differences between rabbit 5-HT$_{1D\alpha}$ and human 5-HT$_{1D\alpha}$ receptors. Similarly, 2-methyl-5-hydroxytryptamine, 5-methyl tryptamine and sumatriptan differ between rabbit 5-HT$_{1D\beta}$ and human 5-HT$_{1D\beta}$ receptors. In addition, ketanserin has a higher affinity for the rabbit 5-HT$_{1D\beta}$ receptor than for the human one, lessening its value as a pharmacological tool to dissect 5-HT$_{1D}$ receptor subtypes in the rabbit (see Zgombick *et al.* 1995).

COMPARISON TO CONTRACTILE RESPONSES OF RABBIT SAPHENOUS VEIN

The binding affinities for the cloned rabbit 5-HT$_{1D\alpha}$ and 5-HT$_{1D\beta}$ receptors were compared to published pK$_A$ values for the contraction of the rabbit saphenous vein (Martin and MacLennan 1990; see Table 3.2). The rank order of affinities of the 5-HT$_{1D\alpha}$ receptor is consistent with that of the rabbit saphenous vein response. In addition, the fact that ketanserin can antagonize the RbSV contraction (pK$_B$ = 7.0) is also consistent with a 5-HT$_{1D\alpha}$, but not a 5-HT$_{1D\beta}$ receptor. Further inspection of potency ratios relative to 5-HT for a larger number of compounds (Table 3.3) illustrates the difficulty in assignment of receptor subtype(s) in this preparation. However, the extremely high potency of methiothepin (pK$_B$ = 9.45) is inconsistent with either a 5-HT$_{1D\alpha}$ or 5-HT$_{1D\beta}$ receptor. Therefore, it appears that a 5-HT$_{1D\alpha}$ receptor may mediate part of the contractile response of the RbSV to sumatriptan. However, none of the agonists studied has sufficient selectivity between the two 5-HT$_{1D}$

Table 3.3 Comparison of potency values (relative to 5-hydroxytryptamine) for binding constants of the cloned rabbit 5-HT$_{1D}$ receptors and for the rabbit saphenous vein

Compound	Potency ratios relative to 5-HT		
	5-HT$_{1D\alpha}$	5-HT$_{1D\beta}$	RbSV[a]
5-Carboxamidotryptamine	0.22	1.02	0.39
5-Hydroxytryptamine	1.00	1.00	1.00
5-CH$_3$-tryptamine	1.51	7.08	4.90
Sumatriptan	5.75	21.38	10.47
α-CH$_3$-5-HT	22.91	48.98	27.54
2-CH$_3$-5-HT	316.23	602.56	263.03
Ketanserin	1.66	74.13	1.32
Methysergide	2.19	11.75	10.00
Methiothepin	17.38	2.04	0.08

[a] Data from Hoyer *et al.* 1994

subtypes in the rabbit to determine the roles of these receptors definitively.

DISCUSSION

Significant progress has been made in the development of serotonin-based therapeutics for acute migraine. During this period, molecular cloning has led to a rapid characterization of serotonin receptor subtypes from many species (Branchek 1993a). A more difficult task has been to relate cloned receptors to those studied in functional models such as vasoconstriction (Kaumann *et al.* 1993). Potential differences in the pharmacology of specific receptors in different species has motivated us to clone 5-HT receptors from several animal genomes.

Because the rabbit saphenous vein has been used in the development of 'sumatriptan-like' 5-HT$_{1D}$ agonists, we chose this species for further characterization. We cloned the 5-HT$_{1D}$ receptors from rabbit and determined that the rabbit 5-HT$_{1D\alpha}$ and 5-HT$_{1D\beta}$ genes display greater than 90% amino acid identity to their human homologues, as observed between human and mammalian receptor counterparts for other biogenic amine G protein-coupled receptors. The translated product of the cloned rabbit 5-HT$_{1D\alpha}$ gene is predicted to be the same length as the human 5-HT$_{1D\alpha}$ receptor. The rabbit 5-HT$_{1D\beta}$ receptor lacks one amino acid in the amino terminus compared with the human counterpart. The observed amino acid differences between the 5-HT$_{1D\alpha}$ and 5-HT$_{1D\beta}$ homologues within the transmembrane region, the presumed ligand recognition site (9 and 11 residues, respectively), are likely to contribute to the observed pharmacological differences. Such an assertion could be tested by site-directed mutagenesis studies as have been performed for many 5-HT receptor subtypes (see Branchek 1993b for review). In comparing the rabbit 5-HT_{1D} receptor profile, it appears that there are significant correlations in the binding profiles between the cloned rabbit and human $5\text{-HT}_{1D\alpha}$ (r = 0.79) and $5\text{-HT}_{1D\beta}$ (r = 0.8) receptors. This characteristic had been reported for the canine and human $5\text{-HT}_{1D\alpha}$ and $5\text{-HT}_{1D\beta}$ homologues (Branchek *et al.* 1995). In comparing these receptor profiles to those obtained from the study of the contractile responses of the rabbit saphenous vein, we have found evidence for a role of the $5\text{-HT}_{1D\alpha}$ receptor in mediating the sumatriptan-induced contraction (Tables 3.2 and 3.3). The rank order of agonist potencies for this response best matches the $5\text{-HT}_{1D\alpha}$ receptor subtype. The affinity of ketanserin is also consistent with its blockade of contraction of the RbSV. However, several agonists have a potency intermediate to the values obtained for the two cloned rabbit 5-HT_{1D} receptors. Finally, methiothepin has an antagonist potency inconsistent with either site. Whether a novel subtype exists in this tissue remains to be determined. Further work on receptor localization and use of better pharmacological tools, such as subtype-selective compounds, should provide more definitive assessment of which 5-HT_{1D}-like receptor(s) is/are involved in mediating this contraction. Ultimately, a clearer understanding of the receptor sites activated by agents used in the clinic may lead to the development of improved therapies for migraine.

Acknowledgements

The authors thank Drs Marlene Cohen and Graeme Martin for helpful discussion, Mr George Moralishuili for the illustrations and Ms Elena Marton for preparing the manuscript. A portion of this work was supported by Eli Lilly and Company.

REFERENCES

Bradley, P.B., Engel, G., Feniuk, W., Fozard, J.R., Humphrey, P.P.A., Middlemiss, D.N., Mylecharane, E.J., Richardson, B.P. and Saxena, P.R. (1986) Proposals for the classification and nomenclature of functional receptors for 5-hydroxytryptamine. *Neuropharmacology*, **25**, 563–576.

Branchek, T. (1993a) More serotonin receptors? *Current Biology*, **3**(5), 315–317.

Branchek, T. (1993b) Site-directed mutagenesis of serotonin receptors. *Medicinal Chemistry Research*, **3**, 287–296.

Branchek, T.A., Bard, J.A., Kucharewicz, S.A., Zgombick, J.M., Weinshank, R.L. and Cohen, M.L. (1995) Migraine: relationship to cloned canine and human 5-HT_{1D} receptors. In: *Experimental Headache Models*, (eds J. Olesen and M.A. Moskowitz), pp. 123–134. Raven Press, New York.

Buzzi, M.G., Moskowitz, M.A., Peroutka, S.J. and Byun, B. (1991) Further characterisation of the putative 5-HT receptor which mediates blockade of neurogenic plasma extravasation in rat dura mater. *British Journal of Pharmacology*, **103**, 1421–1428.

Connor, H.E. and Beattie, D.T. (1996) 5-Hydroxytryptamine receptor subtypes and migraine. In: *Migraine: Pharmacology and Genetics*, (eds M. Sandler, M.D. Ferrari and S. Harnett), pp. 18–31. Chapman & Hall, London.

Connor, H.E., Feniuk, W. and Humphrey, P.P.A. (1989) Characterisation of 5-HT receptors mediating contraction of canine and primate basilar artery by use of GR 43175, a selective 5-HT$_1$-like receptor agonist. *British Journal of Pharmacology*, **96**, 379–387.

Den Boer, M.O., Villalón, C.M., Heiligers, J.P.C., Humphrey, P.P.A. and Saxena, P.R. (1991) Role of 5-HT$_1$-like receptors in the reduction of porcine cranial arteriovenous anastomotic shunting by sumatriptan. *British Journal of Pharmacology*, **102**, 323–330.

Goadsby, P.J. and Edvinsson, L. (1993) The trigeminovascular system and migraine: studies characterising cerebrovascular and neuropeptide changes seen in humans and cats. *Annals of Neurology*, 33, 48.

Hartig, P.R., Branchek, T.A. and Weinshank, R.L. (1992) A subfamily of 5-HT$_{1D}$ receptor genes. *Trends in Pharmacological Sciences*, **13**, 152–159.

Hoyer, D., Clarke, D.E., Fozard, J.R., Hartig, P.R., Martin, G.R., Mylecharlane, E.J., Saxena, P.R. and Humphrey, P.P.A. (1994) International Union of Pharmacology classification of receptors for 5-hydroxytryptamine (serotonin). *Pharmacological Reviews*, **46**, 157–203.

Lee, W.S. and Moskowitz, M.A. (1993) Conformationally restricted sumatriptan analogues, CP-122, 288 and CP-122, 638, exhibit enhanced potency against neurogenic inflammation in dura mater. *Brain Research*, **626**, 303–305.

Kaumann, A.J., Parsons, A.A., Brown, A.M. (1993) Human arterial constrictor serotonin receptors. *Cardiovascular Research* **27**, 2094–2103.

Martin G.R. and MacLennan S.J. (1990) Analysis of the 5-HT receptor in rabbit saphenous vein exemplifies the problems of using exclusion criteria for receptor classification. *Naunyn-Schmiedeberg's Archives of Pharmacology*, **342**, 111–119.

Zgombick, J.M., Schechter, L.E., Kucharewicz, S.A., Weinshank, R.L. and Branchek, T.A. (1995) The 5-HT$_{2A}$ receptor antagonists, ketanserin and ritanserin, discriminated between recombinant human 5-HT$_{1D\alpha}$ and 5-HT$_{1D\beta}$ receptor subtypes: identification of 'selective' 5-HT$_{1D\alpha}$ receptor antagonists. *European Journal of Pharmacology (Molecular Pharmacology Section)*, **291**, 9–15.

DISCUSSION

Connor: Dr Branchek, which receptor do you think mediates contraction of human arteries?

Branchek: We do not have our own data, but from the literature it seems to be the 5-HT$_{1D\beta}$ receptor.

Sandler: Is the 5-HT$_{1D}$ pseudo-gene (Shuck *et al.* 1993) just of evolutionary interest, or does it have a functional role?

Branchek: Pseudo-genes are thought of as evolutionary trash; they were once functional genes, but mutations in the sequence led to a non-functional protein. In general, at least one mutation gives rise to a stop-codon. For the 5-HT$_{1D\alpha}$ receptor (Bard *et al.* 1995), that fragment is transcribed and we found the mRNA in multiple brain samples (we did not look in other tissues), so it is not just an individual difference. If that fragment of the gene is transfected into a cell it does not give rise to any detectable binding signal, so presumably in the organism it is a dysfunctional gene. A pseudo-gene could be long enough to have some activity, but in general they are thought to be dysfunctional.

Moskowitz: Do we know which subtypes are expressed in human coronary vessels? This information is critical to understanding side-effects.

Hamel: We have looked at one coronary artery so far and the 5-HT$_{1D\beta}$ receptor subtype seemed to be clearly expressed (Bouchelet *et al.*, this volume). More studies are needed to get the complete picture.

Branchek: We also looked at that, but the quality of dissection of the preparations we used might not be sufficient to answer the question. With polymerase chain reaction (PCR) studies even minor contamination of an adjacent structure gives a totally different picture and we have had difficulty in detecting signals in human peripheral tissue using *in situ* hybridization, presumably because of post-mortem degradation and low abundance.

Hamel: That is correct. PCR might lead to amplification of signals from various sources. *In situ* hybridization studies on vessels will be the best way to answer these questions. However, in the dissection and cleaning procedure, one can ensure retention of only vascular tissue.

Fozard: There is a 5-HT$_{1D}$ receptor in the endothelium in certain vessels. What is known about its α or β profile?

Hamel: In cultures of human endothelial cells subcloned from capillaries isolated from cortical biopsies, there seems to be a clear expression of the 5-HT$_{1D\alpha}$ subtype (Bouchelet *et al.*, this volume), and we detected the 5-HT$_{1D\beta}$ subtype in two preparations. Thus these receptors seem to be associated with many cell types, cerebral endothelial and smooth muscle cells as well as neurons.

Fozard: Are they present on human coronary endothelium?

Hamel: I have not done that, but endothelial cells and coronary arteries could probably be scraped off easily because these are quite big vessels. There are aortic endothelial cell lines, but I do not know about coronary endothelial cells.

Fozard: Dr Connor, in your work with human coronary vessels, did you scrape them to remove the endothelium first?

Connor: No, but in all my coronary experiments I have not seen any evidence for a 5-HT receptor mediating relaxation.

Bax: *In vivo* infusion of 5-HT into a coronary artery does give relaxation in healthy individuals. However, as soon as a coronary artery becomes atherosclerotic, which usually happens at an early age, the relaxant component disappears. It has not yet been possible to perform *in vitro* experiments with the relaxant receptor.

Fozard: But you could, presumably, detect relaxation with the right conditions?

Bax: Yes. Relaxations are rarely seen *in vitro* because the receptor mediating relaxation is weak compared to the contractile 5-HT$_1$-like receptor.

Connor: Perhaps the endothelial receptor is down at the level of the resistance vessel, which cannot be looked at in isolated tissue experiments.

Ferrari: Would it be different if you perfuse only from the luminal side?

Bax: Perhaps. We are trying to develop that model.

Martin: In some instances 'priming' with an agent such as thromboxane A$_2$ is required in order to unmask 5-HT$_{1D}$ receptor-mediated contraction. This makes it difficult to anticipate *in vivo* reactivity to 5-HT$_{1D}$ agonists based on experience *in vitro*. It is possible that an endothelium-dependent 5-HT$_{1D}$ response requires a similar 'priming' before a functional effect is seen.

Glover: What is known about the localization of the 5-HT$_{1D\beta}$ receptors in the human artery and their relation to serotonergic nerves?

Hamel: The nerves are clearly outside in the adventitia. Nobody has reported nerves going across the smooth muscle. The receptors might be located on both the smooth muscle and endothelial cells of the artery.

Glover: Are the receptors quite dissociated from the nerve?

Hamel: There might be receptors on the endothelium, and these may see a lower concentration of 5-HT. We do not know, but it is possible.

Glover: Does the 5-HT come from nerves, platelets or elsewhere?

Hamel: We do not know.

Connor: I think it is more likely to be from platelets.

Moskowitz: I am not convinced that there is necessarily an endogenous ligand acting under physiological conditions.

Hamel: That is an interesting possibility. The receptor might become functional or manifest only under pathological conditions when the ligand could then gain access to it. This has been suggested for cerebrovascular muscarinic receptors (Shimizu *et al.* 1993).

Bax: Amongst others, Martin and Wilson (1995) have shown that the 5-HT$_7$, receptor may be involved in relaxation. Might a 5-HT$_7$ receptor-mediated effect be hidden in the 5-HT$_{1D}$ effects: a relaxant response hidden within the contractile effect?

Branchek: Sumatriptan will not elicit any response due to a 5-HT$_7$ mechanism because its affinity is several orders of magnitude lower than that of 5-HT or 5-carboxamidotryptamine. Most recent studies used sumatriptan as the agonist, thereby avoiding that complication.

Sandler: We should discuss the 5-HT$_6$ and 5-HT$_7$ receptors in another context because migraine is inextricably bound with depression in a relatively high proportion of cases and we know that the 5-HT$_6$ and 5-HT$_7$ receptors seem to be strongly affected by tricyclic antidepressants and antipsychotic drugs (Monsma *et al.* 1993, Shen *et al.* 1993). These receptors may be involved in the greater migraine story.

Branchek: In either the vasoconstrictor mechanism or the protein plasma extravasation model, an agonist of either the 5-HT$_6$ or 5-HT$_7$ subtype would work in the opposite direction to that expected to be therapeutically beneficial. So this class of agents will probably not be valuable. To target 5-HT$_6$ or 5-HT$_7$ receptors, I suspect one would need antagonists, and I am not aware that those tools exist. The role of these receptors in other neuropsychiatric disorders is widely speculated upon in the literature: the other 'affective' aspects of migraine may indeed be linked to these subtypes.

REFERENCES

Bard, J.A., Nawoschik, S.P., O'Dowd, B.F., George, S.R., Branchek, T.A. and Weinshank, R.L. (1995) The human serotonin 5-hydroxytryptamine$_{1D}$ receptor pseudogene is transcribed. *Gene*, **153**, 295–296.

Bouchelet, I., Cohen, Z., Séguéla, P. and Hamel, E. (1996) Differential expression of sumatriptan-sensitive 5-HT$_1$ receptors in human neuronal and vascular tissues. In: *Migraine: Pharmacology and Genetics*, (eds M. Sandler, M.D. Ferrari and S. Harnett), pp. 55-66. Chapman & Hall, London.

Martin, G.R. and Wilson, R. (1995) Operational characteristics of a 5-HT receptor mediating direct vascular relaxation: identity with the 5-HT$_7$ receptor. *British Journal of Pharmacology*, (Abstract).

Monsma, F.J., Shen, Y., Ward, R.P., Hamblin, M.W., and Sibley, D.R. (1993) Cloning and expression of a novel serotonin receptor with high affinity for tricyclic psychotropic drugs. *Molecular Pharmacology*, **43**, 320–327.

Shen, Y., Monsma, F.J., Metcalf, M.A., Jose, P.A., Hamblin, M.W. and Sibley, D.R. (1993) Molecular cloning and expression of a 5-hydroxytryptamine$_7$ serotonin receptor subtype. *Journal of Biological Chemistry*, **268**, 18200–18204

Shimizu, T., Rosenblum, W.I. and Nelson, G.H. (1993) M3 and M1 receptors in cerebral arterioles *in vivo*: evidence for down regulation or ineffective M1 when endothelium is intact. *American Journal of Physiology*, **264**, 665–669.

Shuck, M.E., Veldman, S.A. and Bienkowski, M.J. (1993) Cloning, sequencing and phylogenetic analysis of a human 5-hydroxytryptamine$_{1D}$ receptor pseudogene. *Gene*, **137**, 339–344.

4

Vascular effects of 5-HT$_{1D}$ receptor agonists and antagonists

Willem A. Bax, Peter de Vries, Antoinette Maassen van den Brink and Pramod R. Saxena

INTRODUCTION

The effect of antimigraine drugs is considered to be mediated via a vasoconstrictor effect in cranial blood vessels, involving the 5-HT$_{1D}$-like subtype of 5-hydroxytryptamine (5-HT, serotonin) receptors (Saxena and Ferrari 1989). Others have suggested involvement of prejunctional 5-HT$_{1D}$ receptors in the trigeminal ganglion (Moskowitz 1992) mediating inhibition of the release of a number of vasodilator, pro-inflammatory peptides, such as calcitonin gene-related peptide (CGRP) (Goadsby and Edvinsson 1993). Novel and traditional antimigraine drugs also constrict peripheral blood vessels (Connor *et al.* 1989, Chester *et al.* 1990, Bax and Saxena 1993) and a significant number of cases has been reported in which the use of antimigraine drugs, like sumatriptan and ergotamine, resulted in myocardial ischaemia (Galer *et al.* 1991, Ottervanger *et al.* 1993). For this reason much effort has been directed towards the development of cranio-selective antimigraine drugs. Interestingly, Kaumann *et al.* (1993) found some evidence that 5-HT$_{1D\beta}$ receptors may mediate coronary vasoconstriction in man, while Rebeck *et al.* (1994) showed the presence of mRNA encoding for 5-HT$_{1D\alpha}$ and not for 5-HT$_{1D\beta}$ receptors in human trigeminal ganglion. Thus, it was suggested that it may be possible to develop antimigraine drugs aimed at prejunctional 5-HT$_{1D\alpha}$ receptors which would be devoid of coronary

Migraine: Pharmacology and genetics
Edited by Merton Sandler, Michel Ferrari and Sara Harnett
Published in 1996 by Chapman & Hall
ISBN 1 86036 006 8

side-effects. On the other hand, careful examination has now revealed that mRNA for 5-HT$_{1D\alpha}$ receptors may be present in canine (Cushing *et al.* 1994) and possibly also in human coronary arteries (p. 63, this volume), whilst mRNA for 5-HT$_{1D\beta}$ receptors or its rat equivalent (5-HT$_{1B}$) has been shown in some human (Bouchelet *et al.*, this volume) and rat (Bruinvels *et al.* 1992) trigeminal ganglion samples. Therefore, it may be postulated that development of an agonist with a selective 5-HT$_{1D\alpha}$ receptor affinity profile will not yield the desired complete cranio-selectivity. Thus, apart from identification of mRNA expressing certain 5-HT receptor subtypes possibly involved in the effect of antimigraine drugs, it may be rewarding to investigate additional receptor subtypes and other functional mechanisms involved in vasoconstrictor effects of antimigraine drugs. Indeed, little is understood about why certain patients report chest symptoms suggesting myocardial ischaemia and coronary vasoconstriction. These patients do not necessarily belong to traditional groups at risk for myocardial ischaemia (Ottervanger *et al.* 1993, Stricker and Ottervanger 1992). Therefore, functional experimental work is essential in analysing the effects of antimigraine drugs. In this chapter, examples of experiments in both cranial and peripheral blood vessels are presented, illustrating that the effects of 5-HT and the antimigraine drug sumatriptan cannot be explained entirely by their action on a single 5-HT receptor subtype. Data are presented that suggest multiple receptor subtypes involved in vasoconstriction of the cranial circulation of anaesthetized pigs, and additional mechanisms mediating sumatriptan-induced vasoconstriction in human isolated coronary arteries.

USE OF THE 5-HT$_{1D}$ RECEPTOR ANTAGONIST GR127935 IN A PORCINE MODEL FOR MIGRAINE

GR127935 has high affinity for both 5-HT$_{1D\alpha}$ (K_i, 1.3 nM) and 5-HT$_{1D\beta}$ (K_i, 0.13 nM) receptors (Skingle *et al.* 1993). GR127935 inhibited sumatriptan-induced inhibition of 5-HT release in guinea-pig dorsal raphe nucleus (Starkey and Skingle 1993), as well as contraction of the canine basilar artery (Skingle *et al.* 1993). In these experiments we studied the effects of GR127935 on the response to sumatriptan and 5-HT of the total carotid blood flow and its arteriovenous anastomotic and capillary fractions in anaesthetized pigs.

Method

The methods used have been described in detail elsewhere (Saxena and Verdouw 1982, Den Boer *et al.* 1991a). In brief, domestic pigs (10–15 kg) were anaesthetized with azaperone (160 mg intramuscularly, im), midazolan hydrochloride (5 mg im) and metomidate (200 mg intravenously, iv), and maintained with continuous iv infusion of pentobarbitone at 20 mg/kg/h. Drugs were administered via a catheter in the inferior vena cava. The right common carotid artery was dissected free and a needle was inserted to allow administration of radioactive microspheres. Blood flow in this vessel was measured by use of an electromagnetic flow meter. The distribution of carotid blood flow was determined five times by injection of the 15 μm microspheres, labelled with either ^{141}Ce, ^{113}Se, ^{95}Nb, ^{103}Ru or ^{46}Sc. At the end of the experiment the animal was killed, and heart, kidneys, lungs and different cranial tissues were dissected. Radioactivity in these tissues was determined using suitable windows discriminating for the different isotopes. Since little or no radioactivity was detected in the heart or kidneys, all microspheres trapped in the lungs reached the lungs from the venous side of the cranial circulation after escaping entrapment in cranial capillaries via arteriovenous anastomotic connections with a diameter allowing for passage of the 15 μm spheres. All data were expressed as mean ± standard error of the mean (SEM). The significance of changes induced by treatment with saline and GR127935 was evaluated by the use of a paired Student's *t*-test. Changes induced by different doses of sumatriptan or 5-HT within one group were evaluated with Duncan's new multiple range test, once analysis of variance (Anova) had revealed that samples represented different populations. A *p* value smaller than 0.05 was considered to denote a significant difference.

Results and discussion

Sumatriptan (30–300 μg/kg iv) dose dependently reduced total carotid blood flow, as well as its arteriovenous anastomotic fraction, without significant modification of the capillary (i.e. nutrient) fraction. GR127935 (0.25 and 0.5 mg/kg) also reduced total carotid blood flow, with a concomitant decrease of the arteriovenous anastomotic fraction and an unchanged capillary fraction. Indeed, Pauwels and Colpaert (1995) have shown that the reported silent 5-HT$_{1D}$ receptor antagonist GR127935 may act as an agonist in cells expressing human cloned 5-HT$_{1D\alpha}$ receptors. In contrast, GR127935 was a silent antagonist at human cloned 5-HT$_{1D\beta}$ receptors. Whether the observed agonist effect of GR127935 in anaesthetized pigs can be explained by a selective agonist effect at 5-HT$_{1D\alpha}$ receptors remains to be established. However, the sumatriptan-induced decrease in the total carotid and arteriovenous anastomotic blood flow (maximal decrease 52 ± 8% and 76 ± 5%, respectively) was attenuated in animals treated with 0.25 mg/kg GR127935, and completely abolished in animals treated with 0.5 mg/kg

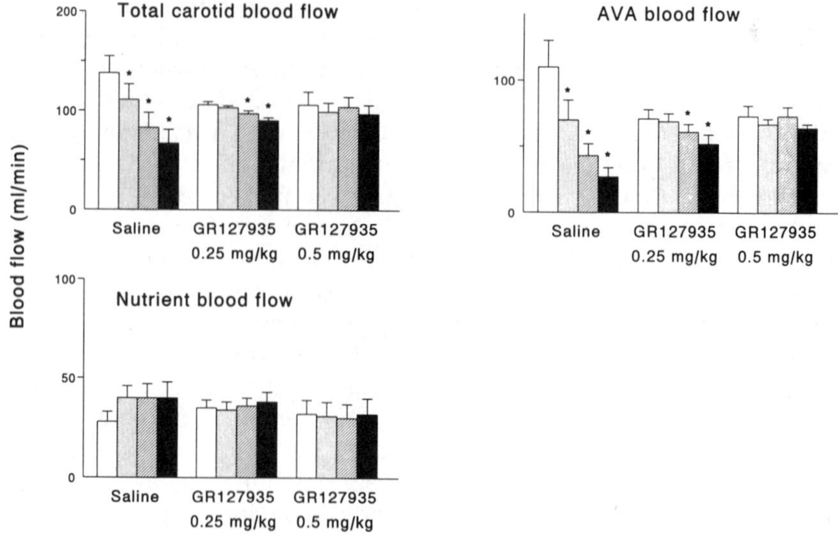

Figure 4.1 Effect of sumatriptan on the total carotid blood flow and its arteriovenous anastomotic (AVA) and nutrient (capillary) fractions in pigs, treated with either saline ($n = 4$) or GR127935 (0.25 and 0.5 mg/kg; $n = 4$ each). From left to right the four bars represent blood flow values before sumatriptan (after treatment with saline or GR127935) and after sumatriptan (30, 100 and 300 µg/kg, respectively). All values are presented as means ± SEM. *, $p < 0.05$ vs baseline.

GR127935 (Figure 4.1). Thus, it may be concluded that GR127935 has a high affinity for the receptor that mediates the cerebrovascular effects of sumatriptan.

To study the effects of GR127935 on the response to 5-HT, a different protocol was used, because 5-HT has a much shorter duration of action. Infusions of 5-HT (2 µg/kg/min for 10 min) were given before and after treatment with GR127935. 5-HT (2 µg/kg/min) did not significantly alter total carotid blood flow (109 ± 13 ml/min vs 103 ± 20 ml/min), but significantly reduced the arteriovenous shunting fraction (80 ± 14 ml/min vs 17 ± 8 ml/min), and induced a concomitant increase of capillary blood flow (28 ± 4 ml/min vs 86 ± 16 ml/min). GR127935 (0.5 mg/kg) resulted in a significant decrease of arteriovenous blood flow, but did not change nutrient blood flow. After GR127935, 5-HT again decreased arteriovenous blood flow, and increased nutrient blood flow, albeit both to a lesser extent than before treatment with GR127935 (Figure 4.2). Since, unlike 5-HT, GR127935 did not increase nutrient blood flow, and since both compounds decreased arteriovenous anastomotic blood flow, it may be concluded that the effects of 5-HT and GR127935 on nutrient

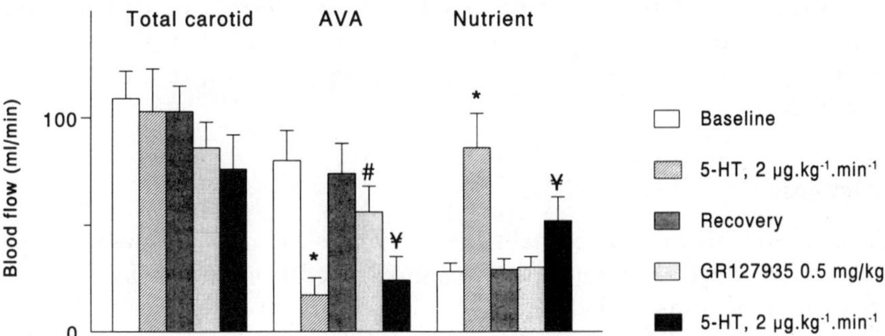

Figure 4.2 Effect of 5-HT (2 µg/kg/min) on the total carotid, arteriovenous anastomotic (AVA) and nutrient blood flow in anaesthetized pigs ($n = 7$), initially and after GR127935 (0.5 mg/kg). Data expressed as mean ± SEM. *, $p < 0.05$ vs recovery blood flow; ¥, $p < 0.05$ vs state after GR127935.

and arteriovenous anastomotic blood flow are mediated via different receptor mechanisms. And although a comparison between the effects of 5-HT and sumatriptan is slightly hampered by the use of a somewhat different protocol, it was shown that the effect of 5-HT remained almost unchanged by treatment with 0.5 mg/kg GR127935, whereas the effect of sumatriptan was virtually abolished by the same dose of GR127935. Thus, it may be suggested that the effects of sumatriptan and 5-HT are mediated in part via different receptor mechanisms. Previously, Den Boer and colleagues showed that the effect of ergotamine and dihydroergotamine was left virtually intact after treatment with the 5-HT_1/5-HT_2 receptor antagonist methiothepin. In contrast, the effect of sumatriptan (Den Boer *et al.* 1991b) or 5-HT (Saxena *et al.* 1986) was blocked completely by methiothepin. Thus, the cerebrovascular effects of 5-HT receptor agonists and antimigraine drugs in anaesthetized pigs are likely to be mediated via multiple receptor subtypes. Knowledge of the full spectrum of receptors and mechanisms mediating the anti-migraine effects of 5-HT receptor agonists will contribute to further improvement of pharmacological treatment of migraine.

ORGAN BATH EXPERIMENTS WITH HUMAN CORONARY ARTERIES: AMPLIFICATION BY THROMBOXANES OF THE CONTRACTILE RESPONSE TO SUMATRIPTAN

Previous studies indicated that contractile responses to 5-HT receptor agonists may be augmented by the presence of low concentrations of thromboxanes (Tx) (MacLennan and Martin 1992, Chester *et al.* 1993). Kaumann *et al.* (1994) showed that the contractile response of human isolated coronary artery segments to sumatriptan may vary. This variability could not be explained by atherosclerosis or disease. We hypothesized that the endogenous production of thromboxanes by coronary artery segments may be a contributing factor to the observed variability.

Methods

The *in vitro* methods used have been described in detail elsewhere (Bax *et al.* 1993, 1994). In brief, hearts were obtained from organ donors who had died of non-cardiac disorders. The hearts were provided by the Rotterdam Heart Valve Bank (Bio Implant Services Foundation) after removal of the valves for transplantation purposes. Ring segments (4 mm) of the right epicardial coronary artery were suspended in 15 ml organ baths containing Krebs bicarbonate solution. The endothelium was left intact.

The endogenous production of thromboxane A_2 by coronary artery was assessed by incubation of segments (length 1–2 cm) in oxygenated Krebs solution (2 ml, 37 °C) for two hours. After incubation, a sample of Krebs solution was removed, and indomethacin (30 μM) was added to stop ongoing cyclooxygenase activity. The concentration of TxB_2, the stable metabolite of TxA_2, was measured by radioimmunoassay (RIA) for TxB_2, and corrected for the weight of the coronary artery segment.

Differences between groups in functional experiments were evaluated with Anova for repeated measurements. Differences in the production of thromboxane were evaluated by using a paired Student's *t*-test. A *p* value smaller than 0.05 was considered to denote a significant difference.

Results and discussion

Sumatriptan induced contraction of human coronary artery segments ($n = 12$) with a magnitude (E_{MAX}, $28 \pm 6\%$ of the response to 100 mM K^+) and potency (pD_2, 6.1 ± 0.1) similar to earlier series (Bax and Saxena 1993). Contraction to sumatriptan was attenuated after incubation of the vascular segment with the thromboxane receptor antagonist SQ30741 (100 nM) ($n = 12$) (Figure 4.3). Since affinity of SQ30741 for 5-HT receptors and other receptors is low, it was postulated that this effect was mediated via a thromboxane receptor for which SQ30741 has high affinity (Schumacher *et al.* 1989). To further investigate this hypothesis we incubated some tissue segments overnight in Krebs bicarbonate solution containing 10 μM aspirin, whereas others were incubated in a Krebs solution not containing aspirin. First, it was shown that the aspirin-treated vessel segments responded with a lower E_{MAX} than the segments not exposed to aspirin, indicating that indeed a cyclo-

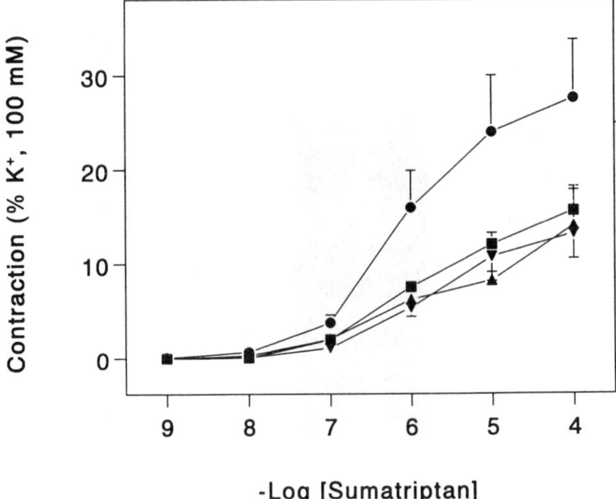

Figure 4.3 Contraction of endothelium-intact human coronary artery segments to sumatriptan. Contraction in the absence of aspirin, without (●) and with (▲) 100 nM SQ30741. Contraction in the presence of 10 μM aspirin, without (■) and with (▼) 100 nM SQ30741 (n = 12). The concentration of sumatriptan refers to mol/l. Data expressed as mean ± SEM.

oxygenase product may be involved in the contractile response. Secondly, it was observed that in the presence of aspirin, SQ30741 no longer attenuated the response to sumatriptan, indicating that the involved cyclooxygenase product was likely to act via a thromboxane receptor (Figure 4.3). Aspirin and SQ30741 did not alter the pD_2 in any of these experiments. Lastly, we measured whether a segment of coronary artery was able to synthesize thromboxanes in detectable amounts. Indeed, thromboxane A_2 was produced by the vessel segments, measured as its stable metabolite, thromboxane B_2. Production of thromboxane A_2 was attenuated by incubation with aspirin (Figure 4.4), which would explain why in the presence of 10 μM aspirin the response to sumatriptan could not be attenuated any further. Thus, a cyclooxygenase product, possibly thromboxane A_2, is involved in the contractile response of human coronary artery segments to sumatriptan. Endogenously produced thromboxane A_2 may be a factor involved in development of chest symptoms after the use of sumatriptan. In addition, these data support previous suggestions that a combined antagonism of 5-HT and thromboxane receptors may be more effective than antagonism of one of these receptors in the treatment of coronary artery vasoconstriction observed in unstable or variant angina pectoris (Willerson *et al.* 1990, Bax *et al.* 1994).

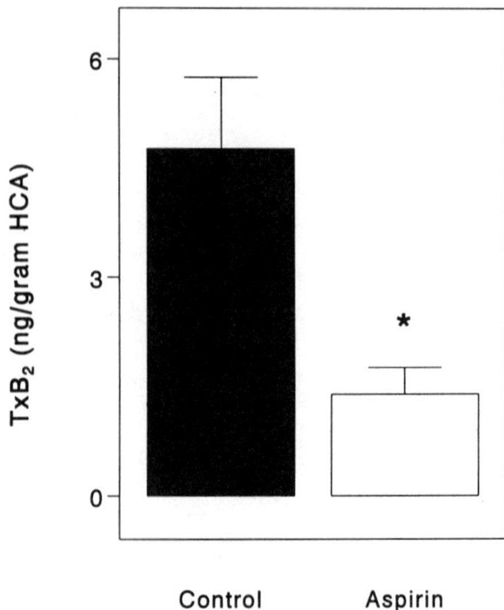

Figure 4.4 Production of thromboxane A$_2$, measured as the stable metabolite thromboxane B$_2$, by segments of human coronary artery (HCA) in the absence (filled bar) and presence (open bar) of 10 μM aspirin ($n = 12$).

SYNOPSIS

The data reported here were selected because they show that the effects (both desirable and undesirable) of antimigraine drugs cannot be explained entirely by the effect of an agonist on a single 5-HT receptor subtype. Further research into the exact vascular effects of 5-HT receptor agonists is likely to result in improvement of current antimigraine drugs from a perspective of antimigraine efficacy, and also from the perspective of further reduction of unwanted side-effects.

Acknowledgements

Supported in part by the Netherlands Heart Foundation, grant nos 89.252 and 93.146. The authors would like to express their sincere gratitude to the Rotterdam Heart Valve Bank (Bio Implant Services Foundation) for their help in supplying us with the human heart tissue, and to J.P.C. Heiligers for expert technical assistence.

REFERENCES

Bax, W.A. and Saxena, P.R. (1993) Sumatriptan and ischaemic heart disease. *Lancet*, **341**, 1419–1420.

Bax, W.A., Renzenbrink, G.J., Van Heuven-Nolsen, D., Thijssen, H.J.M., Bos, E. and Saxena, P.R. (1993) 5-HT receptors mediating contractions of the isolated human coronary artery. *European Journal of Pharmacology*, **239**, 203–210.

Bax, W.A., Renzenbrink, G.J., Zijlstra, F.J., Fekkes, D., Van Heuven-Nolsen, D., Van der Linden, E.A., Bos, E. and Saxena, P.R. (1994) Low dose aspirin inhibits platelet-induced contraction of the human isolated coronary artery; an additional role for 5-HT receptor antagonism against coronary vasospasm? *Circulation*, **89**, 623–629.

Bruinvels, A.T., Landwehrmeyer, B., Moskowitz, M.A. and Hoyer, D. (1992) Evidence for the presence of 5-HT_{1B} receptor messenger RNA in neurons of the rat trigeminal ganglia. *European Journal of Pharmacology*, **227**, 357–359.

Chester, A.H., Martin, G.R., Bodelsson, M., Arneklo-Nobin, B., Tadjkarimi, S., Tornebrandt, K. and Yacoub, M.H. (1990) 5-Hydroxytryptamine receptor profile in healthy and diseased human epicardial coronary arteries. *Cardiovascular Research*, **24**, 932–937.

Chester, A.H., Allen, S.P., Tadjkarimi, S. and Yacoub, M.H. (1993) Interaction between thromboxane A_2 and 5-hydroxytryptamine receptor subtypes in human coronary arteries. *Circulation*, **87**, 874–880.

Connor, H.E., Feniuk, W. and Humphrey, P.P.A. (1989) 5-Hydroxytryptamine contracts human coronary arteries predominantly via 5-HT_2 receptor activation. *European Journal of Pharmacology*, **161**, 91–94.

Cushing, D.J., Baez, M., Kursar, D., Schenck, K. and Cohen, M.L. (1994) Serotonin-induced contraction in canine coronary artery and saphenous vein: role of a 5-HT_{1D}-like receptor. *Life Sciences*, **54**, 1671–1680.

Den Boer, M.O., Villalón, C.M., Heiligers, J.P.C., Humphrey, P.P.A. and Saxena, P.R. (1991a) Role of 5-HT_1-like receptors in the reduction of porcine cranial arteriovenous anastomotic shunting by sumatriptan. *British Journal of Pharmacology*, **102**, 323–330.

Den Boer, M.O., Heiligers, J.P.C. and Saxena, P.R. (1991b) Carotid vascular effects of ergotamine and dihydroergotamine in the pig: no exclusive mediation via 5-HT receptors. *British Journal of Pharmacology*, **104**, 183–189.

Galer, B.S., Lipton, R.B., Solomon, S., Newman, L.C. and Spierings, E.L.H. (1991) Myocardial ischemia related to ergot alkaloids: a case report and literature review. *Headache*, **31**, 446–451.

Goadsby, P.J. and Edvinsson, L. (1993) The trigeminovascular system and migraine: studies characterizing cerebrovascular and neuropeptide changes seen in humans and cats. *Annals of Neurology*, **33**, 48–56.

Kaumann, A.J., Parsons, A.A. and Brown, A.M. (1993) Human arterial constrictor serotonin receptors. *Cardiovascular Research*, **27**, 2094–2103.

Kaumann, A.J., Frenken, M., Posival, H. and Brown, A.M. (1994) Variable participation of 5-HT_1-like receptors and 5-HT_2 receptors in serotonin-induced contraction of human isolated coronary arteries. *Circulation*, **90**, 1141–1153.

MacLennan, S.J. and Martin, G.R. (1992) Effect of thromboxane A_2-mimetic U46619 on 5-HT_1-like and 5-HT_2 receptor-mediated contraction of the rabbit isolated femoral artery. *British Journal of Pharmacology*, **107**, 418–421.

Moskowitz, M.A. (1992) Neurogenic versus vascular mechanisms of sumatriptan and ergot alkaloids in migraine. *Trends in Pharmacological Sciences*, **13**, 307–311.

Ottervanger, J.P., Paalman, H.J.A., Boxma, G.L. and Stricker, B.H.Ch. (1993) Transmural myocardial infarction with sumatriptan. *Lancet*, **341**, 861–862.

Pauwels, P.J. and Colpaert, F.C. (1995) The 5-HT_{1D} receptor antagonist GR127,935 is an agonist at cloned human 5-$HT_{1D\alpha}$ receptor sites. *Neuropharmacology*, **34**, 235–237.

Rebeck, G.W., Maynard, K.I., Hyman, B.T. and Moskowitz, M.A. (1994) Selective 5-HT$_{1D\alpha}$ serotonin receptor gene expression in trigeminal ganglia: implication for antimigraine drug development. *Proceedings National Academy of Science USA*, **91**, 3666–3669.

Saxena, P.R. and Ferrari, M.D. (1989) 5-HT$_1$-like receptor agonists and the pathophysiology of migraine. *Trends in Pharmacological Sciences*, **10**, 200–204.

Saxena, P.R. and Verdouw, P.D. (1982) Redistribution by 5-hydroxytryptamine of carotid arterial blood at the expense of arteriovenous blood flow. *Journal of Physiology (London)*, **332**, 501–520.

Saxena, P.R., Duncker, D.J., Bom, A.H., Heiligers, J. and Verdouw, P.D. (1986) Effects of MDL 72222 and methiothepin on carotid vascular responses to 5-hydroxytryptamine in the pig: evidence for the presence of '5-hydroxytryptamine$_1$-like' receptors. *Naunyn Schmiedeberg's Archives of Pharmacology*, **333**, 198–204.

Schumacher, W.A., Heran, C.L., Allen, G.T. and Ogletree, M.L. (1989) Leukotrienes cause mesenteric vasoconstriction and hemoconcentration in rats without activating thromboxane receptors. *Prostaglandins*, **3**, 335–344.

Skingle, M., Scopes, D.I.C., Feniuk, W., Connor, H.E., Carter, M.C., Clitherow, J.W. and Tyers, M.B. (1993) GR127935: a potent orally active 5-HT$_{1D}$ receptor antagonist. *British Journal of Pharmacology*, **110**, 9P.

Starkey, S.J. and Skingle, M. (1993) 5-HT$_{1D}$ autoreceptors modulate stimulated 5-HT release in the guinea-pig dorsal raphe nucleus. *British Journal of Pharmacology*, **110**, C102.

Stricker, B.H.Ch. and Ottervanger, J.P. (1992) Pijn op de borst door sumatriptan. *Nederlands Tijdschrift voor Geneeskunde*, **136**, 1774–1776.

Willerson, J.T., Golino, P., Eidt, J., Yao, S. and Buja, L.M. (1990) Potential usefulness of combined thromboxane A$_2$ and serotonin receptor blockade for preventing the conversion from chronic to acute coronary artery disease syndromes. *American Journal of Cardiology*, **66**, 48G–53G.

DISCUSSION

Humphrey: Interactions of this sort have been studied over many years. Whether sumatriptan is potentiating thromboxane or thromboxane is potentiating sumatriptan does not matter. What you have is the net effect produced by two agonists mediating a common effect via different receptors. These data do not imply that sumatriptan is releasing thromboxane and causing contractions through that mechanism. Isolated tissues *in vitro* are not physiologically normal tissues and always seem to make prostaglandins of one sort or another, which is why we have always added indomethacin to isolated tissues in our experiments. In these experiments you have a non-physiological tissue which is making prostaglandins, probably PGE$_2$ as well as thromboxane A$_2$, that are acting as background potentiating or sensitizing agents. You may have other agents like nitric oxide, that are working in the opposite direction, so I do not think there is anything unusual here. It is important in that you have measured the thromboxane levels. As you suggest, this may explain the observations of markedly variable contractile responses in isolated human coronary arteries because of the variation in times between removal and when they are studied.

Bax: You may be right, but then you would expect that preservation of the tissue in the laboratory for a longer period of time before the experiment would result in higher thromboxane production and larger contraction to sumatriptan. We did not see that. Furthermore, very fresh coronary artery segments obtained from a healthy person sometimes result in a contractile response that is larger than the response elicited in diseased tissues tested a long time after removal from the heart.

Humphrey: My main point was that as soon as you remove a blood vessel, it is no longer the same as it was *in vivo*. It makes prostaglandins and there will be a background sensitizing tone.

Fozard: Was there a background tone? Did the thromboxane antagonist *per se* relax the tissues?

Bax: No, it did not.

Fozard: Therefore, from these results it appears that the tissues are not making thromboxane in sufficient quantities to maintain tone, yet when you apply sumatriptan there is enough thromboxane to account for 30% of the response.

Humphrey: How do you know what the initial tone was anyway? It is artificial. Presumably there is a level that is continuously there, and you do not know what the 'physiological' baseline should be.

Fozard: If initially a tissue is making sufficient thromboxane to contribute to tone, then that tissue should relax if you add sufficient of the thromboxane antagonist.

Connor: If you can show whether another agonist which produces contraction is blocked by your thromboxane antagonist, that would show the specificity of the interaction you describe.

Bax: We investigated that. The response to endothelin 1 is not blocked by the thromboxane receptor antagonist. Therefore, our data cannot be explained by simply adding the effects of endogenously produced thromboxane and sumatriptan.

Martin: I don't have details from comparisons in human tissue, but we have looked within species in different vessels in which the 5-HT$_{1D}$ receptors mediate contraction. In rabbit saphenous vein 5-HT contractions are mediated exclusively by 5-HT$_{1D}$ receptors; in rabbit femoral artery 5-HT effects are mediated by both 5-HT$_{1D}$ and 5-HT$_2$ receptors in a manner very similar to that observed in human coronary artery. In the presence of threshold concentrations of a thromboxane A$_2$ mimetic, 5-HT effects are augmented, but only at the bottom of the dose–response curve. In other words, 5-HT and thromboxane A$_2$ display threshold synergy, which is a rather common phenomenon. On the other hand, in the femoral artery, one sees the sort of phenomenon that I believe Dr Bax is describing here in the human coronary artery, where super-addition of effects is obtained over the entire range of 5-HT concentrations. We have done no further work on this beyond the level of the receptor, but the results imply that the nature of receptor cross-talk for the same receptor type (i.e. the 5-HT$_{1D}$ receptor) differs depending on the blood vessel, and that this dictates whether or not you will see the sort of response that Dr Bax has described.

This is not a property exclusively related to thromboxane–5-HT$_{1D}$ receptor interactions. From our work it appears that any system which turns on phosphotidyl inositol production will produce exactly the same effect on 5-HT$_{1D}$ receptors. So the super-addition phenomenon is possibly quite widespread, and I would not be surprised if pathologically damaged tissues, in the throes of an inflammatory response, are producing mediators that result in a super-additive response to 5-HT$_{1D}$ receptor agonists.

Bax: We have also looked at potentiation by endothelins, but have had difficulty showing the same sort of potentiation that we observe with thromboxanes. We used thromboxanes because they may well be involved in pathological processes with platelets adhering to vascular endothelium.

Lance: Why would GR127935 be more potent against the effects of sumatriptan than those of 5-HT if they are both working through the same 5-HT$_{1D\beta}$ receptors?

Bax: We do not know, but it would suggest that different receptors may be involved in the two effects. Similarly, the effects of sumatriptan are blocked potently by methiothepin, but the effects of ergotamine or dihydroergotamine are not (Den Boer *et al.* 1991). That suggests that for ergotamine and dihydroergotamine also different receptors would be involved. I do not think we know about all the receptors involved in the effects of all antimigraine drugs.

Lance: So may 5-HT and sumatriptan be acting through multiple receptors?

Bax: Yes, perhaps. However, we should be careful in extrapolating the data obtained in this model to the human *in vivo* situation, and to migraine. On the other hand, this model has been shown to be robust and very predicative of antimigraine drug efficacy.

REFERENCE

Den Boer, M.O., Heiligers, J.P.C. and Saxena, P.R. (1991) Carotid vascular effects of ergotamine and dihydroergotamine in the pig: no exclusive mediation via 5-HT receptors. *British Journal of Pharmacology*, **104**, 183–189.

5

Differential expression of sumatriptan-sensitive 5-HT$_1$ receptors in human neuronal and vascular tissues

Isabelle Bouchelet, Zvi Cohen, Philippe Séguéla and Edith Hamel

INTRODUCTION

In recent years, the treatment of migraine headache has improved dramatically because of the development of the 5-HT$_1$ agonist sumatriptan. At the same time, new pharmacological and molecular tools became available for the identification of the 5-hydroxytryptamine (5-HT, serotonin) receptors targeted by sumatriptan and other related anti-migraine compounds. The efficacy of sumatriptan in aborting acute migraine attack has more than ever focused our efforts towards the identification of the targets (tissues and receptors) through which it can relieve migraine-associated pain. While the controversy over a neurogenic versus a vascular target (Blau 1992, Moskowitz 1992) is still very much alive, the involvement of a 5-HT$_{1D}$ receptor, and more specifically the 5-HT$_{1D\beta}$ subtype (Hamel *et al.* 1993a), at least with regard to cerebral vasoconstriction, has gained credibility since our original suggestion (Hamel and Bouchard 1991). Good evidence has also been provided for

Migraine: Pharmacology and genetics
Edited by Merton Sandler, Michel Ferrari and Sara Harnett
Published in 1996 by Chapman & Hall
ISBN 1 86036 006 8

the involvement of a neuronal 5-HT$_1$-like receptor (probably 5-HT$_{1D}$) in the inhibition of dural trigeminovascular inflammation, but no definitive agreement has been reached yet (see Connor and Beattie, this volume). Two additional issues that deserve consideration while treating migraine sufferers with sumatriptan are its possible interactions with either 5-HT receptors other than those currently associated with cerebral vasoconstriction and/or inhibition of neurogenic inflammation (e.g. 5-HT$_{1F}$), or 5-HT receptors in tissues other than those targeted for treatment, such as brain intraparenchymal microvessels and peripheral blood vessels (e.g. coronary artery). These interactions remain largely unknown but could be instrumental to our understanding of the overall effects of sumatriptan in migraine patients.

This brief review partly addresses these issues by evaluating the selectivity of distribution of sumatriptan-sensitive 5-HT$_1$ receptors (5-HT$_{1D\alpha}$, 5-HT$_{1D\beta}$ and 5-HT$_{1F}$) in human neuronal and vascular tissues.

TRIGEMINAL GANGLION

Presynaptic 5-HT$_{1B}$ (rat) (Buzzi *et al.* 1991) or 5-HT$_{1D}$-like (guinea-pig) (Matsubara *et al.* 1991) receptors have been pharmacologically identified on dural trigeminovascular afferents where they would inhibit release of neuropeptides involved in neurogenic plasma extravasation. The efficacy of sumatriptan and other 5-HT$_{1D}$ agonists has been well documented in this animal model of migraine-associated neurogenic inflammation (see Moskowitz 1992). However, it still remains unclear why 5-HT itself and the 5-HT$_1$ antagonist methiothepin have no effect (see Moskowitz 1992), and why neurogenic inflammation is selective to dural vessels since cerebral vessels at the base and over the convexities of the brain are also innervated by trigeminovascular fibres containing substance P (SP) and calcitonin gene-related peptide (CGRP) (Markowitz *et al.* 1987).

Attempts to identify the molecular subtype(s) of the pharmacological 5-HT$_{1D}$ receptor (Weinshank *et al.* 1992) putatively involved in blockade of neurogenic inflammation have been inconclusive. Both the detection of 5-HT$_{1B}$ receptor mRNA in rat trigeminal ganglion cells by *in situ* hybridization (Bruinvels *et al.* 1992), and the high homology between rat 5-HT$_{1B}$ and human 5-HT$_{1D\beta}$ receptors (Adham *et al.* 1992) originally suggested that human trigeminal ganglia are endowed with 5-HT$_{1D\beta}$ receptors (Bruinvels *et al.* 1992). However, Rebeck and colleagues (1994), using reverse transcriptase-polymerase chain reaction (RT-PCR), occasionally found 5-HT$_{1D\alpha}$ but not 5-HT$_{1D\beta}$ receptor message in post-mortem human trigeminal ganglia. Recently, we performed similar studies and PCR products corresponding to 5-HT$_{1D\alpha}$ and 5-HT$_{1D\beta}$ receptor subtypes were both consistently identified (Figure 5.1) (Bouchelet *et al.* 1995).

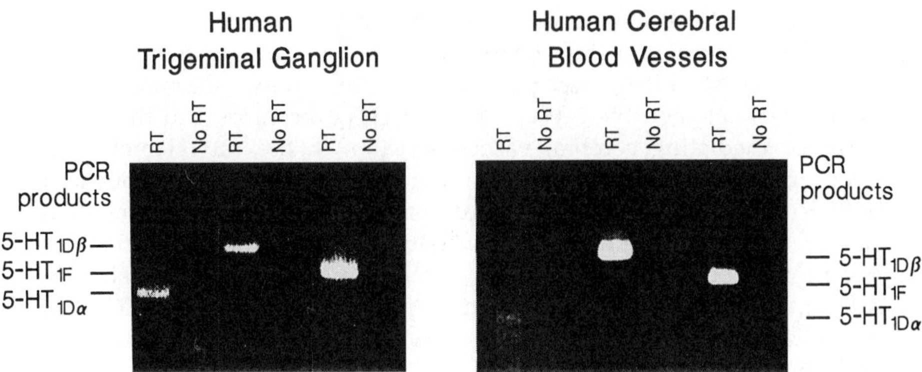

Figure 5.1 Gel electrophoresis of polymerase chain reaction (PCR) products generated from human trigeminal ganglion (left) or cerebral blood vessel (right) cDNA samples submitted (RT) or not (no-RT) to reverse transcriptase. Receptor-specific oligonucleotide primers for 5-HT$_{1D\alpha}$, 5-HT$_{1D\beta}$ and 5-HT$_{1F}$ were used and the PCR products corresponded to the expected sizes of 340, 596 and 482 bp, respectively.

Interestingly, additional *in situ* hybridization studies by Bruinvels and collaborators, with probes specific for rodent or human receptors revealed comparable number of ganglion cells expressing 5-HT$_{1D\alpha}$ and 5-HT$_{1D\beta}$ (or 5-HT$_{1B}$ in rat) receptors in both species (Bruinvels 1993 and personal communication). Our results further suggest that human trigeminal ganglia also express mRNA for the sumatriptan-sensitive 5-HT$_{1F}$ receptor (Figure 5.1) (Bouchelet *et al.* 1995).

These data show that multiple 5-HT$_1$ receptor mRNAs are co-expressed in human trigeminal ganglia. The role of the putative trigeminal 5-HT$_{1F}$ receptor is unknown, but the pharmacological profile of this receptor (Adham *et al.* 1993) makes it an unlikely mediator of the sumatriptan-induced inhibition of neurogenic inflammation. Based on current molecular evidence it is, however, impossible to attest that dural presynaptic trigeminovascular 5-HT$_{1D\alpha}$ receptors are selectively involved in the blockade of neurogenic plasma extravasation.

CEREBRAL BLOOD VESSELS

Sumatriptan was originally identified as a selective agonist at the 5-HT$_1$-like receptor mediating contraction of the dog saphenous vein (Humphrey *et al.* 1988). This compound was soon proven to be beneficial in the treatment of acute migraine headache (Doenicke *et al.* 1988), a finding which generated considerable enthusiasm towards the identification of the 5-HT receptor involved in the contraction of the cerebrovascular smooth muscle. While some authors reported its identity with the 5-HT$_1$-like receptor causing contraction of the dog saphenous vein (Parsons *et al.* 1989), we pointed out the strong pharmacological similarities between the 5-HT$_{1B}$ and/or 5-HT$_{1D}$ receptors and the 5-HT$_1$ receptor mediating cerebral vasoconstriction in the cat (Hamel *et al.* 1989), bovine (Hamel *et al.* 1993b) and human (Hamel and Bouchard 1991) cerebral arteries. Furthermore, using pharmacological correlation analyses and Northern blot hybridization, we identified the 5-HT$_{1D\beta}$ receptor as being responsible for this vasomotor effect (Hamel *et al.* 1993a). In support of this conclusion, Bruinvels *et al.* (1994) used *in situ* hybridization and reported the presence of 5-HT$_{1B}$ (the rodent equivalent of human 5-HT$_{1D\beta}$) receptor mRNA in rat cerebral arteries. Moreover, RT-PCR studies in our laboratory showed the presence of PCR products corresponding to the 5-HT$_{1D\beta}$ subtype while only a faint and occasional signal could be detected for the 5-HT$_{1D\alpha}$ receptor (Figure 5.1). In addition, PCR products corresponding to 5-HT$_{1F}$ receptor mRNA were detected in human cerebral arteries (Figure 5.1) (Bouchelet *et al.* 1995).

Overall, pharmacological data from various laboratories as well as molecular correlates indicate that the primary cerebrovascular target responsible for the sumatriptan-induced cerebral vasoconstriction corresponds to the 5-HT$_{1D\beta}$ receptor subtype. Even though the pharmacological profile of the 5-HT$_{1F}$ receptor (Adham *et al.* 1993) excluded its direct participation in human cerebral vasoconstriction (Hamel *et al.* 1993a), future work should be devoted to identification of its physiological role.

BRAIN INTRAPARENCHYMAL BLOOD VESSELS

Brain intraparenchymal blood vessels may contribute to the initiation of migraine rather than the actual headache phase. However, despite our knowledge that this microvascular bed is innervated by central serotonergic nerve fibres and responsive to intracerebrally released 5-HT (for details, see Cohen *et al.* 1995b), very limited information is available on the possible interaction of circulating sumatriptan with microvascular 5-HT receptors in patients undergoing treatment. Induction of cerebral vasoconstriction (Friberg *et al.* 1991) and increase in blood flow velocity (Caekebeke *et al.* 1992) by sumatriptan in large cerebral arteries from migraine patients have been reported. These studies, however, do not provide any direct assessment of the intracerebral microcirculation which is responsible for the local regulation of cerebral blood flow. In the cat, high doses of sumatriptan exert a direct vasoconstrictor effect on intraparenchymal vessels, while lower doses, equivalent to those used in clinical practice, have no such effect (Kobari *et al.* 1993). These observations suggest that sumatriptan is accessible to 5-HT$_1$-like

Human Brain Microvascular Bed

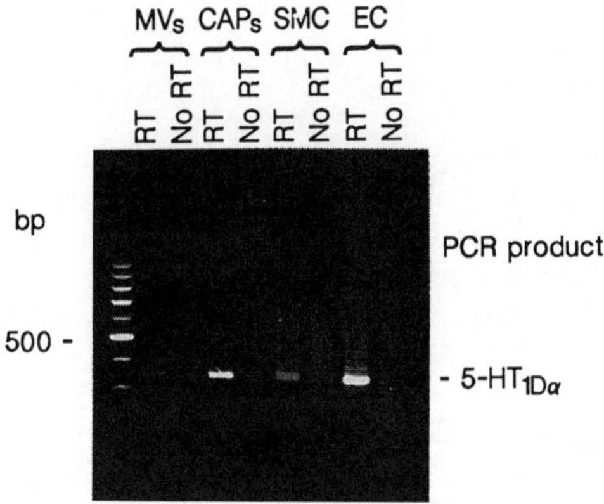

Figure 5.2 Gel electrophoresis of polymerase chain reaction (PCR) products generated from cDNA samples of human microvessels (MVs) and capillaries (CAPs) isolated from post-mortem cortex as well as from cultures of primary smooth muscle (SMC) or subcloned endothelial (EC) cells obtained from temporal cortex biopsies. Samples were submitted (RT) or not (no-RT) to reverse transcriptase before PCR amplification. PCR products corresponded to the expected size of 340 bp for the 5-HT$_{1D\alpha}$ receptor.

receptors on endothelial and/or smooth muscle cells of brain microvessels. Whether this only happens at high doses of sumatriptan or becomes more relevant in migraine patients who might experience changes in blood–brain barrier permeability remains unresolved. In a previous study (Hamel *et al.* 1993a) we failed to detect mRNA transcripts for 5-HT$_{1D\beta}$ receptors in microvessels and capillaries isolated from post-mortem human cerebral cortex, and suggested that these receptors were either not expressed or only at low levels undetectable by Northern blot analysis. Using the more sensitive RT-PCR approach with similar microvascular fractions and with cultures of smooth muscle or endothelial cells generated from human temporal cortex biopsies, we now report the expression of mRNA for the 5-HT$_{1D\alpha}$ receptor in the microvascular bed with a more intense signal in capillaries and endothelial cells (Figure 5.2) (Cohen *et al.* 1995a).

Whether additional 5-HT$_1$-like or other 5-HT receptors are present in human microvascular cells needs to be established. Also, the exact role(s) of these receptors in the regulation of cerebral blood flow and/or blood–brain barrier permeability under normal and pathological conditions deserves further investigation. It is, however, very likely that circulating sumatriptan in patients undergoing acute migraine therapy could interact with endothelial, and possibly, smooth muscle micro-vascular receptors.

CORONARY ARTERY

Since the introduction of sumatriptan in the treatment of acute migraine attack, concerns about its potential coronary side-effects have been raised. In fact, 5-HT-induced contraction in human coronary artery appears to be mediated predominantly by 5-HT$_2$ receptors (Connor *et al.* 1989), but a 5-HT$_1$-like receptor has been associated to the contraction elicited by sumatriptan and/or low concentration of 5-HT (Bax *et al.* 1993). Similar conclusions have been reached in the dog coronary artery with further suggestions that the receptor may share pharmacological similarities with the 5-HT$_{1D\beta}$ subtype (Parsons *et al.* 1992). However, more recent work using molecular biology techniques showed the presence of mRNA corresponding to the 5-HT$_{1D\alpha}$ receptor in dog coronary artery (Cushing *et al.* 1994). Preliminary RT-PCR studies performed in our laboratory with a single distal segment of human coronary artery showed a very strong signal for the 5-HT$_{1D\beta}$ subtype (Bouchelet *et al.* 1995).

Based on pharmacological and molecular data, it appears that the human coronary artery possesses functional 5-HT$_{1D}$ receptors, the molecular identity of which deserves confirmation. Whether this receptor would be activated or not by circulating sumatriptan in patients with suspected or proven coronary diseases remains debatable, but the available data would support the cautious use of sumatriptan in such patients.

SUMMARY

Pharmacology and molecular biology data indicate that 5-HT$_{1D\beta}$ receptors are the primary target for sumatriptan in brain cerebral blood vessels. Such a conclusive answer could not be reached regarding the 5-HT$_{1D}$ receptor targeted by sumatriptan in the inhibition of neurogenic inflammation as both 5-HT$_{1D\alpha}$ and 5-HT$_{1D\beta}$ subtypes are expressed in human trigeminal ganglion. Brain intraparenchymal vessels as well as human brain endothelial and smooth muscle cells were shown to express 5-HT$_{1D\alpha}$ receptors, which could possibly interact with circulating sumatriptan in the process of migraine headache treatment. Also it appears from preliminary molecular data that 5-HT$_{1D\beta}$ receptors at least are expressed in human coronary artery and these might be activated by sumatriptan under pathological conditions. The expression of mRNA for the sumatriptan-sensitive 5-HT$_{1F}$ receptor in human trigeminal ganglion and cerebral blood vessels further emphasizes the importance of clearer definition of the role of this receptor subtype with regards to migraine manifestation and therapy.

Acknowledgements

The authors are grateful to Drs B. Case, A. Olivier and J.-G. Villemure for human post-mortem and surgery material, and to Dr D. Stanimirovic (National Research Council of Canada, Ottawa, Ontario) for culture of human brain endothelial and smooth muscle cells. We also thank Ms A. Woolnough (Fisher Scientific, Canada) and Mr C. Littlefield (MJ Research) for equipment support and Ms L. Michel for preparing the manuscript. This study was supported by a grant from the Québec Heart and Stroke Foundation (E.H.), a grant (MA-9967) and a MRC Scientist Award (E.H.) from the Medical Research Council of Canada, and a McGill Major Studentship (Z.C.).

REFERENCES

Adham, N., Romanienko, P., Hartig, P., Weinshank, R.L. and Branchek, T. (1992) The rat 5-hydroxytryptamine$_{1B}$ receptor is the species homologue of the human 5-hydroxytryptamine$_{1D\beta}$ receptor. *Molecular Pharmacology*, **41**, 1–7.

Adham, N., Kao, H.-T., Schechter, L.E., Bard, J., Olsen, M., Urquhart, D., Durkin, M., Hartig, P.R., Weinshank, R.L. and Branchek, T.A. (1993) Cloning of another human serotonin receptor (5-HT$_{1F}$): a fifth 5-HT$_1$ receptor subtype coupled to the inhibition of adenylate cyclase. *Proceedings of the National Academy of Science USA*, **90**, 408–412.

Bax, W.A., Renzenbrink, G.J., Van Heuven-Nolsen, D., Thijssen, E.J.M., Bos, E. and Saxena, P.R. (1993) 5-HT receptors mediating contractions of the isolated human coronary artery. *European Journal of Pharmacology*, **239**, 203–210.

Blau, J.N. (1992) Migraine: theories of pathogenesis. *Lancet*, **339**, 1202–1207.

Bouchelet, I., Cohen, Z., Case, B., Séguéla, P. and Hamel, E. (1995) Expression of sumatriptan-sensitive serotonin receptors mRNA in human neuronal and vascular tissues. *Society for Neuroscience Abstracts*, **21**, (Part 3), 1853 (#727.11).

Bruinvels, A.T. (1993) Radioligand binding assays, receptor autoradiography and *in situ* hybridisation histochemistry in the mammalian nervous system. In: *5-HT$_{1D}$ Receptors Reconsidered*, Ph.D. thesis. Utrecht University, The Netherlands.

Bruinvels, A.T., Landwehrmeyer, B., Moskowitz, M.A. and Hoyer, D. (1992) Evidence for the presence of 5-HT$_{1B}$ receptor messenger RNA in neurons of the rat trigeminal ganglia. *European Journal of Pharmacology, Molecular Pharmacology Section*, **227**, 357–359.

Bruinvels, A.T., Landwehrmeyer, B., Gustafson, E.L., Durkin, M.M., Mengod, G., Branchek, T.A., Hoyer, D. and Palacios, J.M. (1994) Localization of 5-HT$_{1B}$, 5-HT$_{1D\alpha}$ 5-HT$_{1E}$ and 5-HT$_{1F}$ receptor messenger RNA in rodent and primate brain. *Neuropharmacology* **33**, 367–386.

Buzzi, M.G., Moskowitz, M.A., Peroutka, S.J. and Byun, B. (1991) Further characterization of the putative 5-HT receptor which mediates blockade of neurogenic plasma extravasation in rat dura mater. *British Journal of Pharmacology*, **103**, 1421–1428.

Caekebeke, J.F.V., Ferrari, M.D., Zwetsloot, C.P., Jansen, J. and Saxena, P.R. (1992) Antimigraine drug sumatriptan increases blood flow velocity in large cerebral arteries during migraine attacks. *Neurology*, **42**, 1522–1526.

Cohen, Z., Bouchelet, I., Yong, W.V., Villemure, J.-G., Stanimirovic, D. and Hamel, E. (1995a) Differential expression of serotonin receptors 5-HT1Dα and 5-HT2A mRNA in human brain vessels, vascular cells and astrocytes in culture. *Society for Neuroscience Abstracts*, **21**, (Part 3), 1853, (727.10).

Cohen, Z., Ehret, M., Maitre, M. and Hamel, E. (1995b) Ultrastructural analysis of tryptophan hydroxylase immunoreactive nerve terminals in the rat cerebral cortex and hippocampus: their associations with local blood vessels. *Neuroscience*, **66**, 555–569.

Connor, H.E., Feniuk, W. and Humphrey, P.P.A. (1989) 5-Hydroxytryptamine contracts human coronary arteries predominantly via 5-HT$_2$ receptor activation. *European Journal of Pharmacology*, **161**, 91–94.

Connor, H.E. and Beattie, D.T. (1996) 5-HT receptor subtypes and migraine. In: *Migraine: Pharmacology and Genetics*, (eds M. Sandler, M.D. Ferrari and S. Harnett), pp. 18-31. Chapman & Hall, London.

Cushing, D.J., Baez, M., Kursar, J.D., Schenck, K. and Cohen, M.L. (1994) Serotonin-induced contraction in canine coronary artery and saphenous vein: role of a 5-HT$_{1D}$-like receptor. *Life Sciences*, **54**, 1671–1680.

Doenicke, A., Brand, J. and Perrin, V.L. (1988) Possible benefit of GR43175, a novel 5-HT$_1$-like receptor agonist, for the acute treatment of severe migraine. *Lancet*, **i**, 1309–1311.

Friberg, L., Olesen, J., Iversen, H.K. and Sperling, B. (1991) Migraine pain associated with middle cerebral artery dilatation: reversal by sumatriptan. *Lancet*, **338**, 13–17.

Hamel, E. and Bouchard, D. (1991) Contractile 5-HT$_1$ receptors in human isolated pial arterioles: correlation with 5-HT$_{1D}$ binding sites. *British Journal of Pharmacology*, **102**, 227–233.

Hamel, E., Robert, J.-P., Young, A.R. and MacKenzie, E.T. (1989) Pharmacological properties of the receptor(s) involved in the 5-hydroxytryptamine-induced contraction of the feline middle cerebral artery. *Journal of Pharmacology and Experimental Therapeutics*, **249**, 879–889.

Hamel, E., Fan, E., Linville, D., Ting, V., Villemure, J.-G. and Chia, L.-S. (1993a) Expression of mRNA for the serotonin 5-hydroxytryptamine$_{1Dβ}$ receptor subtype in human and bovine cerebral arteries. *Molecular Pharmacology*, **44**, 242–246.

Hamel, E., Grégoire, L. and Lau, B. (1993b) 5-HT$_1$ receptors mediating contraction in bovine cerebral arteries: a model for human cerebrovascular '5-HT$_{1Dβ}$' receptors. *European Journal of Pharmacology*, **242**, 75–82.

Humphrey, P.P.A., Feniuk, W., Perren, M.J., Connor, H.E., Oxford, A.W., Coates, I.H. and Butina, D. (1988) GR43175, a selective agonist for the 5-HT$_1$-like receptor in dog isolated saphenous vein. *British Journal of Pharmacology*, **94**, 1123–1132.

Kobari, M., Fukuuchi, Y., Tomita, M., Tanahashi, N., Konno, S. and Takeda, H. (1993) Effects of sumatriptan on the cerebral intraparenchymal microcirculation in the cat. *British Journal of Pharmacology*, **110**, 1445–1448.

Markowitz, S., Saito, K. and Moskowitz, M.A. (1987) Neurogenically mediated leakage of plasma protein occurs from blood vessels in dura mater but not brain. *Journal of Neuroscience*, **7**, 4129–4136.

Matsubara, T., Moskowitz, M.A. and Byun, B. (1991) CP-93,129, a potent and selective 5-HT$_{1B}$ receptor agonist blocks neurogenic plasma extravasation within rat but not guinea-pig dura mater. *British Journal of Pharmacology*, **104**, 3–4.

Moskowitz, M.A. (1992) Neurogenic versus vascular mechanisms of sumatriptan and ergot alkaloids in migraine. *Trends in Pharmacological Sciences*, **13**, 307–311.

Parsons, A.A., Stutchbury, C., Raval, P. and Kaumann, A.J. (1992) Sumatriptan contracts large coronary arteries of beagle dogs through 5-HT$_1$-like receptors. *Naunyn-Schmiedeberg's Archives of Pharmacology*, **346**, 592–596.

Parsons, A.A., Whalley, E.T., Feniuk, W., Connor, H.E. and Humphrey, P.P.A. (1989) 5-HT$_1$-like receptors mediate 5-hydroxytryptamine-induced contraction of human isolated basilar artery. *British Journal of Pharmacology*, **96**, 434–449.

Rebeck, G.W., Maynard, K.I., Hyman, B.T. and Moskowitz, M.A. (1994) Selective 5-HT$_{1D\alpha}$ serotonin receptor gene expression in trigeminal ganglia: implications for antimigraine drug development. *Proceedings of the National Academy of Science USA*, **91**, 3666–3669.

Weinshank, R.L., Zgombick, J.M., Macchi, M.J., Branchek, T.A. and Hartig, P.R. (1992) Human serotonin 1D receptor is encoded by a subfamily of two distinct genes: 5-HT$_{1D\alpha}$ and 5-HT$_{1D\beta}$. *Proceedings of the National Academy of Science USA*, **89**, 3630–3634.

DISCUSSION

Edvinsson: In your preparations did you remove the endothelium?

Hamel: No. Our specimens for the human pial vessels and the coronary arteries were the entire blood vessels. They were stripped out of the meninges and/or cleaned carefully, but they were not stripped out of the endothelium.

Edvinsson: We are also doing polymerase chain reaction (PCR) studies. Since we have now removed the endothelium from the vessels we might have new information to discuss soon. When we grow the cells in culture, we see that the expression of the responses may often change or even disappear.

Hamel: Yes, this is a possibility and it is why we have only used very early passages of endothelial cells, while the smooth muscle cells are primary cultures. Similar cultures have also been shown to respond to 5-HT in second messenger assays performed by Dr D. Stanimirovic. We have not got any further in passaging the cells for these studies as we know from other reports that endothelial receptors (e.g. muscarinic) may disappear after numerous passages.

Edvinsson: It differs among receptors. Our experience is that the endothelin and angiotensin receptors disappear after just one or two passages whereas the neuropeptide (NPY) receptor seems more robust. In our work with Dr Branchek the data on human coronary arteries show expression of 5-HT$_{1D\alpha}$, 5-HT$_{1D\beta}$ and 5-HT$_{1F}$ receptors.

Hamel: This is the first coronary artery that we obtained and it was a very small distal segment. It was of a similar size to the pial vessels we were using. The other coronary arteries that we have in the freezer seem to vary in size, but are generally larger. That might explain the difference. Perhaps the 5-HT$_{1D\alpha}$ or 5-HT$_{1F}$ receptors would be seen if we used bigger vessels and had more material to work with.

Edvinsson: In future we should address the role of the post-mortem time. Our preparations came from heart transplantations, so they were fairly fresh. The cerebral vessels were obtained from epilepsy surgery.

Hamel: The earliest vessels we get are four hours post mortem. We have used specimens for up to 24 hours post mortem and we have not seen a correlation with the time after death and the quality of the RNA or the PCR signal.

Edvinsson: As a doctor, one knows that when a patient dies, unlike when a rat is killed, the death process could be 24 hours or more. Many changes may happen during this process.

Hamel: Do you imply that the expression of 5-HT$_{1D\alpha}$ and 5-HT$_{1D\beta}$ receptors in the pial vessels obtained post mortem has something to do with death?

Edvinsson: What you see is a positive finding. It is what you do not see that is the problem. As in electron microscopy, it is difficult to prove absence; a positive finding is more clear-cut.

Hamel: In the pial vessels fresh from the operating room, do you see expression of 5-HT$_{1D\alpha}$ and 5-HT$_{1D\beta}$ receptors? If you do not see these receptors when you do PCR on fresh material and we see them in post-mortem tissue, that would be very puzzling.

Edvinsson: We are not yet ready to do RT-PCR analysis of 5-HT receptors in human brain vessels. We have done that for the NPY and endothelin receptors.

Hamel: I would be surprised if this is a post-mortem phenomenon.

Frants: How will you obtain quantitative data?

Hamel: We do not plan to do quantitative studies at this point. We want to use *in situ* hybridization in the trigeminal ganglion to quantify the relative proportion of cells expressing the α and β subtypes. I would rather do this than quantify the amount of the message. I think that it is more important to know about the specific cells expressing these receptors, their relative abundance and whether they contain calcitonin gene-related peptide (CGRP) or substance P. We may find that the 5-HT$_{1D\alpha}$ receptor, which gives a strong PCR signal in all the trigeminal ganglia that we studied, is the one located in CGRP or substance P immunopositive cells. The 5-HT$_{1D\beta}$ subtype that we also find in the trigeminal ganglion might be associated with blood vessels, microvessels or ganglion cells as well. Its localization might be different to that of the $5\text{-HT}_{1D\alpha}$ receptor and it might not be associated with cells projecting the dura or the pia.

Schoenen: What is the proportion of 5-HT subtype mRNA expression in brain tissue compared to the microvessels?

Hamel: We always run cortex or striatum as controls. In these neuronal tissues, after a 40 cycle PCR, the signal for the $5\text{-HT}_{1D\alpha}$ or $5\text{-HT}_{1D\beta}$ subtype is similar or stronger than that we see in microvessels and cells in culture. The $5\text{-HT}_{1D\alpha}$ signal comes out very strongly in the trigeminals while the $5\text{-HT}_{1D\beta}$ signal may vary in this tissue. The $5\text{-HT}_{1D\beta}$ signal is always very strong in pial vessels while the $5\text{-HT}_{1D\alpha}$ signal is barely detectable. However, PCR is not quantitative. Northern blot analysis is more quantitative. Therefore, that we saw messages for the $5\text{-HT}_{1D\beta}$ and not $5\text{-HT}_{1D\alpha}$ subtype in the pial vessels by Northern blot hybridization (Hamel *et al.* 1993) may be good evidence that the $5\text{-HT}_{1D\beta}$ subtype is a primary receptor in these vessels.

Branchek: Did you try the RNAase protection method? Many people have reverted from RT-PCR to that technique because it is quantitative and you do not need so much material.

Hamel: We have not done that.

Schoenen: Do these data suggest that even finding very selective agents for each receptor subtype would not solve the question?

Hamel: No, I agree that it is important to get a $5\text{-HT}_{1D\alpha}$-specific agent. I think the $5\text{-HT}_{1D\beta}$ subtype is clearly the vascular receptor. The $5\text{-HT}_{1D\alpha}$ subtype might be more related to the trigeminovascular effect. We will not know definitely until we have access to such $5\text{-HT}_{1D\alpha}$-selective compounds.

Schoenen: But the $5\text{-HT}_{1D\alpha}$ receptor is also in the smooth muscle cells.

Hamel: The $5\text{-HT}_{1D\alpha}$ receptor is found in the smooth muscle cells obtained from the intraparenchymal microvessels, but it is also in endothelial cells. This is new information, and we have to know more about the function of this receptor in the microcirculation. However, it does not detract from the fact that the $5\text{-HT}_{1D\alpha}$ receptor is prominent in the trigeminal ganglia as compared to the cerebral blood vessels and a $5\text{-HT}_{1D\alpha}$-selective compound could help discriminate the trigeminal versus vascular effect of sumatriptan in migraine.

Moskowitz: There is a best case/worse case scenario. The best case scenario would be that the ganglion only expresses the $5\text{-HT}_{1D\alpha}$ receptor and the smooth muscle only expresses the $5\text{-HT}_{1D\beta}$ receptor. If ganglia cells synthesize both $5\text{-HT}_{1D\alpha}$ and $5\text{-HT}_{1D\beta}$ subtypes and the smooth muscle synthesizes $5\text{-HT}_{1D\beta}$ receptors (and only $5\text{-HT}_{1D\beta}$ agonists constrict), then it may not matter that the ganglion expresses both 5-HT$_{1D\alpha}$ and 5-HT$_{1D\beta}$ receptor mRNA. Everyone seems to agree that 5-HT$_{1D\alpha}$ mRNA is present in trigeminal ganglia.

Hamel: We are all looking at mRNA, not at the final receptor proteins. We do not know about the amount of proteins present in these tissues. This is also an important issue.

REFERENCE

Hamel, E., Fan, E., Linville, D., Ting, V., Villemure, J.-G. and Chia, L.-S. (1993) Expression of mRNA for the serotonin 5-hydroxytryptamine$_{1D\beta}$ subtype in human and bovine cerebral arteries. *Molecular Pharmacology*, **44**, 242–246.

6

Central and peripheral 5-hydroxytryptamine receptor effects: what have we learnt?

Peter J. Goadsby

INTRODUCTION

Recent developments in 5-hydroxytryptamine (5-HT, serotonin) receptor pharmacology (see Connor and Beattie, this volume) have provided new therapy for patients suffering migraine as well as posing questions about the possible site of action of the new drugs. To understand these developments it is necessary to consider the anatomy and physiology of pain transmission from cranial structures. Since the site of action of antimigraine drugs is not clearly established it is worthwhile considering the possible sites and what is known of the action of antimigraine drugs at these sites. The primary action of an antimigraine drug must be to arrest the headache and as such it is the pain generation and transmission that is of crucial importance.

THE PERIPHERAL PATHWAYS

The trigeminal innervation of pain-sensitive intracranial structures

Surrounding the large cerebral vessels, pial vessels, large venous sinuses and dura mater is a plexus of largely unmyelinated fibres that

Migraine: Pharmacology and genetics
Edited by Merton Sandler, Michel Ferrari and Sara Harnett
Published in 1996 by Chapman & Hall
ISBN 1 86036 006 8

arise from the trigeminal ganglion and in the posterior fossa from the upper cervical dorsal roots. This plexus is well described in monkey (Ruskell and Simons 1987) and cat (Steiger *et al.* 1982, Keller *et al.* 1985). Tracing studies have shown that fibres innervating cerebral vessels arise from within the trigeminal ganglion from neurons that contain substance P (SP) and calcitonin gene-related peptide (CGRP) (Uddman *et al.* 1985), both of which can be released when the trigeminal ganglion is stimulated either in humans or cats (Goadsby *et al.* 1988). Moreover, the cell bodies in the trigeminal ganglion are of bipolar neurons that innervate the large cerebral arteries and dura mater and largely arise from the first or ophthalmic division of the trigeminal nerve (Liu-Chen *et al.* 1983). Stimulation of the cranial vessels, such as the superior sagittal sinus (SSS), is certainly painful in humans (Ray and Wolff 1940, Feindel *et al.* 1960). Human dural nerves that innervate the cranial vessels largely consist of small diameter myelinated and unmyelinated fibres that almost certainly subserve a nociceptive function.

What is the source of pain in migraine?

There are few studies that answer this question directly in humans. Certainly, if the carotid artery is occluded ipsilateral to the side of headache in migraineurs then two-thirds will experience relief, although this does not account for the other one-third (Drummond and Lance 1983). Moreover, distension of major cerebral vessels by balloon dilatation leads to pain referred to the ophthalmic division of the trigeminal nerve (Nichols *et al.* 1993, Martins *et al.* 1993). Vascular structures are, therefore, pain-sensitive but do not provide the entire answer to what generates the pain in migraine.

Plasma protein extravasation and migraine: a model of peripheral drug action

Moskowitz has provided an elegant series of experiments to suggest that the pain of migraine may be a form of sterile neurogenic inflammation (Moskowitz and Cutrer 1993). Neurogenic plasma extravasation can be seen during electrical stimulation of the trigeminal ganglion in the rat (Markowitz *et al.* 1988). Plasma extravasation can be blocked by ergot alkaloids (Markowitz *et al.* 1988), indomethacin, acetylsalicylic acid (Buzzi *et al.* 1989), and the 5-HT$_1$-like agonist, sumatriptan (Buzzi and Moskowitz 1990). The pharmacology of the new abortive antimigraine drugs is outside the scope of this review and interested readers are referred to recent reviews (Feniuk *et al.* 1991) and other work in this volume (see Connor and Beattie, this volume). Suffice to say that sumatriptan is a 5-HT$_{1D}$-like agonist with activity at both α and β

subtypes of that receptor. It is negatively linked to adenylate cyclase and its activation can lead to both hyperpolarization of nerve terminals and vasoconstriction. In addition to plasma protein extravasation (PPE) there are structural changes seen in the dura mater with trigeminal ganglion stimulation and these include mast cell degranulation (Dimitriadou *et al.* 1991) and changes in post-capillary venules, including platelet aggregation (Dimitriadou *et al.* 1992). While it is generally accepted that such changes and particularly the initiation of a sterile inflammatory response would cause pain, it is not clear whether this is sufficient of itself or requires other stimulators or promotors, or both.

The neuronal versus vascular argument

The data concerning PPE and trigeminal ganglion stimulation have, among other discussions, led to the question of the site at which drugs may block this response. Since antimigraine drugs such as dihydro-ergotamine, sumatriptan or 311C90 (zolmitriptan), can block PPE and each have, to varying degrees, vasoconstrictor actions, it has been suggested that this is the basis of the action of these 5-HT_{1D}-like drugs. This argument has been described elsewhere (Humphrey and Goadsby 1994). Essentially it is argued that vasoconstriction itself is sufficient to block PPE, as has been shown in other tissues (Williams and Peck 1977). It is, however, a potent argument against the vasoconstrictor hypothesis that sumatriptan does not block substance P-induced PPE (Buzzi and Moskowitz 1990). Furthermore, the description of conformationally restricted analogues of sumatriptan, such as CP-122,288, which potently block PPE at doses with no vascular effects (Lee and Moskowitz 1993) argues strongly in favour of a neuronal prejunctional site as a possible mediator of the clinical effect of sumatriptan. It can be seen from these studies that there are two potential sites of action of antimigraine drugs in the periphery: the vasculature, being the extracerebral intracranial vessels; and a prejunctional receptor, that is to be found on the nerves that innervate these vessels. We have not learnt definitively from these studies which site should be targeted for therapeutics. Table 6.1 lists and

Table 6.1 What is the antimigraine site?

Model	Sumatriptan	311C90	CP-122,288
PPE (ED_{50} µg/kg)	4.1	2	0.001
pK_i human $5\text{-HT}_{1D\alpha}$	7.9	9.2	8.1
pK_i human $5\text{-HT}_{1D\beta}$	7.9	8.2	7.9
pK_i human 5-HT_{1F}	7.5	7.1	?

PPE, plasma protein extravasation; 311C90, zolmitriptan

compares the effects of sumatriptan, 311C90 and CP-122,288 at two models for drug development, plasma protein extravasation and pharmacological characterization at cloned human receptors. The difference in the effect of the conformationally restricted drug CP-122,288 is not explained by any sub-class of drugs currently known and suggests an action at an as yet unknown receptor. The crucial test of this information will be the clinical study of CP-122,288 in migraine patients.

THE CENTRAL NERVOUS SYSTEM

Experimental cerebral blood flow studies

Experimental evidence suggests that the trigeminovascular system promotes vasodilatation. Nerves that innervate the cerebral vessels through the trigeminovascular system contain almost exclusively vasodilator transmitters, such as CGRP and SP. Available data suggest that lesions of the trigeminal ganglion do not affect resting cerebral blood flow or glucose utilization in the cat (Edvinsson *et al.* 1986). They do, however, affect vasodilator protector mechanisms, such as those seen during hyperaemia following ischaemia or epilepsy (Sakas *et al.* 1989). In addition, it has been shown that in subarachnoid haemorrhage, with threatened cerebrovascular compromise from vasospasm, venous CGRP levels are elevated in humans (Edvinsson *et al.* 1990). Electrical stimulation of the trigeminal ganglion in both humans and the cat leads to increases in extracerebral blood flow and local release of both CGRP and SP (Goadsby *et al.* 1988). In the cat trigeminal ganglion stimulation also increases cerebral blood flow by a pathway traversing the greater superficial petrosal branch of the facial nerve (Goadsby and Duckworth 1987), again releasing a powerful vasodilator peptide, vasoactive intestinal polypeptide (VIP) (Goadsby and Shelley 1990). Interestingly, the VIP-ergic innervation of the cerebral vessels is predominantly anterior rather than posterior and this may contribute to the vulnerability of the region to spreading depression and in part explain why the aura is so very often seen to commence posteriorly. Stimulation of the more specifically vascular pain-sensitive superior sagittal sinus increases cerebral blood flow (Lambert *et al.* 1988) and jugular vein CGRP levels (Zagami *et al.* 1990). Human evidence that CGRP is elevated in the headache phase of migraine (Goadsby *et al.* 1990) and cluster headache (Goadsby and Edvinsson 1994a) supports the view that the trigemino-vascular system may be activated in a protective role in this condition. Taken together the data suggest that the trigeminovascular system is unlikely to be the source of the generation of the aura but is either activated by it, or is activated in parallel by the same process that activates the aura. Moreover, with the recent description of a patient with migraine without aura who had spreading oligaemia in the visual association cortex carefully mapped using position emission tomography (PET) (Woods *et al.* 1994) the whole question of the cerebral circulation may need to be reconsidered and re-examined with the new technology. Studies of these pathways have thus been fruitful but it is important to note that all the animal models mentioned are crude approximations of the very complex pathophysiology of migraine. They must be constantly cross-checked with what is seen in human sufferers.

Selective stimulation of pain-sensitive structures

The sites within the brainstem that are responsible for craniovascular pain have begun now to be mapped. It is without doubt that migrainous pain must find its way into the brain and ultimately to cortex. Central sites may offer both advantages and disadvantages in the treatment of acute attacks of migraine. What is essential is that these sites are characterized and their possible role considered.

Trigeminal nucleus

Nozaki *et al.* (1992) used c-*fos*-immunocytochemistry (a method for looking at activated cells) after meningeal irritation with blood and reported protein expression in the trigeminal nucleus caudalis. After stimulation of the superior sagittal sinus, *fos*-like immunoreactivity is seen in cat in the trigeminal nucleus caudalis and in the dorsal horn at the C1 and C2 levels (Kaube *et al.* 1993c). These latter findings are in accord with similar data from 2-deoxyglucose measurements with superior sagittal sinus stimulation (Goadsby and Zagami 1991) and recent observations of *fos* expression in monkeys (Goadsby *et al.* unpublished data). Taken together they contribute to our view of the trigeminal nucleus extending beyond the traditional nucleus caudalis to the dorsal horn of the high cervical region in a functional continuum that includes a cervical extension that could be regarded as a trigeminal nucleus cervicalis. It has also been shown that cooling of the cord reversibly diminishes firing in the thalamic projection cells of these neurons (Angus-Leppan *et al.* 1992) suggesting that a large portion of the afferent nociceptive information entering the central nervous system traverses these caudal neurons. This concept provides an anatomical explanation for the referral of pain to the back of the head in migraine. Moreover, experimental pharmacological evidence suggests that some abortive antimigraine drugs, such as ergots (Goadsby and Gundlach 1991, Hoskin *et al.* 1996), acetylsalicylic acid (Kaube *et al.* 1993a), sumatriptan (after blood–brain barrier disruption; Kaube *et al.* 1993b), and 311C90 (zolmitriptan); (Goadsby and Edvinsson 1994b) can act at

Table 6.2 Neuroanatomical processing of vascular head pain

Order	Level	Structures
1st	Trigeminal ganglion	Middle cranial fossa
2nd	Trigeminal nucleus	Trigeminal nucleus caudalis
		C1/C2 dorsal horn
	(quintothalamic tract)	
3rd	Thalamus	Ventrobasal complex
		Medial nucleus of posterior group
		Intralaminar complex
Final	Cortex	(?)

these second order neurons to reduce cell activity. These data suggest a possible central site for therapeutic intervention in migraine.

Thalamus

Following transmission in the caudal brainstem and high cervical spinal cord, information is relayed in a group of fibres (the quintothalamic tract) to the thalamus. Processing of vascular pain in the thalamus occurs in the ventroposteromedial thalamus, medial nucleus of the posterior complex and in the intralaminar thalamus (Zagami and Lambert 1990, Zagami and Goadsby 1991). By application of capsaicin to the superior sagittal sinus Zagami and Lambert (1991) have shown that trigeminal projections with a high degree of nociceptive input are processed in neurons, particularly in the ventroposteromedial thalamus and in its ventral periphery. The properties and further higher centre connections of these neurons are the subject of studies which will allow us to build up a more complete picture of the trigeminovascular pain pathways (Table 6.2).

Clinical observations of the trigeminovascular system

Drummond and Lance (1983) have shown that in at least two-thirds of patients there is a significant vascular component to the headache. The level of CGRP is elevated in the external jugular vein blood of migraineurs during headache (Goadsby *et al.* 1990), clearly demonstrating some activation of trigeminovascular neurons during migraine with or without aura. These data have been confirmed in adolescent migraineurs (Gallai *et al.* 1995). Whether the activity is peripherally generated is again uncertain, although it is clear that such changes can in part be seen in both humans and cats with direct stimulation of the trigeminal ganglion.

Possibly the most challenging evidence for understanding the trigeminovascular system and headache comes, as it should, from the clinic. In a well conducted clinical study of patients with migraine with aura the effect of sumatriptan was evaluated with regard to the aura. The drug was administered at the onset of aura in a placebo double-blind parallel groups study as a 6 mg subcutaneous injection, thus assuring absorption. In this setting sumatriptan did not affect the aura length when compared to the placebo group. The most fascinating aspect of the study was that the incidence of headache in the placebo and the treated group was the same, so that despite having good delivery and a suitable drug level with the mean length of the aura being twenty minutes, headache still occurred. It is perhaps even more remarkable that the developed headache responded to a further sumatriptan injection (Bates *et al.* 1994). These data suggest that sumatriptan does not have access to a crucial receptor site during aura and that the interaction of the drug concentration and rate of absorption, along with access to the appropriate site, are the elements of the equation required to terminate the attack. What site in the body does sumatriptan not have access to readily? The obvious suggestion is a site behind the blood–brain barrier which opens up the very exciting possibility that the blood–brain barrier may not be normal in the headache phase of migraine. Indeed, better access to sites within the central nervous system may be an advantage in drug development rather than a drawback.

This review has concentrated upon pain as this is perhaps the greatest complaint of most migraineurs. However, there are a host of other symptoms to consider. It is widely accepted that analgesics, such as aspirin or paracetamol, or non-steroidal anti-inflammatory drugs, such as ibuprofen, are more effective when coupled with an anti-emetic. One of the major advantages of sumatriptan is its efficacy against nausea (Ferrari 1991). It was then of great interest to observe that while 311C90 may derive a benefit in terms of the response to pain by having access to the central nervous system, an initial large study suggests it may not have effects on nausea (Dahlof *et al.* 1994). Figure 6.1 demonstrates the data for nausea two hours after administration of 311C90 in a dose-ranging study. Only at an earlier, initial evaluation, and then perhaps only at high dose, was an anti-nausea effect seen. This will require confirmation, but it is interesting that data for a similarly lipophilic 5-HT$_{1D}$-like agonist, MK-462, demonstrated an anti-nausea effect (Ferrari *et al.* 1994) as would have been expected from the sumatriptan studies. The potencies of various antimigraine drugs are compared in Table 6.3 and one possible difference to account for this may be the fact that 311C90 is relatively more potent at 5-HT$_{1D}$-like receptors than at 5-HT$_{1A}$ when compared with sumatriptan. Given that dihydroergotamine

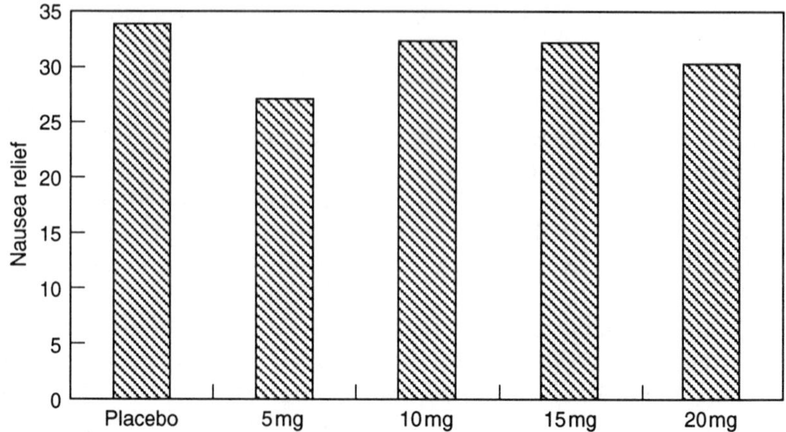

Figure 6.1 Comparison of the effect of increasing doses of 311C90 on patient-reported nausea two hours after administration of test compound during an acute attack of migraine. The number of patients reporting relief of nausea when the placebo group is compared with the four doses of 311C90 (5 mg, 10 mg, 15 mg and 20 mg) is no different for any of the groups.

Table 6.3 What site should be targeted for nausea?

	$5\text{-}HT_{1D\alpha}$	$5\text{-}HT_{1D\beta}$	$5\text{-}HT_{1A}$	*Improves nausea*
Aspirin	−	−	−	No
NSAIDS	−	−	−	No
Ergots	+++	+++	+++	No
Sumatriptan	+++	+++	++	Yes
311C90	+++	+++	+	No(?)
MK-462	+++	+++	++	Yes
CP-122,228	+++	+++	−	?

NSAIDS, non-steroidal anti-inflammatory drugs

is more potent at $5\text{-}HT_{1A}$ receptors and yet often promotes nausea, there seems to be a paradox. It is, however, possible that the optimum activity of an antimigraine drug should not be viewed simplistically as trying to target a single receptor with an absolutely pharmacologically pure compound. Rather we may need to know about the variety of pathophysiological events that take place during a migraine to determine at which receptors and with what potencies the ideal drug would act. Certainly the picture may become much more confusing before becoming clearer.

The treatment of acute attacks of migraine has reached exciting times but this is a two-edged sword. Will conformationally restricted sumatriptan analogues be efficacious in migraine, thus finally concluding the centuries old vascular debate? Will access to the 5-HT$_1$-like receptors in the central nervous system provide a treatment advantage? Is the blood–brain barrier normal in migraine? Can the treatment of nausea or any other manifestation of migraine be separated from the headache by appropriate 5-HT$_1$-like receptor targeting? Current drug developments will answer these and the many clinical questions faced daily in neurology clinics. Perhaps there will be no ideal site but our patients will certainly benefit from the search for one.

Acknowledgements

The author acknowledges the valuable collaboration of H. Kaube, K. Hoskin, K. Keay and Y. Knight in some of the studies reviewed here. The work of the author reported here has been supported by the Wellcome Trust and the Migraine Trust. PJG is a Wellcome Senior Research Fellow.

REFERENCES

Angus-Leppan, H. Lambert, G.A., Boers, P., Zagami, A.S. and Olausson, B. (1992) Craniovascular nociceptive pathways relay in the upper cervical spinal cord in the cat. *Neuroscience Letters*, **137**, 203–206.

Bates, D., Ashford, E., Dawson, R., Ensink, F-BM, Gilhus, N.E., Olesen, J., Pilgrim, A.J. and Shevlin, P. (1994) Subcutaneous sumatriptan during the migraine aura. *Neurology*, **44**, 1587–1592.

Buzzi, M.G. and Moskowitz, M.A. (1990) The antimigraine drug, sumatriptan (GR43175), selectively blocks neurogenic plasma extravasation from blood vessels in dura mater. *British Journal of Pharmacology*, **99**, 202–206.

Buzzi, M.G., Sakas, D.E. and Moskowitz, M.A. (1989) Indomethacin and acetylsalicylic acid block neurogenic plasma protein extravasation in rat dura mater. *European Journal of Pharmacology*, **165**, 251–258.

Connor, H.E. and Beattie D.T. (1996) 5-Hydroxytryptamine receptor subtypes and migraine. In: *Migraine: Pharmacology and Genetics*, (eds. M. Sandler, M.D. Ferrari and S. Harnett, pp. 18–31. Chapman & Hall, London.

Dahlof, C., Diener, H.C., Goadsby, P.J., Massiou, H., Olesen, J., Schoenen, J., Wilkinson, M., Sweet, R.M. and Klein, K.B. (1994) A multicentre, double-blind, placebo-controlled, dose-ranging study to investigate the efficacy and safety of oral doses of 311C90 in the acute treatment of migraine. In: *New Advances in Headache Research*, vol. 4, (ed. F. Clifford Rose), pp. 17–18, Smith Gordon & Co., London.

Dimitriadou, V., Buzzi, M.G., Moskowitz, M.A. and Theoharides, T.C. (1991) Trigeminal sensory fiber stimulation induces morphological changes reflecting secretion in rat dura mater mast cells. *Neuroscience*, **44**, 97–112.

Dimitriadou, V., Buzzi, M.G., Theoharides, T.C. and Moskowitz, M.A. (1992) Ultrastructural evidence for neurogenically mediated changes in blood vessels of the rat dura mater and tongue following antidromic trigeminal stimulation. *Neuroscience*, **48**, 187–203.

Drummond, P.D. and Lance, J.W. (1983) Extracranial vascular changes and the source of pain in migraine headache. *Annals of Neurology*, **13**, 32–37.

Edvinsson, L., McCulloch, J., Kingman, T.A. and Uddman, R. (1986) On the functional role of the trigemino-cerebrovascular system in the regulation of cerebral circulation. In: *Neural Regulation of the Cerebral Circulation*, (ed. C.H. Owman and J.E. Hardebo), pp. 407–18, Elsevier Science, Stockholm.

Edvinsson, L., Juul, R. and Uddman, R. (1990) Peptidergic innervation of the cerebral circulation. Role in subarachnoid hemorrhage in man. *Neurosurgical Reviews*, **13**, 265–272.

Feindel, W., Penfield, W. and McNaughton, F. (1960) The tentorial nerves and localisation of intracranial pain in man. *Neurology*, **10**, 555–563.

Feniuk, W., Humphrey, P.P.A., Perren, M.J., Connor, H.E. and Whalley, E.T. (1991) Rationale for the use of 5-HT1-like agonists in the treatment of migraine. *Journal of Neurology*, **238**, S57–S61.

Ferrari, M.D. (1991) Treatment of migraine attacks with sumatriptan. *New England Journal of Medicine*, **325**, 316–321.

Ferrari, M.D., Terwindt, G.M., Visser, W.H. and Reines, S.A. (1994) A placebo-controlled dose-ranging study of MK-462 versus sumatriptan in migraine. In: *New Advances in Headache Research*, vol. 4, (ed. F. Clifford Rose), pp. 205–207. Smith Gordon & Co., London.

Gallai, V., Sarchielli, P., Floridi, A., Franceschini, M. *et al.* (1995) Vasoactive peptide levels in the plasma of young migraine patients with and without aura assessed both interictally and ictally. *Cephalalgia*, **15**, 384–390.

Goadsby, P.J. and Duckworth, J.W. (1987) Effect of stimulation of trigeminal ganglion on regional cerebral blood flow in cats. *American Journal of Physiology*, **253**, R270–R274.

Goadsby, P.J. and Edvinsson, L. (1994a) Human in vivo evidence for trigeminovascular activation in cluster headache. *Brain*, **117**, 427–434.

Goadsby, P.J. and Edvinsson, L. (1994b) Peripheral and central trigeminovascular activation in cat is blocked by the serotonin (5HT)-1D receptor agonist 311C90. *Headache*, **34**, 394–399.

Goadsby, P.J. and Gundlach, A.L. (1991) Localization of [^{3}H]-dihydroergotamine binding sites in the cat central nervous system: relevance to migraine. *Annals of Neurology*, **29**, 91–94.

Goadsby, P.J. and Shelley, S. (1990) High frequency stimulation of the facial nerve results in local cortical release of vasoactive intestinal polypeptide in the anesthetised cat. *Neuroscience Letters*, **112**, 282–289.

Goadsby, P.J. and Zagami, A.S. (1991) Stimulation of the superior sagittal sinus increases metabolic activity and blood flow in certain regions of the brainstem and upper cervical spinal cord of the cat. *Brain*, **114**, 1001–1011.

Goadsby, P.J., Edvinsson, L. and Ekman, R. (1988) Release of vasoactive peptides in the extracerebral circulation of man and the cat during activation of the trigeminovascular system. *Annals of Neurology*, **23**, 193–196.

Goadsby, P.J., Edvinsson, L. and Ekman, R. (1990) Vasoactive peptide release in the extracerebral circulation of humans during migraine headache. *Annals of Neurology*, **28**, 183–187.

Hoskin, K.L., Kaube, H. and Goadsby, P.J. (1996) Central activation of the trigeminovascular pathway in the cat is inhibited by dihydroergotamine: a c-fos and electrophysiology study. *Brain*, **119**, 101–108.

Humphrey, P.P.A. and Goadsby, P.J. (1994) Controversies in headache. The mode of action of sumatriptan is vascular? A debate. *Cephalalgia*, **14**, 401–410.

Kaube, H., Hoskin, K.L. and Goadsby, P.J. (1993a) Intravenous acetylsalicylic acid inhibits central trigeminal neurons in the dorsal horn of the upper cervical spinal cord in the cat. *Headache*, **33**, 541–550.

Kaube, H., Hoskin, K.L. and Goadsby P.J. (1993b) Sumatriptan inhibits central trigeminal neurons only after blood–brain barrier disruption. *British Journal of Pharmacology*, **109**, 788–792.

Kaube, H., Keay, K., Hoskin, K.L., Bandler, R. and Goadsby, P.J. (1993c) Expression of c-fos-like immunoreactivity in the trigeminal nucleus caudalis and high cervical cord following stimulation of the sagittal sinus in the cat. *Brain Research*, **629**, 95–102.

Keller, J.T., Saunders, M.C., Beduk, A. and Jollis, J.G. (1985) Innervation of the posterior fossa dura of the cat. *Brain Research Bulletin*, **14**, 97–102.

Lambert, G.A., Goadsby, P.J., Zagami, A.S. and Duckworth, J.W. (1988) Comparative effects of stimulation of the trigeminal ganglion and the superior sagittal sinus on cerebral blood flow and evoked potentials in the cat. *Brain Research*, **453**, 143–149.

Lee, W.S. and Moskowitz, M.A. (1993) Conformationally restricted sumatriptan analogues, CP-122,288 and CP-122,638 exhibit enhanced potency against neurogenic inflammation in dura mater. *Brain Research*, **626**, 303–305.

Liu-Chen, L.Y., Han, D.H. and Moskowitz, M.A. (1983) Pia arachnoid contains substance P originating from trigeminal neurons. *Neuroscience*, **9**, 803–808.

Markowitz, S., Saito, K. and Moskowitz, M.A. (1988) Neurogenically mediated plasma extravasation in dura mater: effect of ergot alkaloids. A possible mechanism of action in vascular headache. *Cephalalgia*, **8**, 83–91.

Martins, I.P., Baeta, E., Paiva, T., Campo, T. and Gomes, L. (1993) Headaches during intracranial endovascular procedures: a possible model of vascular headache. *Headache*, **33**, 227–233.

Moskowitz, M.A. and Cutrer, F.M. (1993) Sumatriptan: a receptor-targeted treatment for migraine. *Annual Review of Medicine*, **44**, 145–154.

Nichols, F.T., Mawad, M., Mohr, J.P., Hilal, S. and Adams, R.J. (1993) Focal headache during balloon inflation in the vertebral and basilar arteries. *Headache*, **33**, 87–89.

Nozaki, K., Boccalini, P. and Moskowitz, M.A. (1992) Expression of c-fos-like immunoreactivity in brainstem after meningeal irritation by blood in the subarachnoid space. *Neuroscience*, **49**, 669–680.

Ray, B.S. and Wolff, H.G. (1940) Experimental studies on headache. Pain sensitive structures of the head and their significance in headache. *Archives of Surgery*, **41**, 813–856.

Ruskell, G.L. and Simons, T. (1987) Trigeminal nerve pathways to the cerebral arteries in monkeys. *Journal of Anatomy*, **155**, 23–37.

Sakas, D.E., Moskowitz, M.A., Wei, E.P., Kontos, H.A., Kano, M. and Ogilvy, C. (1989) Trigeminovascular fibers increase blood flow in cortical grey matter by axon-dependent mechanisms during severe hypertension or seizures. *Proceedings of the National Academy of Science USA*, **86**, 1401–1405.

Steiger, H.J., Tew, J.M. and Keller, J.T. (1982) The sensory representation of the dura mater in the trigeminal ganglion of the cat. *Neuroscience Letters*, **31**, 231–236.

Uddman, R., Edvinsson, L., Ekman, R., Kingman, T. and McCulloch, J. (1985) Innervation of the feline cerebral vasculature by nerve fibers containing calcitonin gene-related peptide: trigeminal origin and co-existence with substance P. *Neuroscience Letters*, **62**, 131–136.

Williams, T.J. and Peck, M.J. (1977) Role of prostaglandin-mediated vaso-dilatation in inflammation. *Nature*, **270**, 530–532.

Woods, R.P., Iacoboni, M. and Mazziotta, J.C. (1994) Bilateral spreading cerebral hypoperfusion during spontaneous migraine headache. *New England Journal of Medicine*, **331**, 1689–1692.

Zagami, A.S. and Goadsby, P.J. (1991) Stimulation of the superior sagittal sinus increases metabolic activity in cat thalamus. In: *New Advances in Headache Research*, Vol. 2, (ed. F. Clifford Rose), pp. 169–171 Smith Gordon & Co., London.

Zagami, A.S. and Lambert, G.A. (1990) Stimulation of cranial vessels excites nociceptive neurones in several thalamic nuclei of the cat. *Experimental Brain Research*, **81**, 552–566.

Zagami, A.S. and Lambert, G.A. (1991) Craniovascular application of capsaicin activates nociceptive thalamic neurons in the cat. *Neuroscience Letters*, **121**, 187–190.

Zagami, A.S., Goadsby, P.J. and Edvinsson, L. (1990) Stimulation of the superior sagittal sinus in the cat causes release of vasoactive peptides. *Neuropeptides*, **16**, 69–75.

DISCUSSION

Lance: The thalamus probably plays a much more important part in migraine than we realize. Many patients do not have pain limited to the trigeminal area, let alone the first division. The pain radiates down the face, it radiates to the neck, the shoulder, sometimes to the upper limb, and occasionally even down to the lower limb on the same side, which is surely a spinothalamic distribution resembling a thalamic syndrome. Therefore, we should look closely at the thalamus and central pain-conducting structures as well as the endogenous pain-control pathway.

Goadsby: Certainly. My point is that if differentiating between $5\text{-HT}_{1D\alpha}$ and $5\text{-HT}_{1D\beta}$ receptor subtypes, trying to remove vascular effects and restrict the drugs' spectrum of activity, does not work there are many other options to explore within this pathway.

Branchek: Relevant to the different effects on 5-HT_{1A} and 5-HT_{1D} receptors of the compounds in Table 6.3 is that a small body of literature demonstrates that 5-HT_{1A} agonists appear to be effective against emesis (Okada *et al.* 1994).

Goadsby: The problem is that ergots cause nausea and are very potent at 5-HT_{1A} receptors. But they also work on the dopamine receptor. Perhaps Professor Humphrey was very skilful to have a $5\text{-HT}_{1A/1D}$ receptor agonist in sumatriptan which proved to be more useful than an exclusive 5-HT_{1D} agonist. We may well find out with the conformationally restricted drugs.

Connor: I was surprised that on Table 6.3 you distinguish between the affinity of sumatriptan and 311C90 at the human 5-HT_{1A} receptor.

Martin: Our recent data suggest that for 311C90 (zolmitriptan) the separation of affinities between human recombinant 5-HT$_{1D}$ subtypes and 5-HT$_{1A}$ receptors is wider than for the other drugs presently used in acute therapy.

Diener: I would like to comment on Table 6.3 and the non-steroidal anti-inflammatory drugs. We found that intravenous (iv) aspirin improves nausea and vomiting as well as sumatriptan.

Goadsby: Yes, but the effect of aspirin might not be a 5-HT$_{1A}$ effect. In the sinus model, as well as trigeminal cells, cell groups involved in emesis are active. Part of the stereotypy of a migraine may be the fact that certain aspects of it are wired together. An example may be that 80% of patients with migraine experience stomach symptoms.

Moskowitz: Most people agree that sumatriptan accesses the central nervous system very poorly. In contrast 311C90 does have access. How much more efficacious in migraine is 311C90?

Goadsby: A 311C90/sumatriptan comparative study will answer that question; we cannot draw any conclusions from the data available so far. By comparing a 5 mg 311C90 oral dose and 100 mg oral sumatriptan dose and subtracting the placebo from response in the largest study, one gets an impression that 311C90 might be more efficacious than sumatriptan orally. But there is no injectable form of 311C90 to compare intravenous or subcutaneous administration.

Ferrari: That oral 311C90 is more efficacious than oral sumatriptan might arise from the pharmacokinetics. I agree that the comparison should be made subcutaneously or intravenously. In a head-to-head comparison, it appeared that MK-462 was much more efficacious than sumatriptan, at the cost of greater central side-effects.

Moskowitz: That is one of the potential problems we are concerned about.

Humphrey: Dr Goadsby, when you say that sumatriptan probably does not act through the vasoconstrictor mechanism you refer to the study where it was ineffective when given during the aura (Bates *et al.* 1994). However, even to get to the cerebrovascular smooth muscle, sumatriptan has to cross the blood–brain barrier.

Goadsby: There is no blood–brain barrier for dural vessels.

Humphrey: But these are not the only blood vessels implicated.

Moskowitz: I think Professor Humphrey makes a good point. Either way, it does not argue for or against the vascular mechanisms.

Lance: It is clear from the side-effects of sumatriptan that, in some patients, it does cross the blood–brain barrier. A number of patients complain of somnolence and of feeling 'strange'. These sensations cannot be transmitted by vessels. It could be, as Dr Goadsby intimated, that the blood–brain barrier breaks down in some migrainous patients giving rise to central effects.

Goadsby: The main thing that the study of sumatriptan given in aura suggests to me is that there is a blood–brain barrier change when the headache phase of the migraine starts. That may change the whole picture of what is happening. If this is correct, then sumatriptan may have some access. But it may be subtle rather than an all-or-nothing phenomenon.

Humphrey: It may be a fortunate accident of the pathophysiology that sumatriptan is more selective, given that it does not normally cross the blood–brain barrier. If there is a local disruption of the blood–brain barrier at the site of whatever the lesion is, perhaps that gives you a targeted selectivity (a 'pathophilic' effect?). I agree with Dr Ferrari about the other compounds. It may be that their lipophilicity simply aids absorption from the gut and their efficacy has nothing to do with the central brain penetration.

Goadsby: That is possible. We cannot investigate further without injectable forms of both drugs.

Humphrey: If the blood–brain barrier is disrupted you do not need brain penetration as a pharmacokinetic advantage: they will all cross.

Goadsby: The disruption of the blood–brain barrier may not be a binary event: there may be a small amount of change.

Moskowitz: We should not think of the blood–brain barrier as some fixed partition. Eventually any drug, no matter what its lipid partition coefficient, is going to enter the brain: it is simply a matter of time and concentration. The suggestion Dr Goadsby makes about brainstem is interesting and important. There is a regional hierarchy for disrupting the blood–brain barrier. Disturbing the barrier is relatively easy in the cortex, but in the brainstem this is more problematic.

Goadsby: Trigeminal activation may be permissive in this. We became interested in this question of blood–brain barrier disruption during our sumatriptan studies. We found that it is easier to disrupt the blood–brain barrier with mannitol when you stimulate the trigeminal system than when you do not.

Moskowitz: When the ganglia are stimulated, blood flow increases quite significantly in the terminal area within the caudalis. Therefore you may be delivering a higher fraction of the hyperosmotic agent and this may better disrupt the blood–brain barrier. Effectively you are giving a higher dosage of osmotic agent. The experimental paradigm does not quite address the issue, but it is an interesting observation.

Goadsby: I am talking about stimulation of sagittal sinus rather than ganglion, but you are right; there are always flow changes just associated with metabolism, but they have been associated with migraine as well.

Connor: It is possible to look in a patient at the integrity of the blood–brain barrier during a migraine attack?

Goadsby: I hope that will be done by magnetic resonance imaging (MRI) before too long. I am told that it is theoretically possible to look at water changes with functional MRI.

Lance: George Bruyn referred earlier to the observation by Goltman (1935-1936) of a man with a skull defect that swelled up whenever he had a migraine attack. One of my patients with a similar bone defect describes it standing up like a hard-boiled egg during migraine attacks. This suggests that there is an increase in intracranial pressure that is hard to explain simply by the vasodilatation that has been demonstrated by transcranial doppler and other methods. Computer-aided tomography scanning shows that some patients with severe migraine headaches have cerebral oedema. Both these observations support the idea of some breakdown of the blood–brain barrier, at least in severe cases of migraine.

REFERENCES

Bates, D., Ashford, E., Dawson, R., Ensink, F-B.M., Gilhus, N.E., Olesen, J., Pilgrim, A.J. and Shevlin, P. (1994) Subcutaneous sumatriptan during the migraine aura. *Neurology*, **44**, 1587–1592.

Goltham, A.M. (1935–1936) The mechanism of the brain. *Journal of Allergies*, **7**, 351–355.

Okada, F., Torii, Y., Saito, H. and Matsuki, N. (1994) Antiemetic effects of serotonergic 5-HT$_{1A}$ receptor agonists in Suncus murinus. *Japanese Journal of Pharmacology*, **64**, 109–114.

7

Headache recurrence after subcutaneous sumatriptan

Michel D. Ferrari and W. Hester Visser

INTRODUCTION

Sumatriptan has proved to be a highly effective and generally well-tolerated drug in the acute treatment of migraine. In controlled clinical trials, evaluating the efficacy and tolerability of sumatriptan in single attacks per patient, 6 mg subcutaneous (sc) sumatriptan provided headache relief within two hours in up to 86% of patients and 100 mg oral sumatriptan did so in up to 67% of patients (see Plosker and McTavish 1994). However, in up to 40% of the successfully treated attacks, the headache returned within 24 hours (headache recurrence, HR), necessitating repeated doses of sumatriptan to treat the recurrent headache (Figure 7.1). Interestingly, pre-emptive repeated dosing of sumatriptan did not prevent HR (Ferrari *et al.* 1994a, Rapoport *et al.* 1995).

Remarkably similar rates of HR have been obtained with both older (ergotamine, aspirin) and newer (311C90, MK-462) antimigraine compounds (Ferrari *et al.* 1994b, Visser *et al.* 1996a), suggesting that headache recurrence is a common feature of all acute antimigraine drugs (Ferrari and Saxena 1993, 1995). Little is known, however, about the incidence of HR in clinical practice where patients have unrestricted access to antimigraine drugs. Likewise, there is no information on whether the occurrence of HR is an attack-related phenomenon (i.e.

Migraine: Pharmacology and genetics
Edited by Merton Sandler, Michel Ferrari and Sara Harnett
Published in 1996 by Chapman & Hall
ISBN 1 86036 006 8

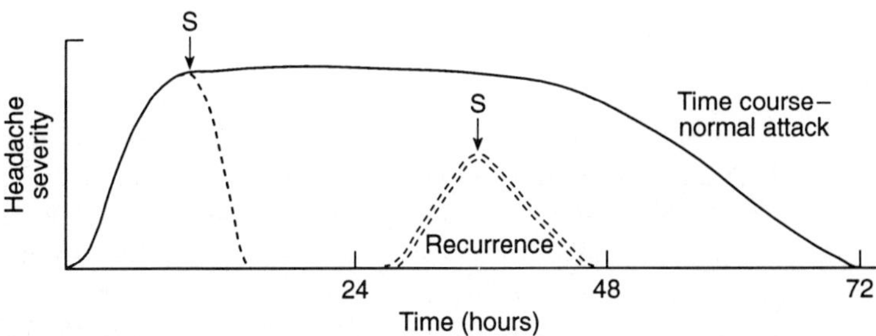

Figure 7.1 Single headache recurrence after sumatriptan, within usual duration of a migraine attack. S, sumatriptan; ——, time course of a normal untreated attack; - - -, time course after sumatriptan; = = =, recurrence of headache.

may vary per attack within a patient), or is patient-dependent (i.e. some patients consistently have HR in all treated attacks, whereas others rarely experience HR). Finally, only limited information is available about whether the incidence of HR changes over time with long-term use of sumatriptan. Answers to these questions are important for the understanding of the mechanisms involved in the pathophysiology and treatment of the migraine attack as well as the HR, and for a better evaluation of the true efficacy of antimigraine drugs.

We therefore evaluated initial relief and HR after oral and sc sumatriptan over more than two years in 869 unselected migraine patients who were attending or had attended our outpatient clinic. We assessed whether the effects of sumatriptan (relief and HR) were consistent over multiple attacks within a patient, and whether these effects had changed over time. This study was part of a large review on the long term efficacy, tolerability and clinical use of sc and oral sumatriptan in clinical practice in The Netherlands (Visser *et al.* 1996b). Here, only the results with respect to HR after sc sumatriptan are presented and discussed.

METHODS

We mailed a questionnaire, consisting of 86 items on the use and effects of sumatriptan, to all 869 migraine (International Headache Society criteria; Headache Classification Committee 1988) patients in our database. Descriptive analyses were carried out on the pooled data for all patients who could be evaluated per item. For analysis of within-patient consistency over multiple attacks, only patients who had treated at least three migraine attacks with sumatriptan were included. For evaluation of change over time, only patients who had treated at least ten migraine attacks were included.

RESULTS

Clinical use

In total 735 (85%) patients filled out and returned the questionnaire. Of these, 453 (62%) patients had used sumatriptan at least once and they comprise the study population. Sumatriptan had been used by 92% for at least one year and by 60% for at least two years: 78% had treated at least ten migraine attacks with sumatriptan. In total 19000 migraine attacks were treated with sc sumatriptan. Of the 453 patients, 111 (25%) had stopped using sumatriptan, mainly because of HR (32%), adverse events (30%) and lack of efficacy (18%).

Headache relief

In total, 77% of patients reported being pain-free within one hour and 89% within two hours after sc sumatriptan. Headache relief was obtained in the majority of attacks in 89% of patients.

Headache recurrence

About 75% of patients indicated they had experienced HR in at least some attacks treated with sc sumatriptan and 40% reported experiencing HR in at least two-thirds of their attacks. Nearly all patients with HR took a repeated dose of sumatriptan to treat the recurrent headache: this was successful in up to 85% of cases. However, in 34% of these patients, the headache almost always returned again (multiple HRs; Figure 7.2) and in 50% the headache returned sometimes. Of those patients who experienced HR in virtually all their attacks, 70% nearly always had multiple HRs.

The time to onset of HR ranged from 1–24 hours after administration of sc sumatriptan. In about half of the patients the time to HR was consistent. The median time to onset was 8–10 hours.

Most patients reported no change over time in efficacy and number of

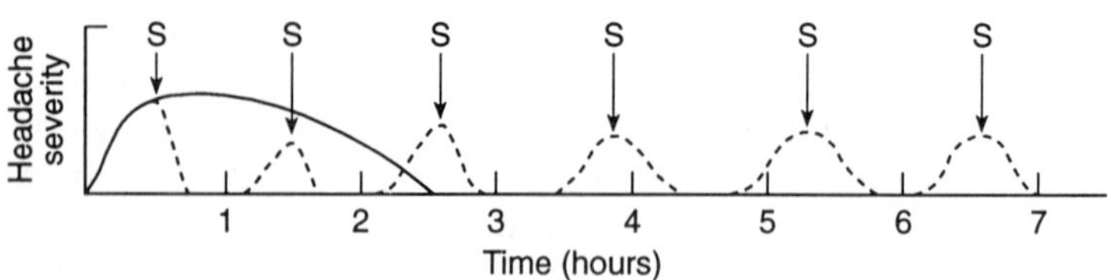

Figure 7.2 Multiple headache recurrences after sumatriptan beyond the usual duration of a migraine attack. S, sumatriptan; ——, time course of a normal untreated attack; - - - -, time course after sumatriptan.

doses used per month. Of the patients who could be evaluated for long-term use with sc sumatriptan, 18% reported reduced efficacy, mainly due to an increase in the number of headache recurrences. Likewise, 20% of the patients reported an increase over time of the number of monthly doses of sumatriptan.

Recurrence of aura

Of the 39 patients who exclusively suffered from attacks of migraine with aura 16 (41%) patients reported that they always or often experienced recurrence of the aura.

DISCUSSION

We studied the clinical use and effects of sc sumatriptan over more than two years, covering 19000 treated attacks, in 453 well-defined migraine patients with unrestricted access to the drug. The response to our survey was very high (85%).

Sumatriptan proved highly and rapidly effective in the majority of patients in most of their attacks. Up to 89% of patients had headache relief in at least two-thirds of their attacks and up to 89% were pain free within two hours. On the other hand, recurrence of the headache, usually within ten hours, occurred in 75% of patients in at least some attacks and in 40% of patients in virtually all their attacks. If patients treated the recurrent headache with a repeated dose of sumatriptan, the majority experienced two or more consecutive HRs. Headache recurrence was also a major reason for patients to discontinue the use of sumatriptan. Of the 25% of patients who stopped using sumatriptan, one third did so because of HR.

Remarkably, the responses to sumatriptan proved rather consistent within patients over multiple attacks as well as over a period of about two years. Only a minority (about 15%) showed varying responses per attack or a change over time. About 40% always had HRs and approximately 45% hardly ever experienced HR. Factors predisposing for HR therefore are patient-dependent rather than attack-related. Identification of these factors, clinical, pharmacokinetic, genetic or environmental, may help to allow personalized optimal clinical management and treatment of migraine patients. Also, it will help in understanding the mechanisms involved in migraine attacks and their treatment.

REFERENCES

Ferrari, MD and Saxena, P.R. (1993) Clinical and experimental effects of sumatriptan in humans. *Trends in Pharmacological Science*, **14**, 129–134.

Ferrari, M.D and Saxena, P.R. (1995) 5-HT$_1$ receptors in migraine pathophysiology and treatment. *European Journal of Neurology*, **2**, 5–21.
Ferrari, M.D., James, M.H., Bates, D., Pilgrim, A.J., Ashford, E.A., Anderson, B.A and Nappi, G. (1994a) Oral sumatriptan: effect of a second dose, and treatment of headache recurrence. *Cephalalgia*, **14**, 330–338.
Ferrari, M.D., Terwindt, G.M., Visser, W.H. and Reines, S.A. (1994b) A placebo-controlled dose-ranging study of MK-462 versus sumatriptan in migraine. In: *New Advances in Headache research*, vol. 4 (ed. F. Clifford Rose), pp. 205–207. Smith Gordon & Co., London.
Headache Classification Committee of the International Headache Society (J. Olesen *et al.*) (1988) Classification and diagnostic criteria for headache disorders, cranial neuralgias and facial pain. *Cephalalgia*, **8** (Suppl. 7), 1–97.
Plosker, G.L. and McTavish, D. (1994) Sumatriptan. A reappraisal of its pharmacology and therapeutic efficacy in the acute treatment of migraine and cluster headache. *Drugs*, **47**, 622–51.
Rapoport, A., Visser, W.H., Ferrari, M.D. *et al.* (1995) Oral sumatriptan in the prevention of headache recurrences after subcutaneous sumatriptan. *Neurology*, **45**, 1505–1509.
Visser, W.H., Klein, K.B., Cox, R.C., Jones, D. and Ferrari, M.D. (1996a) 311C90, a new central and peripherally acting 5-HT$_{1D}$ receptor agonist in the acute oral treatment of migraine: a double-blind, placebo-controlled, dose range finding study. *Neurology*, in press.
Visser, W.H., Vriend de, R.H.M., Jaspers, N.M.W.H. and Ferrari, M.D. (1996b) Sumatriptan in clinical practice; a two year review of 735 migraine patients. *Neurology*, in press.

DISCUSSION

Schoenen: Recurrence depends only on patient factors, not on the kind of treatment. It occurs with every treatment, even placebo. Doesn't this indicate that recurrence is related to a pain trigger continuing some- where during the migraine attack? For any pain, even outside the head, as long as the pain trigger continues any symptomatic treatment is effective for some time and then pain reoccurs. Isn't this an argument in favour of the migraine attack being a protective mechanism for the brain, as suggested some years ago by Professor Lance (1978)? I am not convinced that recurrence of the aura means that this is a new attack. If something continues to happen in the brain parenchyma which, at some time, may produce clinical aura symptoms, and you assume that the migraine attack itself is protective, then the brain parenchyma would need some time to recover. If this process is still going on, then aura symptoms might reoccur also.

Ferrari: If it is true that the aura reoccurs, then my interpretation would be that sumatriptan acts much more proximally than we originally thought, not only at the pain site.

Moskowitz: I would say the opposite. Because the pain generator is unaffected, the final common pathway, which is the pain, is inhibited.

Ferrari: If the pain generator continues, the pain would reoccur, but why would the aura reoccur?

Schoenen: Because the pain 'generator' is present where the aura is generated. You are thinking of a central pain generator, but something has to trigger the pain. This would mean that sumatriptan is working downstream of this trigger and, if this trigger is still there, then you would expect a recurrence.

Goadsby: You should not call it the pain generator, then. We are talking about the migraine generator, and downstream the pain gets treated by sumatriptan, but the migraine generator is still working. The aura can reoccur because the migraine is still there.

Glover: That would fit with the fact that patients report that 'something' continues. The attack generation is still there: the treatment is only downstream.

Lance: Some patients spontaneously have recurrent auras within one attack. I have patients who have two to four auras in a day or a recurrence of aura the next day without being treated by sumatriptan. This might simply be the effect of the migraine generator, that can express itself in an aura or a headache, and most usually in sequence: the aura and then the headache. The sumatriptan acts, as has been said, downstream on the pathway that leads to the pain.

Haan: What is the effect of sumatriptan given during the recurrent aura on that aura or on the headache that follows?

Ferrari: I have not tried that.

Schoenen: We have patients who respond to sumatriptan during the aura and say that their headache is prevented. Is everyone convinced that sumatriptan given during the aura is completely ineffective?

Pilgrim: In the aura study (Bates *et al.* 1994) statistically we did not prevent headache developing. In patients who had an aura which clearly preceded headache, and who had no or mild headache at the time of receiving study medication, there was a small effect, but it was not statistically significant. A substantial proportion of patients who took part in that study had an aura and headache with essentially simultaneous onset. Perhaps we should look at Dr Ferrari's patients to see whether those patients with recurrent aura are the ones who normally have a combined aura and headache in their initial attack, or whether they have the typical pattern of aura preceding a headache.

Ferrari: I would like to stress that recurrence happens with all the acute treatments, even aspirin. The only reason for the emphasis on sumatriptan is that it's been studied after sumatriptan, which is easy to do because sumatriptan turns off the migraine attack so quickly and the recurrence is profound.

Humphrey: What is the recurrence rate after placebo?

Ferrari: It is hard to be sure. All the data on placebo came from just one attack, whereas the sumatriptan data refer to 30–70 attacks over two years. It might occur in one attack after placebo, but I do think that there is a drug-induced action. Why do so many patients have multiple attacks beyond the usual duration of attack? We are seeing more and more patients who have attacks for eight or nine days consecutively, which is not normal.

Humphrey: That needs to be studied. I have not heard of this, even though the drug has been in use for several years. That suggestion contradicts what you said about recurrence happening with all acute treatments and placebo. Is it or isn't it the natural history of the disease? I do not find the fact that a migraine attack reoccurs surprising. When a migraine attack lasts for three or four days, why would one expect one dose of any drug to suffice?

Lance: Unless you switch off the central generator, which we can't yet do.

Humphrey: That is correct. Apparently we're not doing that, and that's why these data are so important. This may be the first evidence that there is a generator and that sumatriptan is only a palliative, switching things off at the other end.

Peatfield: In that case, why would the recurrences go on longer?

Humphrey: Well, we don't know that they do. We have to study that.

Goadsby: Patients not treated with sumatriptan have attacks that last for days. It is not peculiar to any particular treatment.

Lance: If patients who usually have a headache of less than 24 hours are given sumatriptan, and are in the 50% that respond, the headache does not reoccur. In those patients who normally have a headache duration of 72 hours, the headache tends to reoccur any time after 10 hours, commonly the next day. Patients report that the drug works, but that the next day the headache comes back and they need more sumatriptan. My response is to give an ergotamine chaser about 12 hours after sumatriptan, which usually prevents recurrence.

Ferrari: It is true that there is a correlation with the duration of the attack. But it's not true that patients who have attacks lasting one day don't suffer recurrence: they do.

Peatfield: Anecdotally, aspirin has a functional life of about four hours. Is there clinical evidence that the headache after aspirin reoccurs after 12 hours? I find that difficult to believe on pharmacokinetic grounds.

Ferrari: The aspirin data are from the comparison study with sumatriptan. That study wasn't designed to investigate recurrence, but it did occur.

Peatfield: Were patients asked about recurrence at four hours, which is when you would expect recurrence after aspirin on pharmacokinetic grounds?

Pilgrim: There are many problems with drawing conclusions from that study. When it was done recurrence was not an issue of clinical concern. The data were drawn from a question about whether the headache came back within 48 hours. This was at the end of a complicated diary card, and it wasn't well completed. Much of the data was ambiguous. It was probably equally badly completed by both the sumatriptan and the aspirin group, and the fact that we got similar recurrence rates suggests it's a real phenomenon with aspirin, but you can't say accurately when it happens.

Ferrari: I agree. Now we have a drug which is very well studied and we can follow it over multiple attacks, look at within patient consistency, and look at the characteristics between patients.

Pilgrim: The problem with controlled trials involving multiple attacks is the drop-out rate. The longer the trial, the more the drop-outs, so you are selecting a population. The bias becomes much worse when you follow an open population like yours with two years of experience. At the end of two years the population continuing treatment is very different from that at the beginning.

Ferrari: We compared patients who had 3, 10 and 20 attacks and there was no difference in the result. It appears that we were not selecting patients in that way. More important might be that they were coming to a University hospital because they had a problem.

Pilgrim: If the study started after sumatriptan was available for general prescription, the subjects were probably a population who had tried other therapies and had problems with them. So you have a very selected population.

Ferrari: About 80% of the population came to us to be treated with sumatriptan. These were all patients who started in June 1991 when the drug first became available. But I agree they are not a typical selection of migraine patients.

Pilgrim: I would also urge caution about the accuracy of the history of the normal duration of attacks. When we attempted to collect detailed information on the nature of patients' auras in the past and then did a prospective untreated attack before we went into the randomized double-blind trial, we found that the historical data were very different from the one attack studied prospectively. This suggests that patients' historical recollections of the nature and duration of their attack are very inaccurate.

Ferrari: We addressed this methodological question at selection. With respect to recurrence patients seemed to tell the truth. In the prospective study the data were the same. If patients had recurrence, they had multiple recurrences. They were treated, and after 12 hours the headache came back. So they have multiple recurrences: three or four within one attack.

Diener: Three years ago we did a double-blind study with intravenous (iv) aspirin against ergotamine, placebo and sumatriptan in acute migraine attacks. We were not aware that recurrence was a problem when we started, but our impression was that the effect of aspirin lasts about twice as long as sumatriptan and ergotamine. Also, we invite our outpatients to come back if there are recurrences. About 40% of patients return after subcutaneous sumatriptan or dihydroergotamine (DHE), but only about 30% after aspirin iv, which indicates it lasts longer. I have not treated anyone with aspirin who has recurrences beyond the normal length of their attack.

Peatfield: Were you giving these drugs on a random basis or was there some systematic difference?

Diener: There was one systematic difference: private patients have the choice between sumatriptan and the other drugs; non-private patients, about 80% of the population, are given aspirin or DHE.

Peatfield: Was there a systematic difference in which drug was given to which patient? Were you giving aspirin for milder attacks and DHE for the more severe ones?

Diener: Even for a very severe attack patients are given aspirin iv (100 mg).

Humphrey: We must ascertain whether this recurrence is part of the natural history or whether there is some induction or sensitization by sumatriptan. Where there are multiple recurrences, does sumatriptan work multiple times?

Ferrari: Yes.

Humphrey: If sumatriptan is inducing some supersensitivity then the dose of sumatriptan that people take might be expected to steadily increase. As far as I know this does not happen.

Diener: It also does not happen with ergotamine. Some patients have a daily migraine attack and take 0.25 mg ergotamine every day. They do not increase the dose. Other patients increase the dose up to 20 mg a day, but generally patients can use the same amount of ergotamine for 10 years.

Ferrari: We also looked at that. Of our population 20% reported a definite increase in their consumption of sumatriptan over two years. There was also a proportion who reported a decrease.

Peatfield: That could be the natural history of the migraine population.

Ferrari: We often see patients who have multiple recurrences beyond their normal attacks and, although sumatriptan is extremely effective each time, the only way to stop the series of attacks is to endure the attack for 24 hours and not use sumatriptan. Do other clinicians agree?

Haan: I see patients with this problem sometimes, but not often. We advise giving a maximum of two doses of sumatriptan per 24 hours and three injections per attack. After the third injection we stop until the end of the attack.

Peatfield: We don't see this in England. Whether this is because patients are seldom allowed more than one dose per attack, or whether it's a real difference and we're just missing it, I don't know.

Ferrari: We see it with subcutaneous administration but not often with oral doses. You are right that it's because patients are allowed to use sumatriptan on demand. Perhaps if you restrict the number of doses you won't have this problem.

Diener: For ergotamine it takes 10 to 15 years in most patients to develop drug-induced headache. For the patients who increase the dose of acute migraine medication you can see real changes after five years. For sumatriptan you may see dependency more often in the next few years. The people whom we see now are the ones with newly developing sumatriptan headaches. Those we have seen previously were the ones who switched from daily intake of ergotamine to sumatriptan. Now we have the first *de novo* patients who were first given the drug three or four years ago and have reached a point where they use it every second day. Drug-induced headache and dependency may happen with all effective drugs. They perhaps increase the sensitivity of the receptors or of the whole system.

Humphrey: That is my point. First we need to establish that this effect is real. If so, it's probably telling us something very important about migraine itself.

Goadsby: An important issue is whether it happens without drugs! Are we looking at a phenomenon of sumatriptan, ergotamine or any particular drug, or are we looking at part of the natural history of migraine? My impression of the natural history is that sometimes people have very frequent attacks, and sometimes they don't. People had very frequent attacks of migraine before sumatriptan was available.

Ferrari: You do see this phenomenon without drugs. But you don't see it each time. It's only been studied in sumatriptan, but you might encounter this problem in any acute treatment.

Peatfield: Is it possible that the headache attack is a response to some sort of physiological aberration that has to work itself through, and if you block that with sumatriptan it is somehow prolonged in some way?

Moskowitz: After patients with epilepsy have a seizure there is a refractory period during which they tend not to have a seizure. Patients with a full blown headache also tend to have a refractory period. If you suppress the headache with a drug perhaps this refractory period is considerably shortened.

Humphrey: Yes. It may be that the stress of a severe headache somehow does tend to terminate the duration of the attack. And if the headache is ameliorated perhaps it has to go on longer.

Schoenen: Are there data about induced, rather than spontaneous, attacks which are treated? Is there recurrence in induced attacks?

Ferrari: Did a proportion of patients provoked with reserpine have a recurrence?

Lance: Anthony *et al.* (1969) estimated platelet serotonin content, which diminished after injection of reserpine and remained low without further headache. Nattero *et al.* (1976) used iv reserpine therapeutically. After an initial headache, the headache tendency diminished when reserpine was injected every second or third day. It seems that it's a sudden change in the serotonin level that makes the difference, not a sustained low level of serotonin.

Thomsen: We've provoked too few patients to answer this question conclusively. However, we treat those provoked with sumatriptan and it's not my impression that they get a recurrence, but we haven't studied it separately.

Ferrari: Do you continue provocation with nitric oxide while treating the patients? That would be more similar to the clinical situation.

Thomsen: We haven't done that yet.

Goadsby: Do the recurrence data refer to patients whose headaches go away completely and then come back?

Ferrari: Patients tell you they have improvement and then the headache returns. It doesn't necessarily mean that it's completely gone.

Goadsby: This is what confuses me about headache recurrence data. It's very difficult to distinguish whether something goes and returns or if it just fades into the background and then re-emerges.

Ferrari: It profoundly decreases and comes back prominently. I left out all the cases where it was not clear.

Schoenen: Other information would come from those people who are treating migraine attacks with non-drug therapies.

Diener: All my patients tell me that it doesn't work. I think this clearly shows that placebo doesn't work in severe migraine!

Schoenen: Is there often recurrence in those attacks in which patients go to sleep?

Ferrari: There was no difference whether or not the patient went to sleep after an injection of sumatriptan.

Moskowitz: This discussion is important and some excellent points have been raised, but I don't think we shall ever understand migraine if we only focus on the pain. We need to understand the natural history, and that involves much more than headache. The pain is the final event.

Ferrari: I agree. We did look at one parameter other than pain, namely the aura, and were surprised by our results. I urge clinicians to collect data on whether or not this recurrence of aura is true.

REFERENCES

Anthony, M., Hinterberger, H. and Lance, J.W. (1969) The possible relationship of serotonin to the migraine syndrome. *Research and Clinical Studies in Headache*, **2**, 29–59.

Bates, D., Ashford, E., Dawson, R., Ensink, F-B., Gilhus, N.E., Olesen, J., Pilgrim, A.J. and Shevlin, P. (1994) Subcutaneous sumatriptan during the migraine aura. *Neurology*, **44**, 1587–1592.

Lance, J.W. (1978) *Mechanism and Management of Headache*, 3rd Edn, pp. 176–177. Butterworth, London.

Nattero, G., Lisino, F., Brandi, G., Gastaldi, L. and Kemp Genefke, I. (1976) Reserpine for migraine prophylaxis. *Headache*, **15**, 279–281.

8

Recurrent migraine following treatment with 5-HT$_{1D}$ agonists: pharmacokinetic and pharmacodynamic aspects

G.R. Martin and R.S. Martin

INTRODUCTION

Rebound migraine headache following acute intervention with ergots is a long and well established phenomenon, particularly in cases of ergotamine abuse (Saper 1987). Usually, a vicious circle is set up in which increasingly frequent headaches are treated with an ever increasing frequency of drug administration, leading ultimately to dependency. Only cessation of the drug breaks this circle of events. Experience to date with the 5-HT$_{1D}$ receptor agonist sumatriptan indicates that drug-dependent headache is less of a problem with this drug class, although in susceptible patients, i.e. those who have a history of ergotamine abuse, daily intake of sumatriptan appears to sustain ergotamine-dependent headache (Catarci *et al.* 1994).

Against this background of what clearly appears to be a drug-induced condition, there has been much debate concerning headache recurrence in patients receiving sumatriptan (see Ferrari and Saxena 1995). This phenomenon, which still lacks a rigorous definition, is observed as the re-emergence of migraine, with associated symptoms (excepting pro-

Migraine: Pharmacology and genetics
Edited by Merton Sandler, Michel Ferrari and Sara Harnett
Published in 1996 by Chapman & Hall
ISBN 1 86036 006 8

drome or aura), within 24 hours of successfully treating the initial attack. Around 40% of patients experience recurrent migraine with a median time of 12 hours following subcutaneous (sc) sumatriptan (6 mg), slightly fewer (35%) suffer recurrence after oral (po) drug (100 mg), with a median time of 16 hours (see Plosker and McTavish 1994, Ferrari and Saxena 1995). Importantly, a significant proportion (approximately 40%) of patients rarely experience recurrent migraine with sumatriptan, whilst, in comparison, about 10% appear to suffer recurrence after nearly every treated attack. In a comprehensive study of the possible factors underlying patient susceptibility to recurrence, Ferrari and colleagues have excluded significant demographic or clinical distinctions (Jaspers *et al.* 1994, de Vriend *et al.* 1994). Hence, neither the timing of treatment during the attack nor plasma pharmacokinetics appears to differ between patients who suffer recurrence and those who do not (Visser *et al.* 1996).

Although the possibility remains that in some patients sumatriptan might provoke a true drug-induced headache (Osborne *et al.* 1994, Catarci *et al.* 1994), a number of features of the recurrence encourage the view that in most cases it is a re-emergence of the original attack. Firstly, sumatriptan has only a short elimination half-life (plasma $t_{1/2} = 2$ hours; Fowler *et al.* 1991), and hence is unlikely to provide clinically active plasma concentrations of drug for the duration of a migraine attack (up to 72 hours). Secondly, the prodrome or aura are rarely experienced before recurrence, although the headache exhibits the same quality and severity as the original attack. Thirdly, and perhaps most excitingly, a recent study using positron emission tomography has shown that metabolic activity in a localized area of the rostral brainstem is increased during migraine, and remains hyperactive even when headache relief is obtained with sumatriptan (Diener and May, this volume). Such an observation adds credence to anecdotal feedback from patients who comment that in spite of freedom from head pain, they feel as though the migraine attack is still ongoing (see Ferrari and Saxena 1995).

All this implies that sumatriptan, and probably the ergots as well, act simply as a palliative, but it nevertheless begs the question: Is this a limitation imposed by the pharmacological approach, namely 5-HT_{1D} receptor agonism, or is it one that can be countered by careful selection of the physical-chemical, as well as biological, attributes of members of this drug class? Obviously a definitive answer requires detailed mechanistic understanding of the site and mode of action of these drugs. This brief review aims to seek possible clues for the mechanism of recurrence from an examination of some basic aspects of drug pharmacokinetics and pharmacodynamics.

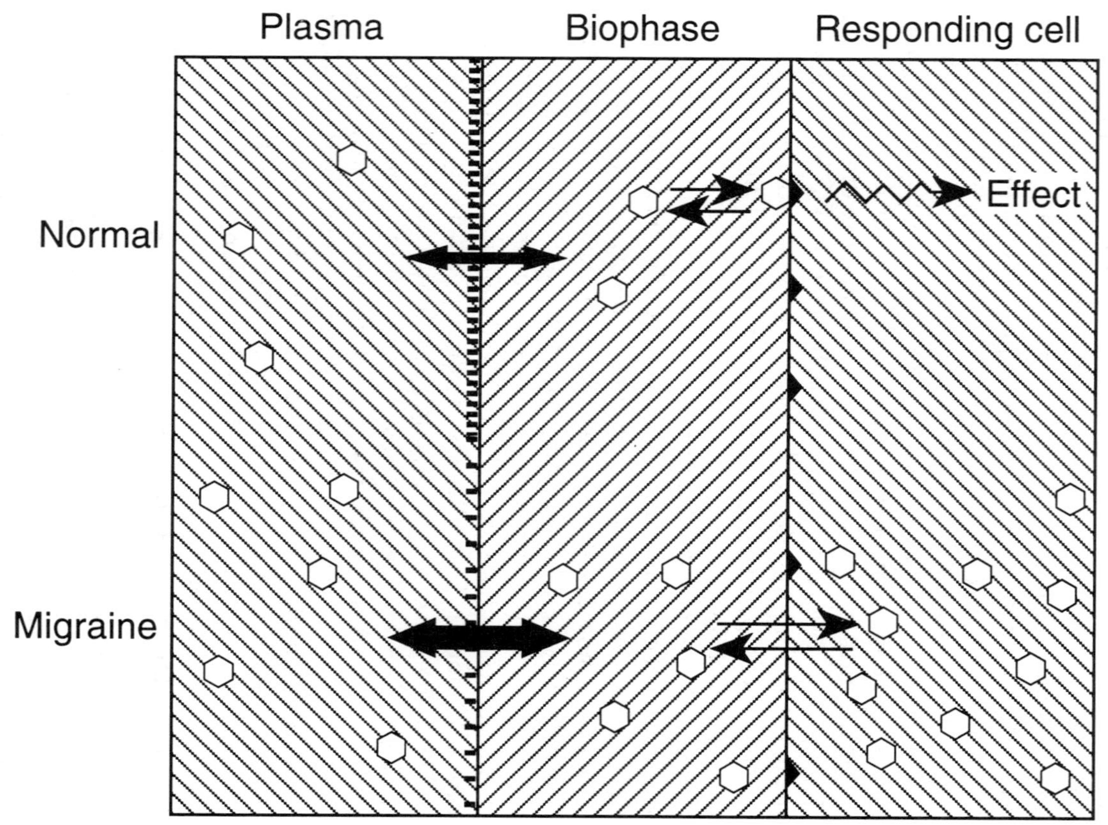

Plasma
Biophase
Responding cell
Normal
Migraine
Effect

FACTORS INFLUENCING DRUG–RECEPTOR INTERACTIONS *IN VIVO*

Figure 8.1 presents a highly simplistic view of the principle factors that might influence the duration of drug effect *in vivo*. These are: a) plasma pharmacokinetics, which dictate the concentration–time relation for drug in the plasma compartment; b) biophase pharmacokinetics, which determine the concentration–time relation for drug in the receptor biophase compartment; and c) kinetics of drug–receptor activation, which determine the persistence of drug effect.

Obviously, post-receptor events are also critical determinants of effect persistence. However, it seems reasonable to assume that receptor–effector coupling is a stable property of the 5-HT$_{1D}$ receptor system, since there is no evidence for acute desensitization. The considerations that follow therefore concentrate on the factors determining drug concentration in the receptor biophase (the drug 'active site') and persistence of drug action at the receptor.

Pharmacokinetic considerations

An excellent review by Ferrari and Saxena (1995) outlined a number of features of sumatriptan recurrent headache which the authors proposed were arguments *against* a simple short plasma half-life hypothesis for recurrence. These were: a) the median time to recurrence (sc = 12 h; po = 16 h) is considerably longer than the two-hour drug plasma elimination half-life; b) a second dose of sumatriptan two hours after the initial dose (2 x 10 mg po) does not prevent the incidence or alter the timing of recurrence (Ashford 1992); c) there are no obvious differences

---

Figure 8.1 Representation of the steps influencing drug action *in vivo*. Three 'compartments' are illustrated: the plasma compartment; a receptor biophase; and a 'diffusion' compartment, access to which is determined by physical-chemical properties of the drug. The drug concentration–time profile in plasma is dictated by measurable plasma pharmacokinetic parameters. In the receptor biophase, the drug concentration–time profile is determined not only by plasma pharmacokinetics, but also by the ease with which drug can move between the compartments. Receptor binding or partitioning of drug is assumed not to alter significantly the biophase concentration, but passage of drug between plasma and biophase is assumed to be influenced by a permeability 'barrier' that is poorly permeable to drug in normal circumstances, but becomes permeable during migraine headache (see text). Finally, persistence of drug effect is governed either by drug–receptor dissociation kinetics (i.e. A.R dissociation rate-limited) or by sequestration into a non-saturable compartment from which slowly diffusing drug sustains the biophase drug concentration (i.e. diffusion rate-limited).

in plasma pharmacokinetics between patients who always get recurrent headache and those who do not (Visser *et al.* 1996); and d) recurrence is also seen in patients taking ergotamine, but with a lower incidence (30%) and with a longer time interval (23 h) (Kirkham *et al.* 1991) despite the fact that ergotamine has a similar plasma half-life to sumatriptan (Orton and Richardson 1982).

However, lack of a clear relation between drug plasma concentrations and recurrence of headache is understandable if the site of drug action, or at least part of it, is not in the plasma compartment, but in a separate compartment (the receptor biophase), access to which is governed by the physical chemistry of the molecule and the permeability of biological 'barriers' separating the two compartments (Figure 8.1). This situation might pertain for sumatriptan. Firstly, the drug is hydrophilic (log $D_{pH7.4}$ = -1.0) and crosses the blood–brain barrier poorly (Humphrey *et al.* 1991). Secondly, although the drug is highly effective at aborting an ongoing headache, it is auspiciously ineffective if given 30–40 min before migraine headache (i.e. during aura; Bates *et al.* 1994) or prophylactically in the treatment of cluster headache (Monstad 1993). Ergotamine, which is a lipophilic molecule (log $D_{pH7.4}$ = $+6.0$) appears to be efficacious in both of these situations. The implication is that a 'barrier' normally exists between the plasma compartment and sumatriptan's site of action and that this 'barrier' becomes permeable to the drug during migraine headache. Support for this proposition comes from elegant animal studies by Goadsby and colleagues showing that intravenous sumatriptan is unable to inhibit cell firing in the trigeminal nucleus caudalis evoked by superior sagital sinus stimulation unless the blood–brain barrier is first disrupted with mannitol (Kaube *et al.* 1993). It is therefore tempting to speculate that a crucial site of action for sumatriptan is within the central nervous system and that access to this site is governed largely by the integrity of the blood–brain barrier.

The impact of a permeability barrier on drug transfer between the plasma compartment and receptor biophase is simulated in Figure 8.2(a) Using published pharmacokinetic parameters for sumatriptan, two conditions are illustrated: low permeability, equivalent, for example, to an intact blood–brain barrier; and a higher permeability representing disruption of the barrier. In the first case, entry of drug into the receptor biophase is much slower than its rate of rise in the plasma compartment and the maximum concentration achieved is very much lower. However, in this simple model, egress of drug out of the biophase is hampered by the same poorly permeable barrier, hence low concentrations of drug are sustained in the biophase compartment for a much longer time than in the plasma. As permeability of the barrier increases, the rate of appearance and disappearance of drug in the biophase more closely approximates that observed in the plasma. It is not difficult to see that in such circumstances plasma profiles of drug are likely to be a poor index of drug concentration in the biophase. Furthermore, differences in integrity of the barrier between subjects would result in very different biophase concentrations of drug in spite of identical plasma profiles.

Figures 8.2(b) and 8.2(c) illustrate a further refinement of the above model, providing an insight into barrier effects on plasma/biophase drug distribution when permeability between the compartments is transiently increased. Here it is envisaged that permeability suddenly rises at the onset of headache and subsequently declines with a time-course that approximates successful treatment with sumatriptan, i.e. 2–4 h. In Figure 8.2(b), drug is given 40 min after the onset of 'headache', when permeability between the plasma and biophase compartments is high but declining. The simulation shows that drug rapidly appears in the biophase and achieves a high concentration that declines slowly. In Figure 8.2(c), drug is given 40 min before the onset of 'headache'. In this case, biophase concentrations of drug rise slowly at first, then increase more rapidly as the permeability barrier breaks down and the 'headache' appears. Peak biophase drug concentrations are lower than those obtained when drug is given 40 min after 'headache' onset and drug is lost from the biophase more rapidly. In summary, these simulations suggest that drug delivery to the biophase is favoured if administration occurs during the permeability increase ('headache') rather than before it. However, whether or not such differences are sufficient to account for different drug effects in the target cell remains speculative.

Pharmacodynamic considerations

Once the drug is in the biophase compartment, interaction with the receptor produces a target cell response, the duration of which might be prolonged by one of two processes (see Figure 8.1): slow drug–receptor ([A.R]) dissociation; or drug sequestration into, followed by slow diffusion from, a non-saturable compartment, e.g. lipophilic partitioning into cells. In both cases the biological half-life of the drug might be expected to exceed the plasma elimination half-life. In this context, it is interesting that the biological effects of ergotamine and dihydroergotamine (DHE), as measured by their vasoconstrictor effects, last considerably longer than expected from their plasma half-life (e.g. Müller-Schweinitzer and Rosenthaler 1987). Conceivably, this might account for the lower incidence of, and the longer median time to, recurrent headache with ergotamine.

In principle, diffusion-limited and dissociation-limited 5-HT_{ID} drug effects can be distinguished experimentally. Details of the method and underlying theory are published elsewhere (Martin *et al.* 1995). The technique uses isolated rings of rabbit saphenous vein to study the time-course of recovery from the vasoconstrictor effects of various 5-HT_{1D} receptor agonists in this vessel (Martin *et al.* 1995). Vascular ring segments, mounted in jacketed organ baths, are superfused with physiological buffer at 37 °C. Initially drug-free, the superfusate is changed to one containing the agonist drug ($10 \times K_A$ or $100 \times K_A$) and vessel constriction is measured as an increase in isometric force. When contracture is at steady-state (about 45 min), the superfusate is exchanged again for drug-free buffer and the tissue response is monitored until the pre-drug state is re-attained. The half-life of the decline in agonist effect ($Rt_{1/2}$) is defined as the time taken for the steady-state contracture to decline by one half (see Figure 8.3).

Interpretation of these data in terms of diffusion or dissociation makes the reasonable assumption that the rate at which [A] (free drug concentration) or [A.R] (drug–receptor complex) declines in the receptor biophase following drug washout is exponential:

$$\text{For diffusion, } [A] = [A]_o.e^{-b.t}$$

$$\text{For dissociation, } [A.R] = [A.R]_o.e^{-b.t}$$

Substitution of each equation into a mathematical model for agonism (Black and Leff 1983) predicts that the decline in agonist effect will also be exponential and that, in the case of diffusion, the value of $Rt_{1/2}$ (see above) is related to the drug concentration applied to the tissue, whereas in the case of dissociation, $Rt_{1/2}$ is concentration-independent:

$$\text{For diffusion:}$$

$$\frac{(Rt_{1/2})_{[100K_A]}}{(Rt_{1/2})_{[10K_A]}} = \frac{\log(100 + 2)}{\log(10 + 2)} = 1.86$$

Figure 8.2 Simulated concentration–time profiles for drug in the plasma compartment and the receptor biophase when a permeability barrier modifies drug transfer between the compartments. Drug concentration and permeability are plotted on dimensionless axes against time in hours. In each panel, the plasma drug profile (O) is simulated using the published elimination half-life (2 h) and T_{max} (14 min) for subcutaneous (sc) sumatriptan. Panel a: biophase concentration–time profiles (open squares and triangles) when permeability (closed squares and triangles) between the plasma compartment and biophase is poor (permeability factor = 0.2; □ and . . . ■ . . .) and when it is increased (permeability factor = 2.0; △ and . . . ▲ . . .). Panels b and c: biophase concentration–time profiles obtained when permeability between the plasma compartment and biophase increases transiently from a poorly permeable resting state (permeability factor = 0.2) to mimic onset of and recovery from migraine headache. In panel b, drug is introduced 40 min after permeability increases. In panel c, drug is introduced 40 min before permeability increases.

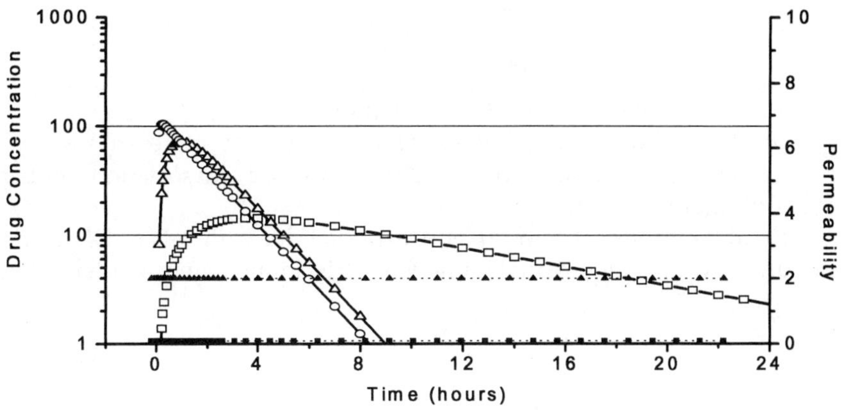

(a)

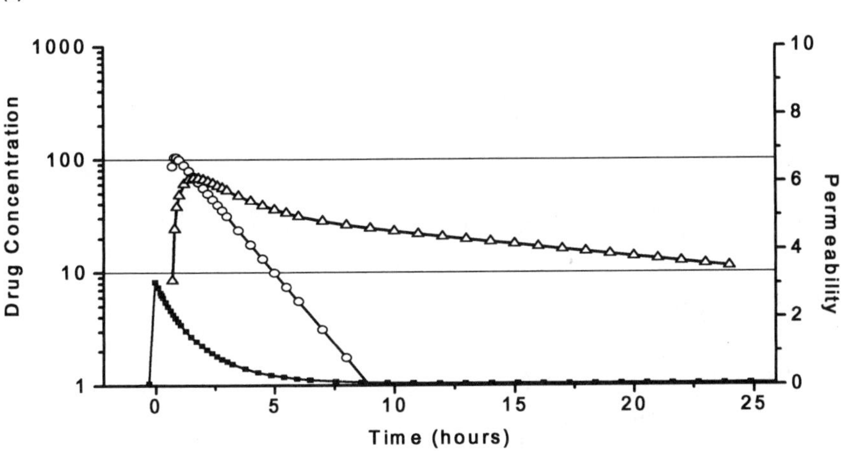

(b)

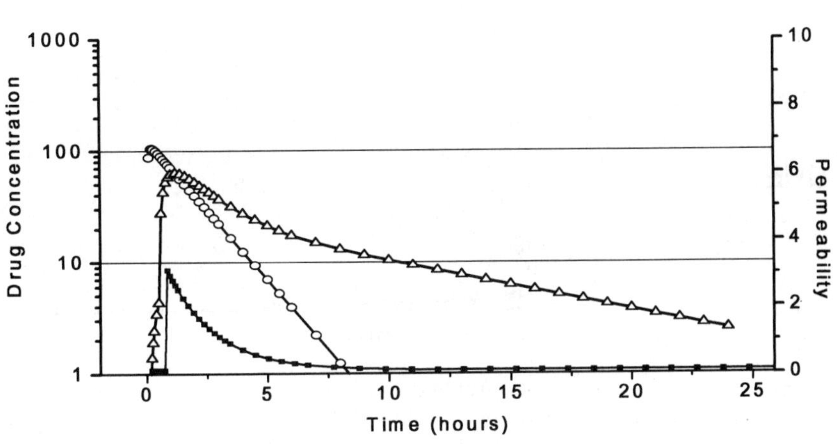

(c)

For dissociation:

$$\frac{(Rt_{1/2})_{[100K_A]}}{(Rt_{1/2})_{[10K_A]}} = \frac{\log(2)}{\log(2)} = 1$$

Hence, the ratio of $Rt_{1/2}$ values obtained at two different agonist concentrations can differentiate diffusion- and dissociation-limited offset of agonist effect.

Typical examples of superfusion experiments with 5-HT, DHE and sumatriptan are shown in Figure 8.3. It is immediately evident that

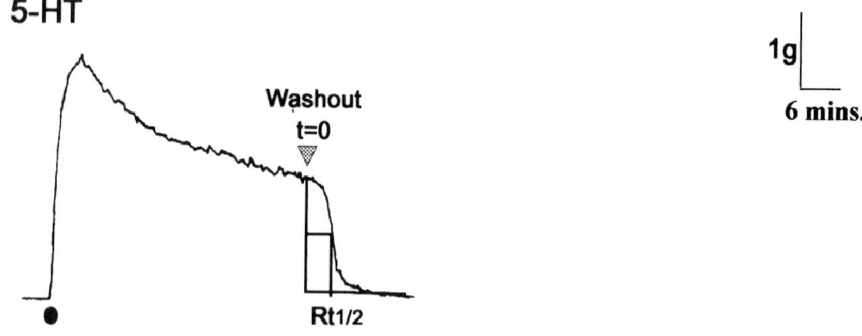

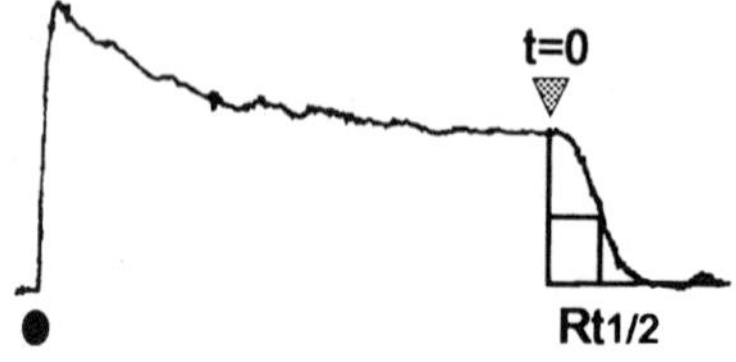

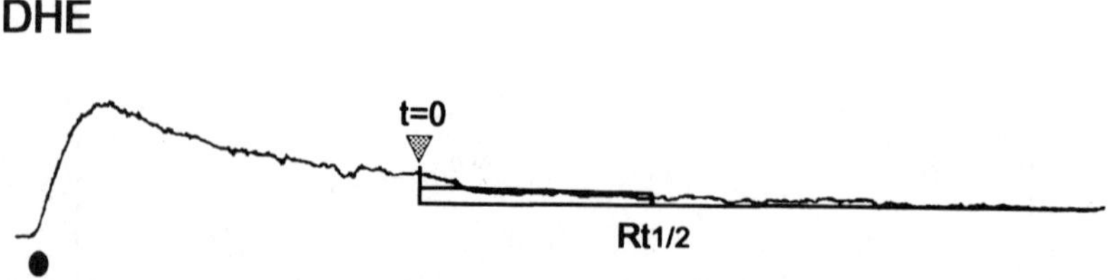

Figure 8.3 Typical examples of onset and offset of effect for 5-hydroxytryptamine (5-HT), sumatriptan and dihydroergotamine (DHE) acting at the 5-HT$_{1D}$ receptor mediating contraction of rabbit saphenous vein.

Table 8.1 Values of washout half-life ($Rt_{1/2}$) for 5-hydroxytryptamine (5-HT), sumatriptan and dihydroergotamine (DHE) at $10 \times K_A$ and $100 \times K_A$ in ring segments of rabbit saphenous vein

Drug	pK_A	$(Rt_{1/2})$ $[100K_A]$ *(min)*	$(Rt_{1/2})$ $[10K_A]$ *(min)*	$Rt_{1/2}$ *ratio*
5-HT	7.1	4.8 ± 0.9	3.1 ± 0.2	1.7
DHE	9.4	26.8 ± 3.7	14.1 ± 2.4	1.9
Sumatriptan	6.2	3.7 ± 0.4	2.6 ± 0.2	1.5
Methysergide	6.8	4.8 ± 0.4	2.2 ± 0.2	2.2

whereas 5-HT_{1D} receptor-mediated responses to 5-HT and sumatriptan are rapidly reversed upon washout, the effect of DHE is much more persistent. However, calculation of $Rt_{1/2}$ values at $10 \times K_A$ and $100 \times K_A$ for each agonist showed that for each drug the half-time for effect washout is concentration-dependent (Table 8.1), indicating that dissociation of A.R is unlikely to contribute significantly to the duration of agonist effect. Instead the $Rt_{1/2}$ ratios were close to the value of 1.86 predicted for diffusion. Interestingly, the non-peptide ergot methysergide behaved more like sumatriptan and 5-HT than DHE (not shown), suggesting that the peptide moiety of the ergots plays an important part in the pharmacodynamic behaviour of these drugs at 5-HT_{1D} receptors.

SUMMARY

Notwithstanding the simplistic nature of the model simulations and the assumptions made in deriving them, features have emerged in this analysis that reflect aspects of clinical experience with sumatriptan. Hence, the concept of an inter-compartment 'barrier' that profoundly influences drug concentrations at the target site offers possible explanations for the lack of any obvious relation between plasma pharmacokinetics and risk of recurrence, the poor efficacy of pre-emptive treatment with the drug, the inability of a second dose of drug to modify the incidence of recurrence (the second dose is administered at a time when permeability has returned to a low level with headache resolution) and the lack of efficacy of a second dose of sumatriptan when the first dose has been ineffective (presumably the subject has not experienced a permeability change sufficient to allow drug into the receptor biophase). Pre-clinical studies of a new antimigraine 5-HT_{1D} agonist (311C90) zolmitriptan) (Martin 1994) show that, unlike sumatriptan, this drug accesses central components of the trigeminovascular system (Goadsby and Edvinsson 1994), implying that it crosses biological 'barriers' more readily. Whether or not this will translate into therapeutic advantage (e.g. in pre-emptive treatment and/or lower incidence of recurrence) awaits the outcome of ongoing clinical trials.

Acknowledgements

Pharmacokinetic and pharmacodynamic models were derived in consultation with Dr Barry Weatherley and Dr John Wood. We gratefully acknowledge their assistance and constructive comments.

REFERENCES

Ashford, E.A. for the Clinical Trial Study Group. (1993) Optimising the dosage regimen for oral sumatriptan – methodology and patients. In: *New Advances in Headache Research*, vol. 3, (ed. F. Clifford Rose). Smith Gordon & Co., London.

Bates, D., Ashford, E. and Dawson, R. (1994) Subcutaneous sumatriptan during the migraine aura. *Neurology*, **44**, 1587–1592.

Black, J.W. and Leff, P. (1983) Operational models of pharmacological agonism. *Proceedings of the Royal Society London (Biology)*, **229**, 141–162.

Catarci, T., Fiacco, F., Argentino, C., Sette, G. and Cerbo, R. (1994) Ergotamine-induced headache can be sustained by sumatriptan daily intake. *Cephalalgia*, **14**, 374–375.

Diener, H.C. and May, A. (1996) PET scan studies in the acute migraine attack. In: *Migraine: Pharmacology and Genetics*, (eds M. Sandler, M. Ferrari and S. Harnett), pp. 109–116, Chapman & Hall, London.

de Vriend, R.H.M., Jaspers, N.M.W.H., Visser, W.H. and Ferrari, M.D. (1994) Clinical differences between responders and non-responders to sumatriptan: a population-based study. In: *New Advances in Headache Research*, vol. 4, (ed. F. Clifford Rose), pp. 243–244. Smith Gordon & Co., London.

Ferrari, M.D. and Saxena, P.R. (1995) 5-HT1 receptors in migraine pathophysiology and treatment. *European Journal of Neurology*, **2**, 5–21.

Fowler, P.A., Lacey, L.F., Thomas, M., Keene O.N., Tanner, R.J.N. and Baber, N.S. (1991) The clinical pharmacology, pharmacokinetics and metabolism of sumatriptan. *European Neurology*, **31**, 291–294.

Goadsby, P.J. and Edvinsson, L. (1994) Central and peripheral trigeminovascular activation in the cat is inhibited by the novel 5-HT$_{1D}$ agonist 311C90. *Headache*, **34**, 394–399.

Humphrey, P.P.A., Feniuk, W., Marriot, A.S., Tanner, R.J.N., Jackson, M.R. and Tucker, M.L. (1991) Pre-clinical studies on the anti-migraine drug, sumatriptan. *European Neurology*, **31**, 282–290.

Jaspers, N.M.W.H., de Vriend, R.H.M., Visser, W.H. and Ferrari, M.D. (1994) Clinical differences between patients with and without headache recurrence after sumatriptan: a population-based study. In: *New Advances in Headache Research*, Vol. 4, (ed. F. Clifford Rose), pp. 256–257. Smith Gordon & Co., London.

Kaube, H., Hoskin, K.L. and Goadsby, P.J. (1993) Inhibition by sumatriptan of central trigeminal neurones only after blood–brain barrier disruption. *British Journal of Pharmacology*, **109**, 788–792.

Kirkham, A.J.T. for the Multinational Oral Sumatriptan and Cafergot Comparative Study Group (1991) A randomised, double-blind comparison of sumatriptan and cafergot in the acute treatment of migraine. *European Neurology*, **31**, 314–322.

Martin, G.R, Martin, R.S. and Wood, J. (1995) Long-acting 5-HT$_{1D}$ receptor agonist effects of dihydroergotamine. Studies using a model to differentiate slow drug-receptor dissociation from diffusion. In: *Experimental Headache Models* (ed. J. Olesen and M.A. Moskowitz), pp. 163–167, Raven Press, New York.

Martin, G.R. (1994) Pre-clinical profile of the novel 5-HT$_{1D}$ receptor agonist 311C90. In: *New Advances in Headache Research*, Vol. 4, (ed. F. Clifford Rose), pp. 3–4. Smith Gordon & Co., London.

Monstad, I. (1993) Pre-emptive oral treatment with sumatriptan during a cluster headache period. *Cephalalgia*, **13**, (Suppl. 13), 35.

Müller-Schweinitzer, E. and Rosenthaler, J.J. (1987) Dihydroergotamine: pharmacokinetics, pharmacodynamics and mechanism of venoconstrictor action in beagle dogs. *Cardiovascular Pharmacology*, **9**, 686–693.

Orton, D.A. and Richardson, R.J. (1982) Ergotamine absorption and toxicity. *Postgraduate Medical Journal*, **58**, 6–11.

Osborne, M.M.J., Austin, R.T.C., Dawson, K.J. and Lange, L. (1994) Is there a problem with long-term use of sumatriptan in acute migraine? *British Medical Journal*, **308**, 113.

Plosker, G.L. and McTavish, D. (1994) Sumatriptan. A reappraisal of its pharmacology and therapeutic efficacy in the acute treatment of migraine and cluster headache. *Drugs*, **47**, 622–651.

Saper, J.R. (1987) Ergotamine dependency – a review. *Headache*, **27**, 435–438.

Visser, W.H., Burggraaf, J., Muller, L.M., Shoemaker, R., Fowler, P.A., Cohen, A.F. and Ferrari, M.D. (1996) Non-response and headache recurrence after sumatriptan not explained by pharmacokinetic differences. *British Journal of Clinical Pharmacology*, in press.

DISCUSSION

Lance: Ergotamine has an interesting action in that it dilates constricted vessels and constricts dilated vessels; its action depends on the intraluminal pressure within the vessel. Might sumatriptan, which has only a vasoconstrictor effect, have to wait for an appropriate degree of vasodilatation, an increase in the intraluminal pressure, before it becomes effective? Is this a possible explanation, other than passing the blood – brain barrier, assuming sumatriptan acts only on vessels and not on neuronal mechanisms?

Ferrari: I don't think that sumatriptan only constricts dilated vessels. It seems also to constrict vessels with normal tone.

Lance: Will it constrict further vessels that are already constricted, assuming some degree of vasoconstriction during the aura phase? Sumatriptan does not seem to prolong or shorten the aura.

Peatfield: The lack of efficacy of sumatriptan given during aura (Bates *et al.* 1994) has nothing to do with the pharmacokinetics. If the drug binds the receptor and simply has to wait for vasodilatation you would expect to begin to see a clinical effect. In fact, it does not seem to be getting to the receptor at which it is active. It is a pity that we do not have any results for zolmitriptan on this issue of treatment during the aura phase.

Lance: Wouldn't that also apply when the drug is present before the blood–brain barrier opens? Sumatriptan has a half-life of two hours and would still be present when the 45-minute aura finished. The vessels are dilating, and the drug is there: why would it not work to prevent the headache then?

Moskowitz: This troubles me as well. Auras can be as short as 20 minutes. I find it difficult to accept that a drug administered 20 minutes before the onset of the headache would necessarily work 20 minutes later based on Dr Martin's arguments.

Peatfield: Might the drug be binding somewhere that is not important in this context, elsewhere in the vascular tree, and therefore be unavailable?

Fozard: One mechanism which may be relevant is the shortening of a drug's action by homologous desensitization. The extent to which sumatriptan desensitizes, either at the receptor or post-receptorial levels, is never discussed in this context. It appeared from Dr Martin's data with the saphenous vein that the constrictor effect was not maintained with the 5-HT$_{1D}$ agonists; it decreased within 20 minutes. Is it possible that the activation of the 5-HT$_{1D}$ receptor in man at the site which is relevant to migraine is desensitizing rapidly, and equally can be reactivated rapidly? I would like to suggest receptor desensitization and reactivation as a possible mechanism that may be relevant to the issue of recurrence.

Martin: At high drug concentrations there is an immediate adaptive response of the tissues, but then the contracture attains a steady-state. These experiments are conducted over at least 45 minutes and there is no evidence during that time for adaptation continuing as an acute desensitization.

Fozard: The degree of adaptation may be crucial. The situation may also be different *in vivo*. I still think receptor desensitization should be considered when we talk about clinical responses with agonists not being maintained.

Pilgrim: We do not really know what happens when sumatriptan is given right at the start of the headache. Many of the patients in the aura study (Bates *et al.* 1994) had a headache for several hours. It may be that sumatriptan does not get to its site of action until some way into the headache phase. Whatever barrier there is may not break down instantly at the point that the headache starts. If sumatriptan is given subcutaneously, plasma levels drop off very substantially in a couple of hours. The patients in the aura study had a typical aura duration of about 30 minutes before the headache started. If that barrier then takes some time to become leaky, there may be very low levels of sumatriptan in plasma by the time that access to the central nervous system is possible.

Goadsby: Unfortunately the only way to sort this out is virtually impossible, namely to give someone the drug before they have their headache or their aura. Perhaps the cluster headache data approach this: the preventative treatment with regular sumatriptan is suggestive of the same phenomenon as the aura study.

Pilgrim: It is also interesting that the time-course of action of sumatriptan given subcutaneously differs greatly in cluster headache and migraine. With cluster headache there is a high level of efficacy by 10 minutes, rather than 60 to 90 minutes with migraine. That suggests that there is something very different about access to the relevant receptors in cluster headache.

Goadsby: The pain of cluster headache builds up very quickly.

Schoenen: Some patients with cluster headaches may get recurrence also.

Martin: I have simply considered the evidence that headache recurrence can have a drug-induced component from the standpoint of a pharmacologist. Indeed, recurrence is evident regardless of the pharmacological approach to headache treatment, as exemplified by octreotide. Whatever the mechanistic basis for the recurrence, it appears to be a discrete event to which certain patients are susceptible. In other patients, the half-life of the drugs may simply be insufficient to cover the duration of the natural attack, leading to breakthrough. The latter case is the only one we can start addressing immediately (with longer-acting drugs), because we don't have a mechanistic understanding of the former. All I have tried to do here is to examine the information we already have about two drug classes, the ergots and sumatriptan, both of which share the same pharmacological mechanism of 5-HT_{1D} receptor agonism. There is a slightly different treatment pattern with these two classes of drug: ergots are given early in an attack, whereas sumatriptan is less effective that way. This must be telling us something important about pharmacokinetic behaviour. My suggestion would therefore be to look for a drug with the pharmacodynamic attributes of ergotamine and an elimination half-life sufficient to ensure cover for around 24 hours. Such a drug should offer greater persistence of effect and, presumably, complete relief to a wider population of patients.

Peatfield: Ergotamine is a confusing drug here because, at minimally higher concentrations than seem to work normally, it interacts with $5\text{-HT}_{2B/2C}$ receptors. Much of the headache obtained the day after an ergot may be induced by an interaction with a quite different serotonin receptor, reflecting the dirtiness of the drug. This could result in oscillation if a quick early benefit is followed by a delayed detriment which is treated with another dose.

Martin: I agree. The pharmacology of the ergots is not as clean as with sumatriptan. However, the elimination half-life is similar for ergot and sumatriptan (it's probably shorter for ergotamine), yet the recurrence incidence is lower with ergotamine. Also, the time to recurrence is longer: for oral therapy it is 23 hours with ergotamine versus 16 for sumatriptan. I would say that's a reflection of the different pharmaco-dynamic behaviour of these two compounds acting through the same receptor–effector system.

Peatfield: If that is partly due to the lipid solubility of the drug rather than functional half-life on the receptors, we need a more lipid-soluble drug.

Humphrey: What is the precise lipid solubility of naratriptan?

Connor: It's slightly more lipid soluble than sumatriptan and its log D is similar to that of zolmitriptan.

Martin: It's not as simple as log D either. Methysergide is a nonpeptide ergot with a high log D, but a washout half-life similar to that for sumatriptan. The difference in pharmacodynamic behaviour of the peptide ergots appears to be accounted for by the peptide tail.

Ferrari: MK-462 is even more lipid soluble and the recurrence data were very high.

REFERENCE

Bates, D., Ashford, E., Dawson, R., Ensink, F-B.M., Gilhus, N.E., Olesen, J., Pilgrim, A.J. and Shevlin, P. (1994) Subcutaneous sumatriptan during the migraine aura. *Neurology*, **44**, 1587–1592.

9

Positron emission tomography studies in acute migraine attacks

H.C. Diener and A. May

INTRODUCTION

Until recently it was supposed that no technique was able to visualize the pathophysiological background of headache or to look for its source. The pioneering work of Olesen *et al.* (1981a, Olesen and Friberg 1991) revealed a focal reduction of regional cerebral blood flow (rCBF) for migraine attacks with aura, usually in the posterior parts of one hemisphere. Since then numerous studies have used different techniques to demonstrate gross changes in cortical perfusion as an explanation for either the aura or the headache in migraine. Positron emission tomography (PET) is the method of choice for quantitative study of metabolic and vascular changes.

The difficulties in performing PET studies are of a clinical as well as a methodological nature. Clinically, patients and attacks are heterogeneous: there are migraine attacks with aura and without aura. It is still a matter of debate whether the aura is just a 'plus' symptom that is absent in migraine without aura or is so mild that patients are not conscious of it. Furthermore in the same patient the aura symptoms may vary from a pure visual aura to long-lasting hemiplegic attacks, and migraine attacks without aura may be intermingled. The headache also varies in severity. From a methodological point of view, it is difficult to motivate a miserable patient who is nauseous or even vomiting to come to the clinic without taking any medication. It is even more difficult to have cyclotron operators, nuclear medicine physicians, radiochemists

Migraine: Pharmacology and genetics
Edited by Merton Sandler, Michel Ferrari and Sara Harnett
Published in 1996 by Chapman & Hall
ISBN 1 86036 006 8

and radiographers constantly available to study acute migraine attacks as they occur.

EARLY PET CHANGES DURING MIGRAINE

Woods *et al.* (1994) published the first report of PET measurements in a patient from the start of a spontaneous migraine attack without aura. The patient was studied while she was participating in a visual activation paradigm and was scanned with 12 successive measurements of rCBF. After the sixth scan she developed unilateral headache, nausea, and photo- and phonophobia. The first decrease in rCBF, noted during the seventh scan was found bilaterally in the visual association cortex. In each subsequent scan, every 12 minutes, the decrease in rCBF spread continuously across the cortical surface at a relatively constant rate, sparing the cerebellum, basal ganglia and the thalamus. The hypo-perfusion involved the middle as well as the posterior cerebral artery territories. The authors estimated the maximal decrease of rCBF to be about 40%, potentially approaching an ischaemic level. However, most of these changes were relatively short-lived, with substantial recovery by the time of the next measurement 12-15 minutes later. This case report is remarkable for two reasons. First, it illustrates for the first time a bilateral spreading hypoperfusion in a spontaneous migraine attack measured with PET. Even more remarkable is the fact that this patient suffered from migraine without aura. This means that the described findings are not in line with the single photon emission computed tomography (SPECT) data from Olesen *et al.* (1981b) who found no changes in rCBF in migraine attacks without aura.

One may speculate that the underlying pathophysiological mechanism in migraine without as well as with aura is the so-called spreading depression of Leão (1944) occurring in different depths of the cortex, as suggested by Lehmenkühler and Richter (1993). However, the typical hyperperfusion in the front line known from animal experiments was not detected in this patient. One explanation is the poor spatial and temporal resolution (about 70 sec) of PET rCBF measurements. On the other hand, the observed changes were relatively short-lived, with substantial recovery in a relatively short time: investigations at a later time would probably miss them. Despite all the logistic problems, there is a clear need to investigate migraine attacks as early as possible to confirm these results.

rCBF DURING MIGRAINE ATTACKS AND IN THE HEADACHE-FREE INTERVAL

In 1994 Friberg *et al.* demonstrated with SPECT that almost 50% of migraine sufferers had interictally abnormal rCBF interhemispherical

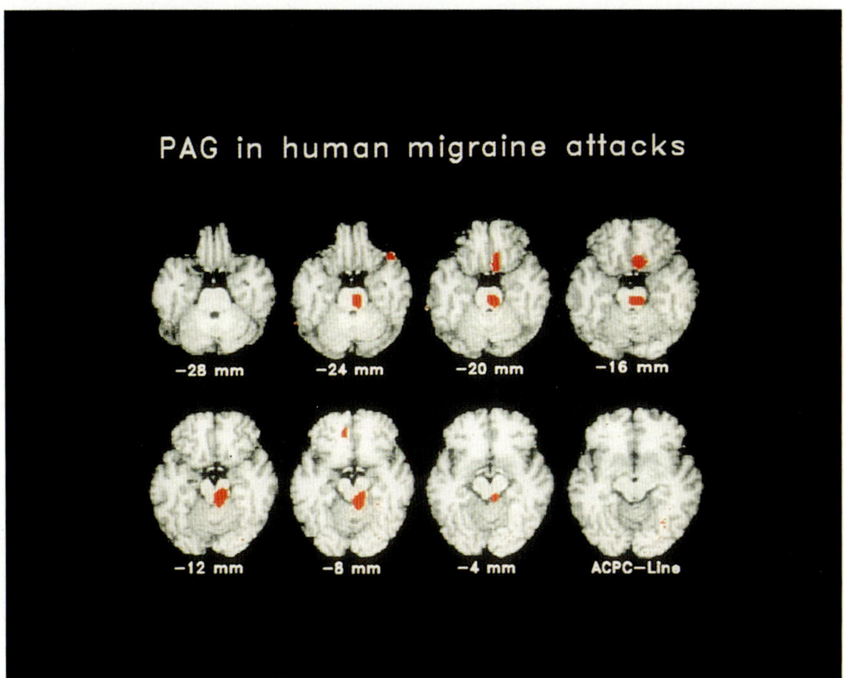

Plate 1 Comparison of acute migraine attack and headache-free interval in nine patients with migraine without aura. The activations during the attack are shown as statistical parametric maps that show the areas of significant regional cerebral blood flow (rCBF) increases ($p < 0.001$) in red superimposed on an anatomical reference image derived from a T1-weighted magnetic resonance image. Numbers refer to the relative distance to the ACPC line (joining the anterior and posterior commissures), which is situated at 0 mm. The anterior part of the brain corresponds to the top of the image, the posterior parts to the bottom. The left side of each image is the right side of the brain. Significant increases in rCBF were detected over several planes in the brainstem slightly lateralized to the left, anterior to the aqueduct and posterior to the cranial nerve nuclei in the periaqueductal grey matter and midbrain reticular formation, as well as in the infero anterocaudal part of the cingulate gyrus (Brodmann area 25). Reproduced with permission from Weiller *et al.* 1995.

asymmetries. These asymmetries were discrete compared to those seen during the aura phase of a migraine attack. The authors concluded that, at least interictally, a cerebrovascular dysregulation exists. It is known, however, that in the experimental animal the stimulation of the trigeminovascular system leads to a pronounced increase in cortical blood flow, possibly mediated through peptidergic projections from the brainstem. By analogy, increased cortical blood flow could be expected during migraine attacks in humans. In a study of 13 patients (3 males, 10 females, age 24–57 years) we investigated the rCBF during spontaneous migraine attacks without aura and in the headache-free interval with the $^{15}CO_2$ inhalation technique using an ECAT 953–15 PET scanner. Patients were included with untreated unilateral migraine headaches during the first six hours of the attack.

Using a region of interest analysis and statistical parametric mapping, no differences in rCBF were found between the hemispheres ipsilateral and contralateral to the headache side. Furthermore, there were no detectable differences in rCBF between repeated measurements during the attack and the headache-free interval. This is in line with the data of Ferrari *et al.* (1995) who found no significant asymmetries of rCBF measured with SPECT outside or during the attack. No significant changes in rCBF ratios were seen during the attack compared with the headache-free interval. Our results are not in accordance with the significant increases of cortical blood flow seen in animal experiments. This may be due to: a) the lack of sensitivity for changes in global cerebral blood flow of the method used; or b) habituation towards the ongoing head pain during a migraine attack. Again there is a clear need to investigate migraine attacks as early as possible to confirm these results.

Sumatriptan is a highly effective drug for the treatment of acute migraine attacks. Its action is believed to be mediated via activation of vascular and neuronal $5\text{-}HT_{1D}$ receptors. Sumatriptan constricts isolated human dural arteries (Humphrey and Feniuk 1991) and middle cerebral arteries (Friberg *et al.* 1991). Therefore, sumatriptan might cause cerebral ischaemia in conditions of reduced cerebral blood flow. Until now, only limited information was available about the quantitative effect of sumatriptan on rCBF in humans. In SPECT no rCBF changes were found after administration of a subtherapeutic dose of sumatriptan in six healthy volunteers (Scott *et al.* 1992) and in seven patients with migraine with aura (Friberg *et al.* 1991). Ferrari *et al.* (1995) detected no rCBF changes in acute migraine attacks without aura treated with 6 mg subcutaneous (sc) sumatriptan in a double-blind, placebo-controlled trial using SPECT.

We studied the effect of sumatriptan in the same 13 patients during spontaneous migraine attacks without aura with the $^{15}CO_2$ inhalation technique using an ECAT 953–15 PET scanner, as before. Again, only patients with untreated unilateral migraine headaches during the first six hours of the attack were included. Region of interest analysis (hemispheres ipsi- and contralateral to the headache side) and statistical parametric mapping revealed no differences in rCBF after treatment with 6 mg sc sumatriptan compared to pretreatment scans. This is in line with the SPECT data of Ferrari *et al.* (1995). Owing to the semiquantitative nature of the $^{15}CO_2$ inhalation technique in PET, slight changes that affect the whole brain cannot be excluded. They seem unlikely in view of the results of Friberg *et al.* (1991) who showed no global effect of sumatriptan on rCBF with the ^{133}Xenon inhalation technique.

We conclude that the treatment of a migraine attack with 6 mg sc sumatriptan is not likely to cause focal or global ischaemia or other rCBF changes in migraine patients.

'MIGRAINE CENTRE' IN THE BRAINSTEM

More important for us was the question whether activation of brainstem nuclei could be visualized with PET during acute migraine attacks. Nine patients (7 females, 2 males; age 29–57) suffering from migraine without aura were studied during a spontaneous, acute right-sided migraine attack (Weiller *et al.* 1995). Headache was classified as migraine without aura according to the Headache Classification Committee of the International Headache Society (1988). All nine patients were studied within six hours of the onset of untreated migraine symptoms. Three of them were on prophylactic treatment with 200 mg metropolol daily.

Each patient had three rCBF measurements: during the acute attack; after the relief of headache and other related symptoms by 6 mg sumatriptan sc; and during the headache-free interval three days to four months later.

Significantly higher rCBF values (+11%) were found during the acute attack compared to the headache-free interval in median brainstem structures over several planes, slightly contralateral to the headache side (see plate 1).   Increased activation was also found in the inferior anterocaudal cingulate cortex as well as in the visual and auditory association cortices during the attack but was not detectable in these areas in the interval scan or after relief from headache and migraine-related symptoms through treatment.

The consistent increases in rCBF in the brainstem (covering periaqueductal grey, midbrain reticular formation and locus coeruleus) persisted, even after sumatriptan had induced complete relief from headache, nausea, and phono-/photophobia. This increase was not seen outside the attack. Therefore, it is unlikely that the observed activation is only due to pain perception or increased activity of the endogenous antinociceptive system. It does not seem to be a consequence of headache or related to the relief from headache, but may be inherent to the migraine attack itself. This could explain why sumatriptan, with its short half-life, and other compounds are effective in mitigating the symptoms of migraine but are sometimes unable to terminate the actual attack and why the headache may reoccur after the effect of the treatment has worn off.

It is beyond the resolution of the PET scanner to attribute foci of rCBF increases to distinct brainstem nuclei. However, the foci of maximum increase coincided, in the Talairach space, with the anatomical location of the dorsal raphe nucleus and the locus coeruleus. Dysfunction of the regulation of these brainstem nuclei involved in antinociception and extra- and intracerebral vascular control provides a far reaching explanation for many of the facets of migraine. It is attractive to consider the observed activation in the brainstem as the first direct visualization of the postulated 'migraine centre' in man.

REFERENCES

Ferrari, M.D., Haan, J., Blokland, J.A.K., Arndt, J.W., Minnee, P., Zwinderman, A.H., Pauwels, E.K.J. and Saxena, P.R. (1995) Cerebral blood flow during migraine attacks without aura and effect of sumatriptan. *Archives of Neurology*, **52**, 135–139.

Friberg, L, Olesen, J., Iversen, H, and Sperling, B. (1991) Migraine pain associated with middle cerebral artery dilatation: reversal by sumatriptan. *Lancet*, i, 13–17.

Friberg, L., Olesen, J., Iversen, H., Nicolic, I. Sperling, B., Lassen, N.A., Olsen, T.S, and Tfelt-Hansen, P. (1994) Interictal 'patchy' regional cerebral blood flow pattens in migraine patients. A single photon emission computerized tomographic study. *European Journal of Neurology*, **1**, 35–43.

Headache Classification Committee of the International Headache Society (J. Olesen *et al.*) (1988) Classification and diagnostic criteria for headache disorders, cranial neuralgias and facial pain. *Cephalalgia*, **8**, (Suppl.7), 19–28.

Humphrey, P.P.A. and Feniuk, W. (1991) Mode of action of the anti-migraine drug sumatriptan. *Trends in Pharmacological Science*, **12**, 444–446.

Leão, A.A.P. (1944) Spreading depression of activity in the cerebral cortex. *Journal of Neurophysiology*, **7**, 391–396.

Lehmenkühler, A. and Richter, F. (1993) Spreading depression in upper and lower depths of the rat cerebral cortex and its possible implications on the type of human migraine. In: *Migraine: Basic Mechanisms and Treatment*, (eds A. Lehmenkühler, K-H. Grotemeyer and F. Tegtmeyer, pp. 267–278. Urban and Schwarzenberg, München.

Olesen, J. and Friberg, L. (1991) Xenon-133 SPECT studies in migraine without aura. In: *Migraine and other Headaches: The Vascular Mechanisms*, (ed. J. Olesen), Vol 1, pp. 237–243. Raven Press, London.

Olesen, J, Larsen, B. and Lauritzen, M. (1981a) Focal hyperemia followed by spreading oligemia and impaired activation of rCBF in classic migraine. *Annals of Neurology*, **9**, 344–352.

Olesen, J, Tfelt-Hansen, P., Henriksen, L. and Larsen, B. (1981b) The common migraine attack may not be initiated by cerebral ischaemia. *Lancet*, **ii**, 438–440.
Scott, A.K., Grimes, S., NG, Critchley, M., Breckenridge, A.M., Thomson, C, and Pilgrim, A.J. (1992) Sumatriptan and cerebral perfusion in healthy volunteers. *British Journal of Clinical Pharmacology*, **33**, 401–401.
Weiller, C., May, A., Limmroth, V., Jüptner, M., Kaube, H., v.Schayck, R., Coenen, H.H. and Diener, H.C. (1995) Brain stem activation in spontaneous human migraine attacks. *Nature Medicine*, **1**, 658–660.
Woods, R.P., Iacoboni, M. and Mazziotta, J.C. (1994) Bilateral spreading cerebral hypoperfusion during spontaneous migraine headache. *New England Journal of Medicine*, **331**, 1689–1692.

DISCUSSION

Lance: The changes demonstrated fit very well with our original animal model (Lance *et al.* 1983) in which we showed the activity of locus coeruleus and raphe affecting the cerebral vasculature.

Bruyn: In your study of nine patients during a migraine attack without aura, your slices were from the lower third of the pons up to the middle half of the mesencephalon (Figure 9.1). The raphe nucleus is included in the area of increased regional cerebral blood flow (rCBF) because you are scanning from the lower third to the rostral direction. The periaqueductal grey is also included in the mesencephalon. I wonder whether the locus coeruleus is included.

Diener: The spatial resolution of positron emission tomography (PET) is not as good as is suggested by the areas of increased flow superimposed on magnetic resonance images. We cannot exactly say which nuclei or areas are represented. All we can say is that this region does contain the locus coeruleus and the dorsal raphe nucleus.

Peatfield: Is it possible to see what is happening in the cortical surface in patients with aura by studying the oxygen extraction ratio, i.e. are we dealing with an ischaemic phenomenon or a physiological reduction in cerebral blood flow where the brain is malfunctioning?

Diener: We did not look at oxygen extraction.

Peatfield: Are you able to do this? Woods *et al.* (1994) did not address this question, although I would judge it to be more fundamental than whether hypoperfusion is moving across the cortical surface.

Moskowitz: Blood flow changes of 10 and 20% are nowhere near the thresholds for ischaemia.

Peatfield: Therefore, should we expect the oxygen extraction ratio to be normal?

Moskowitz: Yes. Ischaemia is an infrequent occurrence.

Peatfield: We need to be told so by someone with the right apparatus.

Moskowitz: Are the raphe projections to neocortex crossed? You reported brainstem flow changes on the opposite side of the headache.

Diener: We were unable to discover this in the literature about humans.

Moskowitz: Animal studies should provide the data. I thought the raphe and locus project ipsilaterally to cortex, yet you observed a contralateral brainstem effect. What is the relationship between the contralateral brainstem and the ipsilateral forebrain?

Schoenen: The afferents may be crossed coming from the ipsilateral forebrain.

Diener: I do not think that the activity we see has much to do with afferents because it is still there when the pain is relieved by treatment. It must have something to do with the generation of the migraine attack itself.

Schoenen: But how long does it last?

Diener: We do not know. The last scan was done two hours after the end of the headache. It is technically impossible to do it later. After two hours the activity is still there: four weeks later it is gone.

Goadsby: If we stimulate a unilateral intracranial vascular structure we see contralateral ventrolateral periaqueductal grey *c-fos* activation. This is consistent with the effect Dr Diener is demonstrating contralateral to the pain signal.

Schoenen: That would be more of an effect of the pain than of a generator.

Goadsby: You could argue that. I do not know.

Schoenen: C-*fos* activation lasts for hours. How can you *a priori* exclude afferents activating a centre which is on the pain-conducting pathways and which stays activated for some time?

Diener: If this were the case I would expect more activity, more caudally, on the ipsilateral side, and there is nothing. The problem is that we are looking at cerebral blood flow rather than neuronal blood flow. As soon as you have inhibitory and excitatory action at the same location the net effect is zero.

Lance: The original monkey work stimulating locus coeruleus did show a predominantly ipsilateral influence. One locus coeruleus inhibits the other. It is possible that in this particular case there may be hyperactivity of one locus, followed by hyperactivity of the other locus. Dr Diener has made an important contribution in demonstrating these brainstem changes. I do not think we can be dogmatic about precisely the nuclei involved or the sequence that they play in the migraine attack, but he has shown a very consistent pattern of activation which should retain one aspect of our focus on the brainstem.

Bruyn: I agree that this is a fundamental observation. It reminds me of Brisaud who called migraine 'Le syndrome du plancher de quatrieme ventricule'. Perhaps over the years we have been looking at the wrong site. Would it be possible to provoke migraine attacks for these studies?

Diener: We wanted to avoid doing that, since we are aware that induced attacks might be different from spontaneous attacks.

REFERENCES

Lance, J.W., Lambert, G.A., Goadsby, P.J. and Duckworth, J.W. (1983) Brain stem influences on the cephalic circulation: experimental data from cat and monkey of relevance to the mechanism of migraine. *Headache*, **23**, 258–265.

Woods, R.P., Iacoboni, M. and Mazziotta, J.C. (1994) Bilateral spreading cerebral hypoperfusion during spontaneous migraine headache. *New England Journal of Medicine*, **331**, 1689–1692.

10

Central 5-hydroxytryptamine supersensitivity in migraine

Vivette Glover, Fayez Ahmed, Neelofar Hussein, Joan Jarman and Richard Peatfield

INTRODUCTION: MIGRAINE AS A BRIEF RECURRENT MOOD DISORDER

It is well established that there is a comorbidity between migraine and both depressive and anxiety disorders. Migraine has many features in common with brief recurrent mood disorders (Glover *et al.* 1993): its brief self-limiting nature; a recurrent pattern; association with particular mood changes; the probable involvement of monoamines, particularly 5-hydroxytryptamine (5-HT); and shared response to certain treatments, particularly with tricyclic antidepressants and monoamine oxidase (MAO) inhibitors. Merikangas *et al.* (1993) found a strong association between migraine with aura and other psychiatric diagnoses, and found that the association was particularly marked with brief recurrent depression. Panic attacks also share several of these characteristics, and the large study of Breslau and Davis (1993) found a particularly increased odds ratio for panic disorder in migraine subjects compared with controls.

We do not yet know what brings on, or stops, any of these conditions, but it may well be that some similar mechanisms obtain. Research on migraine often concentrates on the pathophysiology of the neurovascular

Migraine: Pharmacology and genetics
Edited by Merton Sandler, Michel Ferrari and Sara Harnett
Published in 1996 by Chapman & Hall
ISBN 1 86036 006 8

component of the headache itself rather than the attack in its entirety. A migraine attack usually has several stages, including a prodrome and a refractory period. The prodromal period may be characterized by anxiety, agitation or euphoria. In contrast, the headache phase can also be associated with inertia and depression. It is likely that some of this is mediated by central mechanisms.

There have been many studies of peripheral biological markers in both migraine and affective disorders (Glover *et al.* 1993). During a migraine attack it is well established that there is a release of platelet 5-HT; there is also some evidence for a decreased V_{max} for uptake of 5-HT during an attack. In subjects currently depressed a low V_{max} for 5-HT uptake into platelets is well established; there is also some evidence for low platelet 5-HT content. In contrast, migraine patients, particularly males, have low mean platelet MAO activity, whereas subjects with unipolar depression have been found, as a group, to have raised activity.

The study of peripheral markers is clearly limited in relation to mood disorders, as these most plausibly involve changes in the brain. One way of gaining some insight into central brain chemistry, the so-called window on the brain, is by neuroendocrine challenge tests. In these, a chemical challenge is used which acts on specific monoamine neurons or receptors in the hypothalamus, causing the release of a particular hormone into the blood where it can be measured. Several such challenges have been developed and used in the study of affective disorders. One such probe is *meta*-chlorophenylpiperazine (*m*-CPP) which is a general 5-HT receptor agonist, possibly with particular potency at 5-HT$_{2C}$ receptors. *m*-CPP has been shown to induce migraine in susceptible subjects (Brewerton *et al.* 1988). Another such probe is the drug ($\pm$)-fenfluramine. This was shown in an early study to induce headache in subjects prone to 'essential headache' (del Bene *et al.* 1977). This drug causes the release of 5-HT, which then causes the release of both prolactin and cortisol into the bloodstream (Coccaro *et al.* 1989, Power and Cowen 1992, Bond *et al.* 1995). Several studies have found that subjects with depression have a blunted response to such a challenge compared with controls (Power and Cowen 1992), although whether this is primarily linked with depression or other associated features, such as a history of suicide attempts or violent impulsive aggression, is less clear (Coccaro *et al.* 1989). In contrast, panic subjects between attacks were found to have an augmented prolactin response (Targum and Marshall 1989). ($\pm$)-Fenfluramine induced significant anxiety after two hours in the panic patients, but not in the controls.

As part of an ongoing study, we have employed a ($\pm$)-fenfluramine challenge in migraine subjects and matched controls to examine any difference in the central response to a 5-HT-releasing agent.

(±)-FENFLURAMINE CHALLENGE STUDY

The migraine subjects, all headache-free at the start of testing, and free from psychoactive or migraine medication for at least four weeks, had no history of depressive or anxiety disorder, as assessed by the Schedule for Affective Disorders and Schizophrenia – Lifetime version (SADS-L) questionnaire. Blood samples were taken at baseline and at hourly intervals for the next five hours, and were stored at −70°C for later prolactin and cortisol assays. Each subject also kept an hourly record of the development of their symptoms, including headache, nausea, photophobia and phonophobia.

The (±)-fenfluramine induced migrainous symptoms (headache with associated nausea, photophobia and phonophobia) in five out of the seven migraine subjects who kept a record of their symptoms, with an onset starting at one hour and peaking at two to three hours (Figure 10.1). The migraineurs also showed a significantly greater response in prolactin rise than the controls (Figure 10.2). There was no significant difference in their cortisol responses, although these were also raised in the migraine group.

These results have shown that (±)-fenfluramine can induce migrainous symptoms in susceptible subjects and that this was significantly different from its effect in a control population. The prolactin response

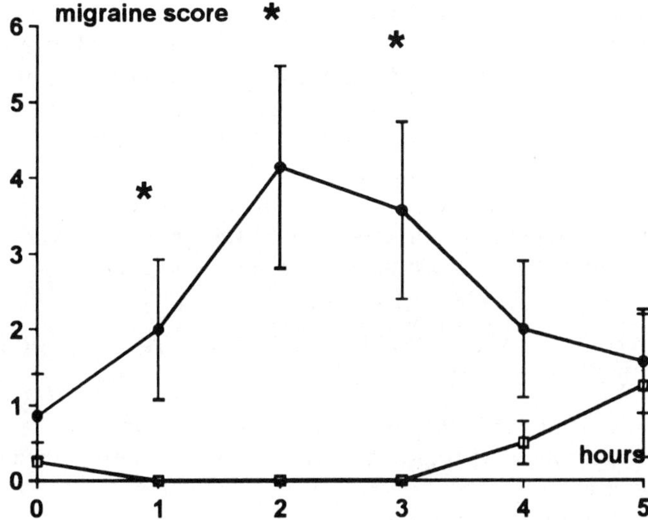

Figure 10.1 The effect of fenfluramine challenge on development of migraine symptoms (headache, nausea and photo- and phonophobia) in migraine subjects (●, *n* = 7) and controls (□, *n* = 4). * *p* < 0.05 Mann Whitney U test.

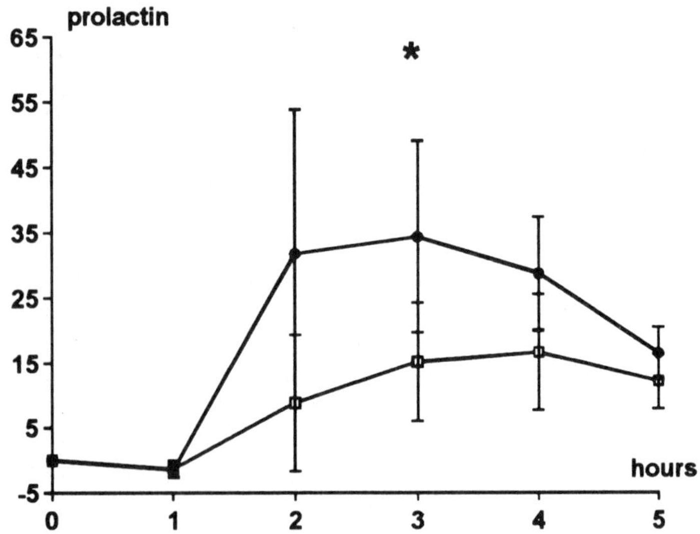

Figure 10.2 The effect of fenfluramine on plasma prolactin concentration (ng/ml) in migraine subjects (●, $n = 8$) and controls (□, $n = 6$). * $p < 0.05$ Mann Whitney U test.

was also significantly different in the migraine group compared with the controls, and suggests that the migraine group had a central 5-HT supersensitivity, as proposed over 20 years ago by Sicuteri (1972). This is in contrast to the findings in depression, but similar to those in panic subjects (Power and Cowen 1992). One may ask whether the increase in prolactin observed in migraine subjects after (±)-fenfluramine challenge is an indirect result of the migraine attack, rather than a direct difference in response to the drug. This is possible but unlikely, as we have previously shown that red wine which caused a severe migraine attack in susceptible subjects had no effect on plasma prolactin levels in those individuals who developed attacks (unpublished observations).

DIFFERENCES BETWEEN (±)-FENFLURAMINE AND *m*-CPP IN MIGRAINE INDUCTION

These results with (±)-fenfluramine are in marked contrast to those that have been described with *m*-CPP (Brewerton *et al.* 1988, Gordon *et al.* 1993), and it is instructive to consider these differences. The effects of different 5-HT probes in neuroendocrine challenge test are given in Table 10.1. The migraine symptoms after (±)-fenfluramine started to occur one hour after the administration of the drug and peaked two to three hours after the challenge. This is in contrast to the headache or

Table 10.1 Effects of 5-HT challenge probes on migraine and biological indices

Challenge substance	Site of action on 5-HT system	Biological effects	Migraine inducer/ time of onset	Comment	Reference
Fenfluramine	Release ↑ Re-uptake ↓	Prolactin ↑ Cortisol ↑ Temperature ↑	Yes 2–3 h	Greater prolactin increase in migraine and panic subjects than in controls. Anxiety induced in panic subjects.	Targum and Marshall (1989), Coccaro *et al.* (1989), Power and Cowen (1992), Bond *et al.* (1995)
m-CPP	Receptor agonist ?especially 5-HT$_{2C}$	Prolactin ↑ Cortisol ↑ Temperature ↑ Anxiety ↑	Yes 5–8 h	No difference between migraine and control subjects in prolactin increase. Correlation between headache and cortisol increase in both controls and migraineurs. No correlation with prolactin increase.	Brewerton *et al.* (1988), Gordon *et al.* (1993)
Buspirone	5-HT$_{1A}$ partial agonist	Temperature ↓ Anxiety ↓ ACTH ↑ Cortisol ↑ Prolactin ⟷	No	Temperature and anxiety effects presynaptic. ACTH and cortisol effects postsynaptic. Hypothermic response attenuated in depression.	Cowen *et al.* (1994)
Sumatriptan	5-HT$_{1D}$ agonist	Temperature ↓ ACTH ↑ Cortisol ↑ β-endorphin ↑ Prolactin ⟷	Migraine blocker	Temperature reduction shown in guinea-pig.	Skingle *et al.* (1994), Facchinetti *et al.* (1994)

m-CPP, *m*-chlorophenyl piperazine; ACTH, adrenocorticotropic hormone.

migraine induced by *m*-CPP, which occurred from five to eight hours after administration (Brewerton *et al.* 1988, Gordon *et al.* 1993), although the plasma drug levels peaked much earlier. Brewerton *et al.* (1988) suggest that the delayed *m*-CPP effect may be due to a rebound supersensitivity. This difference in time-course between the migraine-inducing properties of these two drugs suggests that they are operating by different mechanisms, and that the ($\pm$)-fenfluramine effect is not due to a direct stimulation of the postsynaptic receptors stimulated by *m*-CPP. The two drugs also differ in that whereas the rise in prolactin induced by *m*-CPP, that occurred from one to three hours after the drug administration, was similar in migraine subjects and controls (Gordon *et al.* 1993), with ($\pm$)-fenfluramine, as shown here, the migraine subjects showed a significantly greater response than controls.

These results suggest that the difference between migraine subjects and controls does not lie in central postsynaptic, particularly 5-HT_{2C} receptors. This is supported by the recent positron emission tomography (PET) scan study which found no difference in 5-HT_2 cortical receptors between migraine subjects and controls (Chabriat *et al.* 1995). Rather the difference may lie in their readiness to release 5-HT in response to some trigger. We have failed to find any such difference in ($\pm$)-fenfluramine- or red wine-induced release of 5-HT from the platelets of migraine subjects and controls (Jarman *et al.* 1995). However, it remains quite possible that there is a difference in the releasing properties of 5-HT neurons, both centrally and peripherally, and that subjects prone to migraine are more ready to release 5-HT from presynaptic stores.

REFERENCES

Bond, A., Feizollah, S. and Lader, M. (1995) The effects of D-fenfluramine on mood and performance, and on neuroendocrine indicators of 5-HT function. *Journal of Psychopharmacology*, **9(1)**, 1–8.

Breslau, N. and Davis, G. (1993) Migraine, physical health and psychiatric disorder: a prospective epidemiologic study in young adults. *Journal of Psychiatric Research*, **27**, 211–222.

Brewerton, T.D., Murphy, D.L., Mueller, E.A. and Jimerson, D.C. (1988) Induction of migraine-like headaches by the serotonin agonist m-chlorophenylpiperazine. *Clinical Pharmacology and Therapeutics*, **43**, 605–609.

Chabriat, H., Tehindrazanarivelo, A., Vera, P., Samson, Y., Pappata, S., Boullais, N. and Bousser, M. (1995) 5-HT_2 receptors in cerebral cortex of migraineurs studied using PET and 18F-fluorosetoperone. *Cephalalgia*, **15**, 104–108.

Coccaro, E.F., Siever, L.J., Klar, H.M. *et al.* (1989) Serotonergic studies in patients with affective and personality disorder. *Archives of General Psychiatry*, **46**, 587–599.

Cowen, P.J., Power, A.C., Ware, C.J. and Anderson, I.M. (1994) 5-HT_{1A} receptor sensitivity in major depression. A neuroendocrine study with buspirone. *British Journal of Psychiatry*, **164**, 372–379.

Del Bene, E., Anselmi, B., Del Bianco, P.L., Fanciullacci, M., Galli, P., Salmon, S. and Sicuteri, F. (1977) Fenfluramine headache: a biochemical and monoamine receptorial human study. In *Headache: New Vistas*, (ed. F. Sicuteri), pp. 101–109. Biomedical Press, Florence.

Facchinetti, F., Nappi, R.E., Sances, G., Fioroni, L., Nappi, G. and Genazzani, A.R. (1994) The neuroendocrine effects of sumatriptan, a specific ligand for 5-HT$_1$-like receptors. *Clinical Endocrinology*, **40**, 211–214.

Glover, V., Jarman, J. and Sandler, M. (1993) Migraine and depression: biological aspects. *Journal of Psychiatric Research*, **27**, 223–231.

Gordon, M.L., Lipton, R.B., Brown, S.-L., Nakrasieve, C., Russell, M., Pollack, S.Z., Korn, M.L., Merriam, A., Solomon, S. and van Praag, H. (1993) Headache and cortisol responses to m-chlorophenylpiperazine are highly correlated. *Cephalalgia*, **13**, 400–405.

Jarman, J., Glover, V. and Sandler, M. (1991) Release of [^{14}C]5-hydroxytryptamine from human platelets by red wine. *Life Sciences*, **48**, 2297–2300.

Jarman, J., Pattichis, K., Peatfield, R., Glover, V. and Sandler, M. (1995) Red wine induced release of ^{14}C-5-hydroxytryptamine from platelets of migraine patients and controls. *Cephalalgia*, in press.

Merikangas, K., Merikangas, J. and Angst, J. (1993) Headache syndromes and psychiatric disorders: association and familial transmission. *Journal of Psychiatric Research*, **27**, 197–210.

Power, A. and Cowen, P. (1992) Neuroendocrine challenge tests: assessment of 5-HT function in anxiety and depression. *Molecular Aspects of Medicine*, **13**, 205–220.

Sicuteri, F. (1972) Headache as a possible expression of deficiency of brain 5-HT (central denervation supersensitivity). *Headache*, **12**, 69–72.

Skingle, M., Higgins, G.A. and Fenuik, W. (1994) Stimulation of central 5-HT$_{1D}$ receptors causes hypothermia in the guinea pig. *Journal of Psychopharmacology*, **8**, 14–21.

Targum, S. and Marshall, L. (1989) Fenfluramine provocation of anxiety in patients with panic disorder. *Psychiatry Research*, **28**, 295–306.

DISCUSSION

Goadsby: If a group of migraineurs fast overnight and are then simply given a placebo, what happens?

Glover: We have yet to do that. In *m*-chlorophenylpiperazine (*m*-CPP) studies, the placebo had no effect on prolactin release. I predict the same will be true here.

Lance: This throws light on hypothalamic function in migraineurs. The release of 5-hydroxytryptamine (5-HT) would be generalized throughout the body, so are you using this as an index of 5-HT supersensitivity and the ability to release 5-HT throughout the body or specifically in the hypothalamus?

Glover: The fenfluramine will act everywhere. The prolactin will be an index of what is happening in the hypothalamus.

Sandler: At what receptor does the 5-HT released by fenfluramine act?

Glover: That is not well established. It has been suggested to be the 5-HT$_2$ or 5-HT$_{2C}$ receptor (Goodall *et al.* 1993).

Fozard: Animal behavioural studies suggest that it is the 5-HT$_{2C}$ or 5-HT$_{2B}$ receptor. When food intake is inhibited, for example, it was recently shown to be 5-HT$_{2B}$.

Peatfield: Does fenfluramine have any direct action?

Fozard: Not at these sorts of doses. At low doses, fenfluramine is a highly selective releaser from 5-HT-containing neurons in animals. The difference in time-course between fenfluramine and that reported for *m*-CPP by Brewerton *et al.* (1988) is fascinating for someone like me who argues that broadly the same mechanism(s) are involved. As Professor Lance said, 5-HT release is generalized with fenfluramine: it may come from many cell types including platelets and/or central neurons, whereas *m*-CPP goes specifically into the circulation and acts directly to stimulate the 5-HT receptors. There is no evidence that at the plasma concentrations found in man *m*-CPP has an indirect mode of action. These are very different situations and that may have a bearing on the different time-courses. Another point is that both challenge tests involve 'single-dose' clinical pharmacology. Perhaps if one used a range of doses one might have a convergence of the time-courses in certain circumstances.

Sandler: I do not find the time-lag surprising. Looking at the many triggers for migraine (Sandler 1995), such as *m*-CPP, fenfluramine, red wine or chocolate, we have found great differences in time-course. For example, in double-blind trials, we found the time-courses were three hours for red wine (Littlewood *et al.* 1988) and about 12 hours for chocolate (Gibb *et al.* 1991). For nitric oxide (NO), which I also consider to be just a trigger, there was also a significant delay between taking nitroglycerin and onset of headache in predisposed subjects (Olesen *et al.* 1993, Thomsen *et al.* 1993). I would say that the basic difference between migraine sufferers and normal subjects lies in their sensitivity to triggers (Sandler 1995). Some people are susceptible to one, some to another. There may well be some as yet unidentified triggering mechanisms associated with all migraine episodes. Presumably the difference in time before headache onset reflects the length of the chain in the cascade of events leading to the final common path.

Fozard: That is precisely why I was surprised, because if 5-HT receptor activation is triggering the attack following both fenfluramine and *m*-CPP, I would expect more similar time-courses.

Glover: That is right. I think they are all triggers and that the time-course may be some indication of the position in the cascade, presuming that the drugs get to the site equally quickly.

Schoenen: The time-lag with fenfluramine still appears short compared to the other chemical triggers where there is a delay of three to four hours.

Peatfield: In chocolate it is almost certain that the agent is covalently bound with some lipid. Much of the 12-hour delay probably reflects the need to turn the chocolate into a vasoactive substance in the gut.

Lance: Injection of reserpine, which releases serotonin from body stores, rapidly produces a typical migraine in a migrainous patient within three hours. In a non-migrainous patient it just gives a dull ache.

Thomsen: With fenfluramine, does the migraine develop slowly or is there a sudden onset?

Glover: We have not asked patients that. We simply asked them to fill in questionnaires every half hour and added up the scores. We should ask them in more detail what they feel.

Schoenen: It would be helpful to know if the 'migrainous symptoms' induced by fenfluramine fulfilled the International Headache Society (IHS) criteria for a migraine attack (Headache Classification Committee 1988). Everyone working with NO, tyramine or fenfluramine should agree on common diagnostic criteria. NO produces a headache very quickly, but a migraine attack only later. It is different to have just a headache. One can think about sensitization in some structure centrally or peripherally that induces headaches, but not necessarily a migraine attack.

Thomsen: Perhaps you could ask 'Is it like your normal migraine?', and request that patients fill out a headache diary, allowing classification according to the IHS criteria.

Glover: Yes. We should ask them that, and about any differences.

Peatfield: What is important is the fact that these patients are more sensitive.

Moskowitz: Combining the positron emission tomography techniques that Professor Diener described (Diener and May, this volume) and your administration of fenfluramine to see if any brain changes anticipate the pain might provide an interesting model for common migraine.

REFERENCES

Brewerton, T.D., Murphy, D. L., Mueller, E.A. and Jimerson, D.C. (1988) Induction of migraine-like headaches by the serotonin agonist m-chlorophenylpiperazine. *Clinical Pharmacology and Therapeutics*, **43**, 605–609.

Diener, H.C. and May, A. (1996) Positron emission tomography studies in acute migraine attack. In *Migraine: Pharmacology and Genetics*, (eds M. Sandler, M.D. Ferrari and S. Harnett) pp. 109–116. Chapman & Hall, London.

Gibb, C.M., Davies, P.T.G., Glover, V., Steiner, T.J., Clifford Rose, F. and Sandler, M. (1991) Chocolate is a migraine-provoking agent. *Cephalalgia*, **11**, 93–95.

Goodall, E.M., Cowen, P.J., Franklin, M. and Silverstone, T. (1993) Ritanserin attenuates anorectic, endocrine and thermic responses to D-fenfluramine in human volunteers. *Psychopharmacology*, **112**, 461–466.

Headache Classification Committee of the International Headache Society (J. Olesen *et al.*) (1988) Classification and diagnostic criteria for headache disorders, cranial neuralgias and facial pain. *Cephalalgia*, **8** (Suppl. 7), 1–97.

Littlewood, J.T., Gibb, C., Glover, V., Sandler, M., Davies, P.T.G. and Clifford Rose, F. (1988) Red wine as a cause of migraine. *Lancet*, **i**, 558–559.

Olesen, J., Iversen, H.K. and Thomsen, L.L. (1993) Nitric oxide supersensitivity: a possible molecular mechanism of migraine pain. *NeuroReport*, **4**, 1027–1030.

Sandler, M. (1995) Migraine to the year 2000. *Cephalalgia*, in press.

Thomsen, L.L., Iversen, H.K., Brinck, R.A. and Olesen, J. (1993) Arterial supersensitivity to nitric oxide (nitroglycerin) in migraine sufferers. *Cephalalgia*, **13**, 395–399.

11

The pharmacology of food and drink

R.C. Peatfield, N. Jarrett and V. Glover

An association of headache with food stuffs such as cheese and chocolate, and with red wine, is well established in the lay literature. Systematic surveys of patients attending the Princess Margaret Migraine Clinic have established that about 18–19% of patients report sensitivity to cheese and/or chocolate, and usually to both (Peatfield *et al.* 1984). In a more recent epidemiological survey (Peatfield 1995) the 18% of migraine patients sensitive to all alcoholic drinks were distinguished from a further 12% sensitive only to red wine, but not to white wine or clear spirits. There was a statistically significant but imperfect correlation between red wine and food sensitivity and it was extremely rare for a diet-sensitive patient to be tolerant of all forms of alcohol (Peatfield 1995).

It has proved difficult to reproduce this epidemiological finding in an experimental context (see Kohlenberg 1982). Data drawn from elimination diets, for example, are particularly open to suggestibility and bias. The first convincing provocation study was done by Hanington (1970), in which she administered tyramine and lactose capsules separately to a group of diet-sensitive patients and found that headache was induced on 78% of occasions by tyramine and 6% of occasions by lactose. It is now clear that tyramine cannot be the only responsible substance in foods, as it is not found in sufficient quantity in many incriminated foods, such as red wine (Hannah *et al.* 1988). A blinded study of red wine compared with diluted vodka did show a significant association

Migraine: Pharmacology and genetics
Edited by Merton Sandler, Michel Ferrari and Sara Harnett
Published in 1996 by Chapman & Hall
ISBN 1 86036 006 8

with headache ($p < 0.001$ Fisher's exact test, two-tailed) (Littlewood *et al.* 1988) and a smaller study of chocolate compared with placebo chocolate also demonstrated a convincing association with headache (Gibb *et al.* 1991).

Our recent studies at the Princess Margaret Migraine Clinic have been largely concerned with alcoholic drinks, partly because their biochemistry seems to be a little easier to elucidate, and partly because of the wider implications in controlling alcohol consumption (Tannock *et al.* 1993). In all these studies we have deliberately selected patients who are not sensitive to alcohol as such: they can all drink white wine and clear spirits in social quantities, but not red wine or, sometimes, beer.

The possible mechanisms of this response have been discussed in detail elsewhere (Peatfield *et al.* 1995). Our finding of a lower activity of platelet phenolsulphotransferase P in susceptible subjects (Littlewood *et al.* 1982) has been confirmed by Launay *et al.* (1988), whereas platelet monoamine oxidase is no lower in diet-sensitive subjects (Glover *et al.* 1981). Littlewood *et al.* (1985) demonstrated an inhibition of phenolsulphotransferase *in vitro* by red wine consistent with the consumption *in vivo* of a single glass. Jarman *et al.* (1991) showed that serotonin (5-hydroxytryptamine) could be released from pre-loaded platelets by red wine, which could also be demonstrated *in vivo* (Pattichis *et al.* 1994, 1995). Unfortunately the platelets of migraine patients sensitive to red wine did not prove more sensitive than those from non-dietary migraine patients when studied *in vitro* (Jarman *et al.* 1995). In a small study of six red wine-sensitive patients (Peatfield *et al.* 1995), we compared a Chianti, which had greater serotonin-releasing properties, with a Valpolicella. No difference was seen in the induction of headache by the wines, in five of six subjects in each case, although the size of this study and the modest chemical difference between the two wines selected does not permit a definite conclusion.

The mechanism of red wine-induced headaches might instead involve a direct interaction with one or more 5-hydroxytryptamine receptors. An obvious candidate is the 5-HT$_{2C}$ receptor. Although no abnormalities were identified in the cortical distribution of this receptor in a small group of unselected migraine patients (Chabriat *et al.* 1995), it is believed to be the site of action of *m*-chlorophenylpiperazine (*m*-CPP), a metabolite of trazodone found by Brewerton *et al.* (1988) to induce headaches in susceptible subjects. (See Curzon and Kennett 1990, Fozard 1992, Fozard and Kalkman 1994). Stimulation of this receptor among others is believed to cause vasodilatation via an endothelium-dependent nitric oxide-mediated pathway (Glusa and Richter 1993). It has been demonstrated that migrainous subjects are excessively sensitive to glyceryl trinitrate, a supplier of nitric oxide, which is further evidence of the involvement of this pathway in the mechanisms

Table 11.1 Pharmacology of red wines (diluted 1:20)

Wine	Grape	Percentage inhibition of ^3H-5-HT binding to 5-HT$_{2C}$ receptors	5-HT release from platelets (% of control)
Thornhill	Zinfandel	82	125
Cono Sur	Cabernet Sauvignon	54	129
La Veritiere	Sangiovese	47	138
Chateau La Tour St. Bonnet	Merlot	47	<110
Chateauneuf du Pape	Grenache etc.	69	<110
Barossa	Pinot Noir	66	<110

of migraine (Olesen *et al.* 1994). It has also been established that red wine contains vasodilating substances, residing in the pigments, which act via a nitric oxide-mediated pathway (Fitzpatrick *et al.* 1993), a mechanism suggested for the low prevalence of cardiovascular disease in habitual wine drinkers.

We have screened a wide variety of red wines for their ability to bind to the 5-HT$_{2C}$ receptor found in the pig choroid plexus (Pazos *et al.* 1984). All the red wines studied inhibit the binding of ^3H-5-HT to these 5-HT$_2$ receptors, ranging from 82% for a Californian Zinfandel to 47% for an Italian Sangiovese. There is no correlation between 5-HT$_{2C}$ receptor binding and the ability of these wines to release 5-HT from pre-loaded platelets (Table 11.1).

We hope to study two of these wines with widely different properties in these two *in vitro* models in a further series of red wine-sensitive subjects. We have also been undertaking some control experiments in medical students able to consume alcohol without undue headache. Ten subjects were given the Italian Sangiovese wine previously studied *in vitro* (5 ml/kg). This induced a modest increase in body temperature while prolactin levels were unchanged and cortisol levels reduced a little, whereas vodka diluted to supply the same amount of alcohol induced no change in temperature, although cortisol levels were again reduced slightly. Stress levels, as measured by a McKay and Cox questionnaire, were reduced by the vodka but not by red wine, which would suggest that red wine contains an additional anxiogenic agent. In contrast, *m*-CPP induces an increase in temperature, cortisol and prolactin, even in control subjects. It remains uncertain, of course, whether *m*-CPP is interacting with central as well as vascular 5-HT receptors. Also, sensitive subjects usually start to develop a headache within three hours of consuming red wine, whereas the response to m-CPP may be delayed, with a peak headache at 8–12 hours (Brewerton *et al.* 1988).

We have, therefore, yet to provide conclusive evidence that red wines interacting more strongly with any particular subtype of serotonin receptor are more likely to induce headaches *in vivo*. Intensive efforts are still being made to identify the precise headache-inducing substance or substances in alcoholic drinks.

REFERENCES

Brewerton, T.D., Murphy, D.L., Mueller, E.A. and Jimerson, D.C. (1988) Induction of migraine-like headaches by the serotonin agonist *m*-chlorophenylpiperazine. *Clinical Pharmacology and Therapeutics*, **43**, 605–609.

Chabriat, H., Tehindrazanarivelo, A., Vera, P., Samson, Y., Pappata, S., Boullais, N. and Bousser, M.G. (1995) 5-HT$_2$ receptors in cerebral cortex of migraineurs studied using PET and ^{18}F-fluorosetoperone. *Cephalalgia*, **15**, 104–108.

Curzon, G. and Kennett, G.A. (1990) *m*-CPP: a tool for studying behavioural responses associated with 5-HT$_{1C}$ receptors. *Trends in Pharmacological Sciences*, **11**, 181–182.

Fitzpatrick, D.F., Hirschfield, S.L. and Coffey, R.G. (1993) Endothelium-dependent vasorelaxing activity of wine and other grape products. *American Journal of Physiology*, **265**, H774–778.

Fozard, J.R. (1992) 5-HT$_{1C}$ receptor agonism as an initiating event in migraine. In: *5-Hydroxytryptamine Mechanisms in Primary Headache*, (eds J. Olesen and P.R. Saxena), pp. 200–212. Raven Press, New York.

Fozard, J.R. and Kalkman, H.O. (1994) 5-Hydroxytryptamine (5-HT) and the initiation of migraine: new perspectives. *Naunyn-Schmiedeberg's Archives of Pharmacology*, **350**, 225–229.

Gibb, C.M., Davies, P.T.G., Glover, V., Steiner, T.J., Clifford Rose, F. and Sandler, M. (1991) Chocolate as a migraine-provoking agent. *Cephalalgia*, **11**, 93–95.

Glover, V., Peatfield, R., Zammit-Pace, R., Littlewood, J., Gawel, M., Clifford Rose, F. and Sandler, M. (1981) Platelet monoamine oxidase activity and headache. *Journal of Neurology, Neurosurgery and Psychiatry*, **44**, 786–790.

Glusa, E. and Richter, M. (1993) Endothelium-dependent relaxation of porcine pulmonary arteries via 5-HT$_{1C}$-like receptors. *Naunyn-Schmiedeberg's Archives of Pharmacology*, **347**, 471–477.

Hanington, E., Horn, M. and Wilkinson, M. (1970) Further observations of the effects of tyramine. In: *Background to migraine: 3rd Migraine Symposium*, (ed. A.L. Cochrane), pp. 113–119. Heinemann, London.

Hannah, P., Glover, V. and Sandler, M. (1988) Tyramine in wine and beer. *Lancet*, **1**, 879.

Jarman, J., Glover, V. and Sandler, M. (1991) Release of (^{14}C) 5-hydroxytryptamine from human platelets by red wine. *Life Sciences*, **48**, 2297–2300.

Jarman, J., Pattichis, K., Peatfield, R., Glover, V. and Sandler, M. (1996) Red wine induced release of (^{14}C) 5-hydroxytryptamine from platelets of migraine patients and controls. *Cephalalgia*, in press.

Kohlenberg, R.J. (1982) Tyramine sensitivity in dietary migraine: a critical review. *Headache*, **22**, 30–34.

Launay, J.M., Soliman, H., Pradalier, A., Dry, J. and Dreux, C. (1988) Activités PST plaquettaires: le 'trait' migraineux? *Therapie*, **43** 273–277.

Littlewood, J., Glover, V., Sandler, M., Petty, R., Peatfield, R. and Clifford Rose,

F. (1982) Platelet phenolsulphotransferase deficiency in dietary migraine. *Lancet*, **i**, 983–986.

Littlewood, J.T., Glover, V. and Sandler, M. (1985) Red wine contains a potent inhibitor of phenolsulphotransferase. *British Journal of Clinical Pharmacology*, **19**, 275–278.

Littlewood, J.T., Gibb, C., Glover, V., Sandler, M., Davies, P.T.G. and Clifford Rose, F. (1988) Red wine as a cause of migraine. *Lancet*, **i**, 558–559.

Olesen, J., Thomsen, L.L. and Iversen, H. (1994) Nitric oxide is a key molecule in migraine and other vascular headaches. *Trends in Pharmacological Sciences*, **15**, 149–153.

Pattichis, K., Louca, L.L., Jarman, J. and Glover, V. (1994) Red wine can cause a rise in human whole blood 5-hydroxytryptamine levels. *Medical Science Research*, **22**, 381–382.

Pattichis, K., Louca, L.L., Jarman, J., Sandler, M. and Glover, V. (1995) 5-Hydroxytryptamine release from platelets by different red wines: implications for migraine. *European Journal of Pharmacology*, **292**, 173–177.

Pazos, A., Hoyer, D., and Palcios, J.M. (1984) The binding of serotonergic ligands to the porcine choroid plexus: characterisation of a new type of serotonin recognition site. *European Journal of Pharmacology*, **106**, 539–546.

Peatfield, R.C. (1995) Relationships between food, wine, and beer precipitated migranous headaches. *Headache*, **35**, 355–357

Peatfield, R., Glover, V., Littlewood, J.T., Sandler, M. and Clifford Rose F. (1984) Prevalence of diet-induced migraine. *Cephalalgia*, **4**, 179–183.

Peatfield, R., Hussein, N., Glover, V. and Sandler, M. (1995) Prostacyclin, tyramine and red wine. In: *Experimental Headache Models*, (eds J. Olesen and M.A. Moskowitz), pp. 267–276. Raven Press, New York.

Tannock, C., Bullock, R. and Peatfield, R.C. (1993) Problem drinkers do not get headache. *Cephalalgia*, **13**, 365.

DISCUSSION

Sandler: If you are trying to find a role for the 5-HT$_{2C}$ receptor in migraine, then the claim of Brewerton *et al.* (1988) that *m*-chlorophenylpiperazine (*m*-CPP) initiates attacks in some migraineurs but not controls is a key plank in your platform. Unfortunately, Gordon *et al.* (1993) were unable to replicate this work completely.

Fozard: Gordon *et al.* (1993) used half the dose of *m*-CPP used by Brewerton *et al.* (1988) in a placebo-controlled challenge study. They observed late-occurring headache in five of eight migraineurs and four of ten normal subjects with *m*-CPP, compared with three of eight migraineurs and one of ten normal subjects following placebo. Thus, the trend was similar despite the small size of the study sample.

Glover: They induced headache with *m*-CPP with the same long time-course in both migraine subjects and controls. They found no difference in the prolactin response between migraineurs and controls. The cortisol response to *m*-CPP preceded the headache and was associated with headache severity and duration.

Fozard: There are at least four other reports that *m*-CPP can trigger late-onset severe headache (see Fozard 1992). None of these studies specifically involved migraine patients. It is, therefore, interesting that the same proportion of subjects developed headache in those reports as the proportion of the patients with no predisposition to migraine that developed headache in the Brewerton *et al.* (1988) study.

Sandler: I do believe *m*-CPP to be a trigger in some migrainous patients, but it is only one among many different triggers. Dr Fozard, why do you consider it to be so important?

Fozard: The findings with *m*-CPP should be put in the context of other clinical findings, in particular that very low doses of compounds like methysergide and pizotifen and high doses of propranolol are effective in preventing migraine. The common denominator here is activation or blockade of the 5-HT$_{2B}$ receptor. This site is present on the endothelial cell, is linked to nitric oxide (NO) synthesis and, as I show in my chapter (Fozard, this volume), provides a plausible basis for an involvement of 5-HT in the initiation of migraine.

Thomsen: I think you have to move further down the cascade to find a common final pathway. I agree that it might be nitric oxide and subsequent events. Our studies, for example, are concerned with nitroglycerin, which does not have an effect on 5-HT$_{2C}$ receptors but activates the nitric oxide cascade.

Peatfield: There is no problem there. Our task is not to explain headache in general. Clearly this pharmacology does not apply to every headache patient. We have to explain why the red wine-sensitive patient is sensitive to red wine. Further down the pathway there are likely to be other ways of breaking into it which may apply to every headache patient, or only to some. Perhaps every headache patient is sensitive to NO donors such as nitroglycerin, but only some headache patients have sufficient 5-HT$_{2C}$/5-HT$_{2B}$ receptors to be sensitive to red wine in normal quantities.

Schoenen: From your clinical data, do you have the impression that this sensitivity to a trigger may change? Is there a relationship, for example, between frequency of attacks and ability to provoke a migraine with this kind of chemical trigger? Many of my patients say that when they are in remission from migraine, because they have had treatment or are pregnant, for example, they can drink red wine without getting a migraine.

Peatfield: In a cascade of transmitters and other chemical substances, one can envisage a block further down the pathway that prevents these patients getting headache, when they have taken a prophylactic agent or are pregnant, for example.

Schoenen: Another explanation might be that there is sensitization centrally or in the trigeminal pathway which makes these people more sensitive to a trigger.

Peatfield: I do not see a problem there either. I have not addressed the question of where this receptor is, whether it is neuronal or vascular. It could be in the trigeminal nucleus.

Where is this delay thought to come from? Is there a delay in the stimulation of the 5-HT$_2$ receptor? Is there a built-in cascade of responses that take six to eight hours? Ought we to be hunting for some aspect of serotonin pharmacology that takes this length of time?

Fozard: This is a difficult question to which I have no satisfactory answer. My feeling is that neurogenic inflammation does take time to develop, and may be an important factor. Also, natural migraine itself probably takes a similar time to develop. I do not see a basic difference between the time course involved in an attack provoked by NO or histamine or m-CPP and the development of a natural migraine attack. I suspect that the neurogenic inflammation evolves slowly until it triggers sufficient of the sensory fibres to result in headache.

Sandler: I still feel uneasy about this 5-HT$_2$ receptor. The 5-HT$_{1D}$ receptor is the only receptor for which we have convincing evidence of its involvement in migraine.

Fozard: I agree that 5-HT$_{1D}$ receptor activation appears to be beneficial in the treatment of migraine. However, that does not necessarily give information about what might be missing in the condition. If one uses a selective antagonist, however, and interrupts a natural process, one can begin to draw preliminary conclusions about the involvement of an endogenous agonist. This is a major strength of the hypothesis that 5-HT$_{2B}$ receptors are involved in the initiation of migraine (Fozard, this volume).

Moskowitz: The evidence about 5-HT's involvement in pathogenesis seems just as much against it as for it.

Sandler: We need more 5-HT data. There are radiolabelled markers that are fairly specific for the 5-HT$_{1D}$ site, such as [^{125}I]GTI (serotonin-5-O-carboxymethylglycyl-[^{125}I] tyrosinamide) (Boulenguez *et al.* 1991, Bruinvels *et al.* 1994). Could we not manufacture a positron emission tomography (PET) scan version of that and find out what is happening during a migraine attack?

Humphrey: There are two issues. Firstly, the therapeutic value of a 5-HT receptor agonist might be a coincidence. Secondly, I agree that there is no definitive evidence that 5-HT is involved in the pathophysiology. However, we do know that when 5-HT is released by reserpine migraine-like symptoms occur in migraineurs. Some years ago I noted that the 5-HT uptake blockers also cause headaches in individuals

(Humphrey 1991), but I do not know whether they cause migraine in migraineurs. Their effects may be related to 5-HT release, but perhaps more localized to the brain. I am not sure whether it is the 5-HT which is released centrally or peripherally that causes the migraine-like attack.

Moskowitz: Isn't fluoxetine (Prozac) used for treatment of migraine?

Humphrey: Yes, but this is analogous to reserpine. Reserpine provokes a migraine-like headache and then there is a period of remission, as if a new state of tone (5-HT?) is reached when a migraine cannot occur.

Goadsby: Fluoxetine is helpful in a particular group of people who end up in the 'very difficult headache' clinic. However, the only solid evidence about these uptake inhibitors is that they are not useful in migraine.

Merikangas: Anecdotally, fluoxetine often exacerbates migraine. People with both migraine and depression may do better on another class of antidepressant.

Schoenen: Fluoxetine is very widely used. We see many patients who are taking it and they do not report a worsening of migraine.

Sandler: It seems that depressed people are more sensitive to pain (e.g. Blumer and Heilbronn 1982). Therefore, treatment with antidepressants may allow them to tolerate their migraine headache with relative equanimity.

Peatfield: But then you would think that depressed patients with pain would respond better to these drugs than patients who are not depressed, but that is not the case. Some earlier papers suggested that these drugs were better for tension-type headaches than for migraine. Is this still borne out and what rationale can we offer? Is tension headache really a manifestation of a depressive state, or is there something different about it?

Goadsby: That has been best studied in patients with 'chronic daily headache', some of whom benefit from fluoxetine. However, chronic daily headache is not well defined.

Diener: After a German newspaper ran a headline saying that these new drugs have almost no side-effects, many patients using amitriptyline for tension-type headache asked for fluoxetine. Most reported that fluoxetine was less effective than amitriptyline.

Lance: Zimelidine was almost guaranteed to produce a migrainous headache or make migraine worse. The modern serotonin uptake inhibitors may be beneficial, depending possibly upon the degree of depression, but they are certainly not as helpful for chronic tension headache or migraine as the old tricyclics.

Patrick Henri from Bordeaux said that the French suffer more from migraine after white wine than red wine, which is contrary to our experience in Australia and the UK, where most people blame red wine. Is this generally observed in France?

Tournier-Lasserve: This is not a scientific observation, but I think it is true. In France, neurologists recommend migraineurs not to drink white wine.

Peatfield: Are these people alcohol sensitive? They may drink more white wine than red and therefore say white wine triggers migraine, but can they drink red wine in equivalent alcohol quantities and not get a headache? Epidemiologists should ask migraineurs if they get migraine after every form of alcohol. I suspect that the gene that produces alcohol sensitivity might be quite common in France, whereas the gene that causes specific red wine sensitivity may well be exclusive to an Anglo-Saxon population.

Schoenen: What do we know about the central effects on the brain of chemicals (including red wine) able to trigger attacks? Have there been studies of cerebral blood flow and metabolism?

Peatfield: Part of the problem is the alcohol-induced effect. To do PET scan studies either one would have to remove the alcohol from red wine, which might alter the pharmacological trigger, or one would have to give patients a pure alcohol preparation and subtract its effect from that of the red wine. I am sure that within red wine there are pharmacologically active substances which are triggers, and I am proposing that they are connected with serotonin.

Schoenen: I was also thinking about fenfluramine, tyramine, nitric oxide, etc.

Peatfield: I am sure that some of these substances are getting into the brain.

Sandler: Does red wine release prolactin?

Glover: *In vitro*, red wine acts similarly to fenfluramine: it causes release of 5-HT from platelets and from synaptosomes. But *in vivo* in the same fenfluramine model we failed to show an increase in prolactin after red wine ingestion. We have no evidence that it acts like that centrally. It may still act to release 5-HT peripherally. We have evidence that red wine causes an increase in whole blood 5-HT, which white wine does not. We think it is released from the intestine.

Peatfield: We gave an anxiety questionnaire to the medical students. When they took red wine, they became more anxious, which suggests there is some anxiogenic element within red wine that is not in vodka.

Diener: Is there a negative relationship between migraine and alcoholism?

I have never seen a chronic alcoholic who had migraine, whereas 30% of people with cluster headache are chronic alcoholics.

Peatfield: Were these patients of the 'got to have a drink before breakfast' type, or were they liver-failure patients?

Diener: They were admitted to psychiatric institutions for alcohol withdrawal.

Merikangas: We examined rates of alcoholism among the relatives of people with migraine, depression, alcoholism, anxiety and normal controls. We found a very low risk of alcoholism in the relatives of migraineurs compared to those of all the clinical groups and those of the controls as well. That suggests that there may be something protective against the development of alcoholism in these families. Your observation is also borne out by epidemiological studies, such as the Zurich cohort study in which we see much lower rates of alcoholism in people with migraine than in the general population (Merikangas *et al.* 1990)

Diener: This is not connected with pain-avoiding behaviour because cluster headache patients drink alcohol even if they know that they will provoke a headache.

Peatfield: Presumably the psychoactive action of alcohol in these patients to make them 'hooked' is so powerful that it would even overcome the discomfort induced by alcohol in a patient with cluster headache.

Merikangas: Some patients on 'antabuse' continue to drink even though the drug makes them sick.

Peatfield: There is something very powerful which is not seen in the patients with liver failure whom we saw who were excessive social drinkers. They are not 'hooked' and would not be referred to a psychiatrist because they do not feel that there is anything addictive about their behaviour.

Tournier-Lasserve: It might be difficult to correlate the analysis of risk of alcoholism among relatives of migraineurs compared to the general population. It depends enormously on how and where the migraineurs are seen. A migraineur going to a neurologist is not the same type of patient as the alcoholic in a psychiatric institution. We should be extremely careful in the epidemiogenetics of migraine to consider where we find the patients, what age they are, etc.

Merikangas: We looked specifically at people whom we identify from the population at large as well as those who came for treatment, because we were interested in that very question, to see if the aggregation of migraine and these other disorders in families was different for those who saw a neurologist, which is 2% of the general population. We found no difference in the family history of migraine among people from the population and those who came for treatment.

Peatfield: Among patients who come to me for treatment it is very unusual to find a patient who **only** gets headaches triggered by these food stuffs and red wine. Such people do not need a doctor to tell them to avoid the triggers. Most patients have spontaneous attacks as well as triggered attacks. They come to me because they still have spontaneous attacks although they avoid their triggering factor. There is some sort of circuit that fires the attack, which can be acted on by a trigger, but in that sub-group of patients still continues when not acted on by a trigger. I am sure that another group of people only get attacks with the trigger and never need to see a doctor. The majority of migraineurs have no such trigger: they do not have this particular abberation that makes them sensitive to red wine.

Ferrari: What happens if a patient provokes a migraine attack by drinking wine and then drinks wine the next day?

Peatfield: Anecdotally, they are often more resistant to a second challenge. It would be hard to get a large sample of sensitive patients for that kind of study.

Moskowitz: How do you see the dietary triggers in the context of the other migraine triggers, such as exercise, bright lights, too much or too little sleep, fasting and menstruation?

Peatfield: I envisage a circuit generated within the brainstem, as Professor Lance has been suggesting for many years, which fires from time to time, and external factors can act on that. I am arguing that most dietary triggers go through a serotonergic mechanism. Hypoglycaemia, I am sure, functions slightly differently. It is clear that NO donors act much closer to the final common pathway. Virtually all migraineurs (80%) are sensitive to NO donors, while only 15% to 18% are food-and/or wine-sensitive.

Moskowitz: What do you see as the sequence here? Does something enter the system, get into the circulation, and activate the pain system directly or indirectly through metabolites, or after the substance is ingested, does something go through the circulation, enter the brain and then secondarily affect a cascade that is universal for all the trigger mechanisms?

Glover: I would say that there are many different points of entry. Stress presumably acts at the locus coeruleus or raphe. Probably our thinking is too linked to the serotonergic system. One can't force absolutely everything into that.

Sandler: About ten years ago, we found that phenolsulphotransferase is profoundly inhibited by red wine and not so much by white wine (Littlewood *el al.* 1985). One can envisage a scenario where phenolsulpho-transferase acts as an enzymic barrier to a variety of phenolic toxins. In that case, when red wine inhibits this enzyme, toxic flavonoids, for example, might enter the bloodstream.

Merikangas: What about ice-cream headaches?

Peatfield: They are probably vascular phenomena, physiological responses to vasoconstriction.

Merikangas: Don't migraineurs have a higher risk?

Peatfield: Migraineurs have sensitive blood vessels. The pharmacological mechanism is unclear, but I do not see a problem. It is probably a mistake to try to incorporate every known trigger into the same mechanism. Sex hormone receptors are widespread and I do not think it is helpful to start looking at serotonin for a mechanism of menstrual migraine.

Moskowitz: If all these various triggers ultimately reach a sequence of events with more-or-less typical features, it is important to identify the threads that connect them. How and where are they finally acting to trigger headache?

Lance: We did a large trial of 90 adult migraine patients not specifically selected for dietary migraine, although 40% did claim specific dietary triggers (McQueen *et al.* 1989). After elimination diets and challenges by the dieticians (double-blind for the clinician), those remaining in the study were prescribed 'good' or 'bad' diets. Both groups had exactly the same number of headaches per month. Also, my patients with specific food triggers have the same number of migraine attacks when they avoid the triggers as before. The only thing that they agree precipitates attacks is alcohol, specifically red wine. Otherwise, in adults, I think the question of dietary migraine is very suspect.

Sandler: Migrainous patients may well be more sensitive than the general population to different kinds of triggers (Sandler 1995). One could even include the electrical events of a migraine aura as a trigger leading to the headache phase.

Goadsby: If you accept that there are people who have migraine equivalent, the aura is not much of a trigger. I suggest that it is not a trigger: it just happens to occur in some patients, irrespective of whether at the start, in the middle or at the end of the headache. The aura is an epiphenomenon of another process happening in the brain.

Moskowitz: We don't have the data for that yet. I disagree with you because I think the coincidence between the sidedness of the aura and the onset of a headache cannot be dismissed, despite the fact that there is not a 100% correlation. For 85% of attacks, if there is a right-brain event, a right-sided headache develops. One could contend that the other 15% is equally important, but I don't think that is the correct way to think about it now. From experimental animal data, it is clear that recurrent events in the cortex, such as spreading depression, can lead to activation of ipsilateral pain pathways that are part of the trigeminal neurovascular system (Moskowitz *et al.* 1993). C-*fos* expression can be blocked by transecting the primary afferents innervating the meninges, or by injecting sumatriptan. We must look seriously at the cortex for events that anticipate headache.

Goadsby: A single spreading depression was not a significant trigger. You used between six and nine spreading depressions to get the signal in the trigeminal system. That is excessive compared to the average migraine which does not have six to nine auras before the headache.

Moskowitz: The average migraine aura lasts 30 to 40 minutes, whereas in a rat the average spread across cortex at 3 mm per minute is shorter than that. That is why we induced multiple spreading depressions in our rodent experiments. We have offered the following hypothesis to explain how neurophysiological events in cortex can activate the trigeminal system. The brain is an organ which normally sequesters chemicals which are nociceptive, such as potassium or arachidonate metabolites, including protons. The brain exquisitely regulates its extracellular environment so that substances coming out of nerve cells and glia are equally balanced by inactivation and uptake. Venous drainage does not normally participate in this input/output equation. The supposition is that during spreading depression (or whatever underlies the aura), levels in the perivascular space increase to concentrations sufficient to discharge perivascular C-fibres. After 20–40 minutes, these levels are sufficient to cause headache. Martin Lauritzen and Richard Kraig have shown enhanced levels of K^+ and arachidonate in extracellular space during repeated spreading depressions (Kraig and Cooper 1987, Lauritzen *et al.* 1990).

Goadsby: The fact remains that that is not an explanation for the 15% of people who have contralateral pain, unless you say, of course, that they have silent aura. It also does not satisfy patients with migraine equivalent. How can this be such a pronounced stimulation if they do not get pain?

Lance: In a careful prospective study Jensen *et al.* (1986) found that as many patients developed the headache on the side contralateral to the aura, as on the other, inappropriate side, which does not support this particular theory. Only recently did Olesen *et al.* (1990) find there to be three out of 38 patients in whom the headache was on the inappropriate side.

Moskowitz: The preliminary observations made by my colleague Michael Cutrer at the Massachussetts General Hospital suggest that between 80% and 85% of cases have the correct side affected. As to why some patients may have the headache on the wrong side, there are instances in medicine in which pain occurs, particularly in relation to visceral pain, on the 'wrong' side of the body. Oliver Cope (1963) discusses the pain associated with acute appendicitis. He provides an example of appendiceal inflammation causing pain referred to the left testicle. How may a right-sided inflamed appendix cause unilateral pain on the 'wrong' side? We don't know. The spinal cord anatomy associated with visceral innervation is not as precisely defined as pain arising in the cutaneous distribution. I suggest that we shouldn't be dogmatic, given our current state of knowledge about innervation patterns, and reject ideas simply because a minority of patients present with headache on the 'wrong' side.

Goadsby: By analogy, patients with migraine equivalent would resemble patients with acute appendicitis with an inflamed appendix but no pain.

Lance: My point is that you can have patients with migrainous aura but no headache and patients with headache but no migrainous aura. Therefore, to deduce that one depends on the other because, in about 10% of patients, fortification spectra precede the headache is faulty reasoning: 90% of patients have the headache without a classical aura. This does not detract from Professor Moskowitz's work which is an important model for understanding the genesis of pain and headache. What I criticize is the link between aura and migraine.

Moskowitz: I do believe there are many syndromes which make up the migraine problem. Let me suggest an explanation for how headache might develop without aura. The afferents that innervate the brain are on the surface, a few millimetres below the pia mater. The most sensitive ones are at the level of the circle of Willis at the base of the brain. Let us suppose that the events triggering headache emanate from the hypothalamus. How would you recognize an event within the hypothalamus as strictly brain in origin? Patients may be hungry, show a change of emotion or water balance. None of us would recognize in ourselves this as a disturbance in the hypothalamus. I suggest that there may be other areas in the brain which may truly be silent, or not so silent, which can then give rise to a headache through a mechanism described above. We need to examine brain regions (particularly those draining into the meninges) that contain the primary afferents for those triggering events relating to the onset of pain. Migraine aura is suggested as one triggering event. Headache in the epilepsies may have a similar pathogenesis. My main point is that we cannot abandon the neurobiological basis of pain, and that pathophysiology must incorporate those principles. Most importantly, the proposed hypotheses are in fact testable.

Lance: But 25% of patients do indeed get those hypothalamic symptoms as a regular premonitory symptom before the headache.

Moskowitz: That may well tell us that there are other trigger sites besides primary visual and sensory cortex that cannot be well studied with our present imaging techniques.

Lance: We agree then that we can add hypothalamic structures as well!

Peatfield: In our series (Peatfield *et al.* 1981) that seems to have initiated this argument about the proportions of patients with ipsilateral and contralateral aura symptoms and headache, there were many patients who were dysphasic and had sensory symptoms in the non-dominant hand, which suggests that there is more than one part of the brain involved. I think the spreading depression is probably patchy and most patches are asymptomatic or almost so. Most of my patients whom I classify as having a classical migraine speak of a few blobs in the visual fields before an attack: it is very unusual to get the 'typical' scintillating scotoma migrating across the visual field.

Moskowitz: What is required to provoke focal symptoms from an area of brain? We know that neuronal packing density in the primary occipital area is quite high. If a small area is involved, a rather significant fraction of neurons (and visual space) may be abnormal. The representation for language and for speech are more diffusely represented. A narrow wave of abnormal neurophysiological activity affects a relatively small percentage of that area subserving a particular function. The abnormality would not necessarily manifest: it would be clinically silent. If we wish to understand the triggering events, we should examine the human brain with respect to its neurophysiological activity. It would be beneficial to develop techniques that are more specific than blood flow.

Lance: The observation by Woods *et al.* (1994) that a patient without a typical aura but with a little blurring of vision had precisely the same changes on PET scanning as one would expect in a patient with classical aura means there may indeed be a sub-clinical type of aura going on bilaterally in some patients. Many patients with migraine complain of a generalized blurring of vision or photopsia, not the classical aura, but only 10% get the real spectrum of zigzags. Some who become confused, lose their memory and are generally impaired may have spreading depression or a vasoconstrictive process before or during the headache. Our views have met in the hypothalamus. Perhaps we can meet on the cortex as well!

Schoenen: As well as the PET study (Woods *et al.* 1994) there is various evidence that the brain doesn't function normally during migraine attacks. Barkley *et al.* (1990) have shown depression of activity with magneto-encephalography. We have shown a depressed cortical alpha activity during migraine attacks without aura (Schoenen *et al.* 1987). Another argument was implicit in my earlier question. All these triggers can activate the brain. It is most unlikely that the three-hour delay is just due to the building up of neurogenic inflammation. I would suggest that this might be due to an activation of the brain parenchyma triggering a cascade which leads to a migraine attack. I have one reservation, however, which comes from my clinical experience that most of my patients who have migraine with aura have a much lower frequency of attacks than those who have migraine without aura or both types of migraine attack. That is where we should think about something, as I said earlier, that is sensitizing the trigeminovascular system, or the trigeminal pathway.

Peatfield: I think that that must be due to selection. I would like to see those data reproduced in a population-based sample.

Schoenen: The Danish population-based study (Rasmussen and Olesen 1992) clearly shows that this is not due to patient selection.

Lance: It is also my impression that the more frequent the migraine becomes, the less the aura.

Peatfield: But isn't it the aura patients who come to see you? We see many patients who have one or two auras and are terrified by them.

Goadsby: I don't think so. General practitioners are comfortable with aura patients: their attacks are less frequent and are quite easy to treat. In contrast, patients without aura have more frequent attacks and they are referred for management.

Peatfield: Some general practitioners do not believe that migraine can take place without an aura. Patients are referred for a diagnostic assessment because they have very frequent headaches. I suspect there is a selection bias.

REFERENCES

Barkley, G.L., Tepley, N., Simkins, R., Moran, J. and Welch, K.M.A. (1990) Neuromagnetic fields in migraine: preliminary findings. *Cephalalgia*, **10**, 171–176.

Blumer, D. and Heilbronn, M. (1982) Chronic pain as a variant of depressive disease. *Journal of Nervous and Mental Diseases*, **7**, 381–393.

Boulenguez, P., Chauveau, J., Segu, L., Morel, A., Delaage, M. and Lanoir, J. (1991) Pharmacological characterization of serotonin-O-carboxymethyl-glycyltyrosinamide, a new selective indolic ligand for 5-hydroxytryptamine (5-HT)$_{1B}$ and 5-HT$_{1D}$ binding sites. *Journal of Pharmacology and Experimental Therapeutics*, **259**, 1360–1365.

Brewerton, T.D., Murphy, D.L., Mueller, E.A. and Jimerson, D.C. (1988) Induction of migraine-like headaches by the serotonin agonist *m*-chlorophenyl-piperazine. *Clinical Pharmacology and Therapeutics*, **43**, 605–609.

Bruinvels, A.T., Landwehrmeyer, B., Probst, Al, Palacios, J.M. and Hoyer, D. (1994) A comparative autoradiographic study of 5-HT$_{1D}$ binding sites in human and guinea-pig brain using different radioligands. *Molecular Brain Research*, **21**, 19–29.

Cope, O. (1963) *Some Observations on the Acute Abdomen*, Oxford University Press.

Fozard, J.R. (1992) 5-HT$_{1C}$ receptor agonism as an initiating event in migraine. In: *5-Hydroxytryptamine Mechanism in Primary Headache*, (eds J. Olesen and P.R. Saxena), pp. 200–212. Raven Press, New York.

Fozard, J.R. (1996) 5-Hydroxytryptamine and nitric oxide: the causal relationship between two endogenous precipitants of migraine. In: *Migraine: Pharmacology and Genetics*, (eds M. Sandler, M.D. Ferrari and S. Harnett), pp. 167–179. Chapman & Hall, London.

Gordon, M.L., Lipton, R.B., Brown, S.L. Nakraseive, C., Russell, M., Pollack, S.Z., Korn, M.L., Merriam, A., Solomon, S. and van Praag, H.M. (1993) Headache and cortisol responses to *m*-chlorophenylpiperazine are highly correlated. *Cephalalgia*, **13**, 400–405.

Humphrey, P.P.A. (1991) 5-Hydroxytryptamine and the pathophysiology of migraine. *Journal of Neurology*, **238**, 538–544.

Jensen, R., Tfelt-Hansen, P., Lauritzen, M. and Olesen, J. (1986) Classic migraine. A prospective reporting of symptoms. *Acta Neurologica Scandinavica*, **73**, 359–362.

Kraig, R.P. and Cooper, A.J.L. (1987) Bicarbonate and ammonia changes in brain during spreading depression. *Canadian Journal of Physiology and Pharmacology*, **65**, 1099–1104.

Lauritzen, M., Hansen, A.K., Kronborg, D. and Wieloch, T. (1990) Cortical spreading depression is associated with arachidonic acid accumulation and preservation of energy charge. *Journal of Cerebral Blood Flow and Metabolism*, **10**, 115–112.

Littlewood, J.T., Glover, V. and Sandler, M. (1985) Red wine contains a potent inhibitor of phenolsulphotransferase. *British Journal of Clinical Pharmacology*, **19**, 275–278.

McQueen, J., Loblay, R.H., Savain, A.R., Anthony, M. and Lance, J.W. (1989) A controlled trial of dietary modification in migraine. In: *New Advances in Headache Research*, (ed. F. Clifford Rose), pp. 235–242. Smith Gordon & Co., London.

Merikangas, K.R., Angst, J., Isler, H. (1990) Migraine and psychopathology: results of the Zurich cohort study of young adults. *Archives of General Psychiatry*, **47**, 849–853.

Moskowitz, M.A., Nozaki, K. and Kraig, R.P. (1993) Neocortical spreading depression provokes the expression of c-*fos* protein-like immunoreactivity within trigeminal nucleus caudalis via trigeminovascular mechanisms. *Journal of Neuroscience*, **13**, 1167–1177.

Olesen, J., Friberg, L., Skyhøj Olsen, T., Iverson, H.K., Lassen, N.A., Anderson, A.R. and Karle, A. (1990) Timing and tomography of cerebral flow, aura and headache during migraine attacks. *Annals of Neurology*, **28**, 791–798.

Peatfield, R.C., Gawel, M.J. and Clifford Rose, F. (1981) Asymmetry of the aura and pain in migraine. *Journal of Neurology Neurosurgery and Psychiatry*, **44**, 846–848.

Rasmussen, B.K. and Olesen, J. (1992) Migraine with aura and migraine without aura: an epidemiological study. *Cephalalgia*, **12**, 221–228.

Sandler, M. (1995) Migraine to the year 2000. *Cephalalgia*, **15**, 259–264.

Schoenen, J., Jamart, B. and Delwaide, P.J. (1987) Topographic EEG mapping in common and classic migraine during and between attacks. In: *Advances in Headache Research*, (ed. F. Clifford Rose), pp. 25–33. John Libbey, London.

Woods, R.P., Iacoboni, M. and Mazziotta, J.C. (1994) Bilateral spreading hypoperfusion during spontaneous migraine. *New England Journal of Medicine*, **331**, 1689–1692.

12

5-HT$_{1D}$ and GABA$_A$ receptors in migraine

Michael A. Moskowitz

In 1990, migraine became the first neurological condition to be treated successfully with a receptor-selective drug. This drug, sumatriptan, binds with high affinity to serotonin$_{1D}$ (5-HT$_{1D}$) receptors. This receptor also mediates the effects of less selective antimigraine drugs such as dihydroergotamine and ergotamine tartrate. The 5-HT$_{1D}$ recognition site, however, should not remain unique for too long as other relevant receptors have been proposed as therapeutic targets in migraine, including NK$_1$ (neurokinin$_1$), NPY$_2$ (neuropeptide Y$_2$), α_2-adrenergic, somatostatin, μ opioid, histamine$_3$, and GABA$_A$ (gamma-amino butyric acid$_A$) receptors. This partial list (circa 1995) continues to expand.

We present here a brief summary of work (mostly from my own laboratory) describing the importance of two distinct receptors in migraine therapy, 5-HT$_{1D}$ and GABA$_A$.

5-HT$_{1D}$ RECEPTORS

A large body of data addresses the mechanism by which 5-HT$_{1D}$ receptors relieve migraine headaches (Moskowitz 1992; Humphrey and Feniuk 1991, Ferrari and Saxena 1993). Two mechanisms have been proposed. The first is based primarily upon 5-HT$_{1D}$-mediated constriction of vascular smooth muscle within cephalic vessels (Humphrey *et al.* 1988). The second is based upon neurogenic mechanisms and the

Migraine: Pharmacology and genetics
Edited by Merton Sandler, Michel Ferrari and Sara Harnett
Published in 1996 by Chapman & Hall
ISBN 1 86036 006 8

binding of 5-HT$_{1D}$ agonists to receptors expressed on trigeminal nerve endings innervating the meninges. Evidence for the latter is as follows.

In animal models, 5-HT$_{1D}$ receptor agonists (sumatriptan and the ergot alkaloids) block the development of neurogenic inflammation (NI) within the meninges (Saito *et al.* 1988, Buzzi and Moskowitz 1990) and block the expression of c-*fos* within lamina I,II$_o$ of trigeminal nucleus caudalis by inhibiting impulse transmission (Nozaki *et al.* 1992, Moskowitz *et al.* 1993). Sumatriptan's effects on neurogenic inflammation are partly reversed by pretreatment with GR127935, a selective 5-HT$_{1D}$ receptor antagonist (Yu *et al.*, unpublished work, 1995).

5-HT$_{1D}$ receptor-induced blockade of oedema does not depend upon the development of vasoconstriction *per se*. If it did, oedema from many different causes would be blocked. In experimental animals, oedema elicited by electrical trigeminal nerve stimulation, or systemic or intraganglionic capsaicin injection seem particularly susceptible (Markowitz *et al.* 1987). In contrast, sumatriptan does not decrease plasma protein leakage following administration of α-methyl-serotonin (a 5-HT$_2$ receptor agonist) or substance P (SP). However, oedema is blocked selectively by pimozide (after α-methyl-5-HT) and by an NK$_1$ receptor antagonist (after SP). Blockade is thus receptor and stimulus dependent.

Blockade of neurogenic inflammation may be selective within the 5-HT$_{1D}$ receptor family. The 5-HT$_{1D}$ receptor is comprised of at least two closely related receptors encoded by distinct genes (Hartig *et al.* 1992). The mRNA encoding 5-HT$_{1D\alpha}$ receptor protein is expressed by trigeminal neurons (Rebeck *et al.* 1994). In contrast, 5-HT$_{1D\beta}$ mRNA was not detectable using reverse transcriptase-polymerase chain reaction in human or guinea-pig trigeminal ganglia, despite the demonstration of 5-HT$_{1D\beta}$ sequence amplification in human striatum using the same oligonucleotide probe. Hamel and colleagues (1993) found that 5-HT$_{1D\beta}$ receptors, homologues to 5-HT$_{1B}$ receptors in rat and mice, are expressed selectively within human pial vascular smooth muscle. Existing drugs do not show more than 15-fold discrimination between the α and β receptor subtypes. According to current postulates, drugs selective for the α subtype would block impulses within the trigeminal nerve without causing constriction of pial or coronary vessels. On the other hand, 5-HT$_{1D\beta}$ receptor agonists would constrict vascular smooth muscle without blocking neurogenic inflammation or neurotransmission. Testing subtype-selective drugs in migraine patients can resolve this issue.

Data from my lab are consistent with the notion that 5-HT$_{1D}$ receptors on meningeal axons inhibit SP and calcitonin gene-related peptide (CGRP) release during stimulation. In fact, inhibition of CGRP release was reported in animals during trigeminal stimulation (Buzzi *et al.* 1991) and in migraineurs after sumatriptan administration (Goadsby and

Edvinsson 1993). It is difficult to conceive how vasoconstriction inhibits neuropeptide release from sensory fibres, as some have proposed, or blocks neurogenic inflammation or pain transmission. Blockade of NI may reduce pain because NI can sensitize primary afferent fibres. Moreover, NI may promote throbbing pain by sensitizing primary afferents to haemodynamic events which are not usually noxious.

5-HT$_{1B}$ knock-out mice

As noted above, 5-HT$_{1B}$ receptors in rats and mice are the homologues to human 5-HT$_{1D\beta}$ receptors. We have adapted and validated the trigeminal electrical stimulation model in mice in order to study mutant mice lacking expression of the 5-HT$_{1B}$ receptor subtype. Rene Hen of Columbia University, New York developed the knock-out using well-established techniques of homologous recombination (Saudou *et al.* 1994).

We found that plasma leakage is similar in vehicle-treated wild-type and mutant mice, rats and guinea-pigs. In rats, but not guinea-pig, (guinea-pigs, like humans, lack 5-HT$_{1B}$ receptors), a specific 5-HT$_{1B}$ receptor agonist, CP-93,129 selectively blocks plasma protein extravasation (Matsubara *et al.* 1991). Thus, when CP-93,129 was injected 10–15 min before electrical stimulation in rats, oedema decreased considerably, whereas in guinea-pigs, CP-93,129 was ineffective even at high doses (1400 mg/kg). We have observed that CP-93,129 blocks plasma protein extravasation in the wild-type, but not the 5-HT$_{1B}$ knock-out mouse. If the 5-HT$_{1D\alpha}$ gene is expressed in the mutant trigeminal ganglia, we anticipate that sumatriptan will block oedema formation in both mutant and wild-type mice. If 5-HT$_{1B}$ receptors are expressed exclusively, then the expectation is that sumatriptan and CP-93,129 will be inactive.

In summary, our findings establish important 5-HT$_{1D}$ receptor-mediated neurogenic effects which develop independently from vascular smooth muscle constriction. Moreover, it appears that 5-HT$_{1D\alpha}$ subtype-selective compounds offer distinct therapeutic advantages over existing compounds.

Immediate early response genes

Using a model of early immediate response gene expression (c-*fos*), we have also shown that sumatriptan and ergot alkaloids block trigemino-vascular transmission. C-*fos* transcription factor serves as a marker of neuronal activation within lamina I,II$_o$ of the trigeminal nucleus caudalis (Nozaki *et al.* 1992, Cutrer *et al.* 1995), and is not expressed by quiescent neurons. (Lamina I,II$_o$ contain the termination sites of small unmyelinated C-fibres and the second order neurons projecting to the spinothalamic tract.) Cells expressing *c-fos* appear in lamina I,II$_o$ especially after tonic noxious stimuli, such as capsaicin or formalin injection, in tissues such as nasal mucosa (Anton *et al.* 1991) or fore paw (Presley *et al.* 1990), or after injecting autologous blood or carrageenin into the cisternal space. The number of cells expressing the gene usually corresponds to the intensity of the stimulus (amount, not volume, of injectate). Sumatriptan, ergot alkaloids, and analgesics such as morphine block *c-fos* expression, as do valproic acid (F.M. Cutrer, unpublished work 1995) and prior surgical transection of trigemino-vascular afferents.

Because intense vasoconstriction develops with headache after intracisternal blood or capsaicin, sumatriptan is more likely to block headache pain by potent neurogenic mechanisms. It follows that constriction and pain relief can be dissociated. For example, there are anecdotal reports that sumatriptan relieves pain during intense vaso-constriction caused by subarachnoid haemorrhage. Hence, our models appear more consistent with the predominance of a neurogenic, possibly 5-HT$_{1D\alpha}$ receptor-mediated, mechanism. This suggests that 5-HT$_{1D}$ receptor agonists would possess the potential to block pain associated with diverse causes of headache, such as alcohol withdrawal (hangover headache) or certain forms of meningitis, regardless of vessel calibre. Anecdotal reports support this possibility as well. Our model predicts that so-called 'antimigraine drugs' are not specific for migraine because they relieve headaches other than migraine (e.g. cluster headache).

GABA RECEPTORS

Valproic acid is reportedly useful for acute and prophylactic treatment of migraine headaches (Jensen *et al.* 1994, Kozubski and Sokolowski 1994, unpublished work). It blocks GABA transaminase activity and increases glutamic acid decarboxylase activity to enchance the action of endo-genous GABA. Valproic acid is one of eight drugs that block neurogenic inflammation within rodent meninges (the remaining seven are sumatriptan, dihydroergotamine, chronic methysergide, ketorolac, aspirin (poorly), indomethacin and corticosteroids). When administered in therapeutically relevant doses (≤ 3 mg/kg), valproate blocks plasma protein extravasation induced by electrical trigeminal stimulation and chemical stimulation (capsaicin). It should be noted that GABA$_A$ agonists cause weak arteriolar vasodilation and **not** constriction. Administering the selective GABA$_A$ antagonist bicuculline reverses valproate's effect whereas the GABA$_B$ antagonist, phaclofen, does not. Moreover, muscimol (a GABA$_A$ agonist), but not baclofen (a GABA$_B$

agonist), inhibits plasma protein extravasation by bicuculline, but not by phaclofen-reversible mechanisms (W.S. Lee *et al.* 1995, unpublished work).

GABA$_A$, a heteropentomeric receptor, possesses allosteric modulatory sites for both neurosteroids (including progesterone metabolites) and benzodiazepines, among others. Binding to these sites facilitates the actions of endogenous GABA and enhances chloride ion conductance. The fact that progesterone metabolites and benzodiazepines (V. Limmroth 1995, unpublished work) block meningeal oedema formation further implicates the GABA$_A$ receptor subtype as an important mediator. Not surprisingly, we found that bicuculline but not phaclofen reversed the effects of progesterone metabolites in the inflammation model. Importantly, bicuculline methiodide (a hydrophilic analogue which does not cross the blood–brain barrier) reversed the actions of neurosteroids and valproate, suggesting that crossing the blood–brain barrier is not necessary for the blockade of meningeal plasma protein extravasation. Hence, the detrimental central nervous system effects of administered GABA$_A$ agonists and valproate may be circumvented by developing CNS impermeable drugs (V. Limmroth *et al.* 1995, unpublished work).

The above evidence suggests that the activation of GABA$_A$ receptors blocks NI. However, the receptor location differs from 5-HT$_{1D}$. In 1988, we postulated that ergot alkaloids blocked NI by prejunctional mechanisms based upon their inhibition of NI induced by capsaicin or electrical stimulation and inactivity against plasma extravasation following substance P (Saito *et al.* 1988). Molecular evidence has since substantiated this assertion (see above). Valproate, muscimol and progesterone metabolites, in contrast, significantly suppress plasma protein extravasation caused by SP administration both in normal animals and in those deficient in capsaicin-sensitive fibres. Together these results indicate that GABA receptors are expressed on cellular elements within the vessel wall unrelated to small calibre trigeminovascular afferents. Initial attempts to identify this location indicate that prior surgical parasympathectomy (sphenopalatine ganglionectomy) completely blocks the anti-oedema effects of valproate, muscimol and progesterone metabolites, whereas the response to sumatriptan is unaltered in these animals. Hence, we have tentatively assigned the location of GABA$_A$ receptors to parasympathetic axons innervating the meninges.

SUMMARY

We have shown that there is considerable potential for developing safer and more effective migraine treatments based on existing knowledge of serotonin and GABA receptor pharmacology.

Acknowledgements

Some of the studies described in this report were supported by NIH Grant NS21558 and by a Bristol-Myers Squibb Unrestricted Award for Research in Neuroscience.

REFERENCES

Anton, F., Herdegen, T., Peppel, P. and Leah, J.D. (1991) C-fos-like immuno-reactivity in rat brainstem neurons following noxious chemical stimulation of the nasal mucosa. *Neuroscience*, **41**, 629–641.

Buzzi, M.G. and Moskowitz, M.A. (1990) The antimigraine drug, sumatriptan (GR43175), specifically blocks neurogenic plasma extravasation from blood vessels in dura mater. *British Journal of Pharmacology*, **99**, 202–206.

Buzzi, M.G., Carter, W.B., Shimizu, T., Heath, H. III and Moskowitz, M.A. (1991) Dihydroergotamine and sumatriptan attenuate levels of CGRP in plasma in rat superior sagittal sinus during electrical stimulation of the trigeminal ganglion. *Neuropharmacology*, **30**, 1193–1200.

Cutrer, F.M., Moussaoui, S., Garret, C. and Moskowitz, M.A. (1995) The nonpeptide NK_1 antagonist, RPR-100–893, decreases c-fos expression in trigeminal nucleus caudalis following noxious chemical meningeal stimulation. *Neuroscience*, **64**, 741–750.

Ferrari, M.D. and Saxena, P.R. (1993) Clinical and experimental effects of sumatriptan in humans. *Trends in Pharmacological Sciences*, **14**, 129–133.

Goadsby, P.J. and Edvinsson, L. (1993) The trigeminovascular system and migraine: studies characterizing cerebrovascular and neuropeptide changes seen in humans and cats. *Annals of Neurology*, **33**, 48–56.

Hamel, E., Fan, E., Linville, D., Ting, V., Vellemure, J.-G. and Chia, L.-S. (1993) Expression of mRNA for the serotonin 5-hydroxytryptamine 1Dβ receptor subtype in human and bovine cerebral arteries. *Molecular Pharmacology*, **44**, 242–246.

Hartig, P.R., Branchek, T.A. and Weinshank, R.L. (1992) A subfamily of 5-HT receptor genes. *Trends in Neuroscience*, **13**, 152–159.

Humphrey, P.P.A. and Feniuk, W. (1991) Mode of action of the anti-migraine drug sumatriptan. *Trends in Pharmacological Sciences*, **12**, 444–446.

Humphrey, P.P.A., Feniuk, W., Perren, M.J., Connor, H.E., Oxford, A.W., Coates, I.H. and Butina, D. (1988) GR 43175, a selective agonist for the 5-HT1D-like receptor in dog isolated saphenous vein. *British Journal of Pharmacology*, **94**, 1123–1132.

Jensen, R., Brinck, T. and Olesen, J. (1994) Sodium valproate has a prophylactic effect in migraine with aura: a triple-blind, placebo-controlled crossover study. *Neurology*, **44**, 647–651.

Markowitz, S., Saito, K. and Moskowitz, M.A. (1987) Neurogenically mediated leakage of plasma protein occurs from blood vessels in dura mater but not brain. *Journal Neuroscience*, **7**, 4129–4136.

Matsubara, T., Moskowitz, M.A. and Byun, B. (1991) CP-93,129, a potent and selective 5-HT_{1B} agonist blocks neurogenic plasma extravasation within rat but not guinea-pig dura mater. *British Journal of Pharmacology*, **104**, 3–4.

Moskowitz, M.A. (1992) Neurogenic versus vascular mechanisms of sumatriptan and ergot alkaloids in migraine. *Trends in Pharmacological Sciences*, **13**, 307–311.

Moskowitz, M.A., Nozaki, K. and Kraig, R.P. (1993) Neocortical spreading depression provokes the expression of c-fos protein-like immunoreactivity within trigeminal nucleus caudalis via trigeminovascular mechanisms. *Journal of Neuroscience*, **13**, 1167–1177.

Nozaki, K., Mislowitz, M.A. and Boccalini, P. (1992) CP-93,129, sumatriptan, dihydroergotamine block c-fos expression within rat trigeminal nucleus caudalis caused by chemical stimulation of the meninges. *British Journal of Pharmacology*, **106**, 409–415.

Presley, R.W., Menétrey, D., Levine, J.D. and Basbaum, A.I. (1990) Systemic morphine suppresses noxious stimulus-evoked fos protein-like immuno-reactivity in the rat spinal cord. *Journal of Neuroscience*, **10**, 323–335.

Rebeck, G.W., Maynard, K.I., Hyman, B.T. and Moskowitz, M.A. (1994) Selective 5-HT$_{1D\alpha}$ serotonin receptor gene expression in trigeminal ganglia: implications for antimigraine drug development. *Proceedings of the National Academy of Science USA*, **91**, 3666–3669.

Saito, K., Markowitz, S. and Moskowitz, M.A. (1988) Ergot alkaloids block the neurogenic extravasation in dura mater: proposed action in vascular head-aches. *Annals of Neurology*, **24**, 732–737.

Saudou, F., Amara, D.A., Dierich, A., LeMeur, M., Ramboz, S., Segu, L., Buhot, M.D and Hen, R. (1994) Enhanced aggressive behavior in mice lacking 5-HT$_{1B}$ receptor. *Science*, **265**, 1875–1878.

DISCUSSION

Sandler: These knock-out mice are irritable and very aggressive animals.

Moskowitz: According to Saudou *et al.* (1994) if the animals are reared alone they become very aggressive. We do not isolate the animals; we keep them all in groups of five or six.

Sandler: This extreme isolation-induced aggression is particularly inter-esting to me because Levi-Montalcini and her colleagues (*Aloe et al.* 1986) noted a massive release of nerve growth factor into the bloodstream in normal mice made aggressive by isolation.

Moskowitz: Dr Hen tells me they are also very sexually active.

Connor: How might the GABA receptors on the parasympathetic nerves modify the extravasation response?

Moskowitz: I do not know. One can imagine, based on the constituents within the parasympathetic system, such as nitric oxide synthase, acetylcholine, and vasoactive intestinal polypeptide (VIP), that it is a modulatory effect on primary afferent function. I do not have any data to address that.

Goadsby: How did you perform the c-*fos*/GABA experiments?

Moskowitz: In the c-*fos* experiments the animal is anaesthetized and prepared. Because of surgical trauma, we then quiesce the animals by keeping them anaesthetized with the intracisternal catheter in place for six hours, during which time the c-*fos* expression presumably rises and then falls to a low baseline level. Then the animal is given valproic acid, or another blocking agent, followed at the appropriate time by 100 μl of a 0.1 μM solution of capsaicin injected intracisternally. After two hours we perfuse the animal and cut serial sections throughout the caudalis. Someone blinded to the treatment group counts cells individually. We have developed a statistical method which allows us to count 16 sections within the caudalis to then estimate total c-*fos* activity.

Goadsby: How does the parasympathetic system affect that c-*fos* expression? Are you suggesting that the parasympathetic nerves in some way normally inhibit the effect of capsaicin on stimulating c-*fos* and then, when you block them with valproate, that is taken away?

Moskowitz: Yes. We postulate that there would be some modulatory effect of the parasympathetic system on the functioning primary afferents.

Glover: From your reasoning, wouldn't you expect benzodiazepines to have more effect on migraine attacks?

Moskowitz: Intravenous benzodiazepines have been tried with some anecdotal success. It was originally thought to be working by putting people to sleep. Zolpidem is more effective in blocking neurogenic extravasation. It may relate to the issue of dosage and efficacy.

Edvinsson: Did you perform the sphenopalatine ganglionectomy experiments unilaterally? How long was the post-operative time?

Moskowitz: We have done it unilaterally and bilaterally ten days before the experiments. We performed immunohistochemistry afterwards to show that the VIP-immunoreactive fibres were depleted.

Hamel: Where would the GABA come from? Also, when you do the sphenopalatine lesioning, do you see a hypersensitivity to your GABA agonist? Unless I am mistaken, GABA is present in the sphenopalatine ganglia.

Moskowitz: It is present in nerve fibres that surround meningeal vessels and in endothelial cells, and glutamic acid decarboxylase is present. Sometimes we did see, but not consistently, more neurogenic inflammation in the sphenopalatine lesion animals than in controls. That was the only irregularity that we saw. As expected, the sumatriptan response was quite robust.

Goadsby: Several years ago, looking at dura with Violetta Dimitriadou, our impression was that stimulation of the sphenopalatine itself produced plasma extravasation (unpublished data). I have therefore wondered how much of the plasma extravasation when the trigeminal ganglion is stimulated is directly antidromic and how much is through the trigeminal vascular reflex.

Moskowitz: The basic observation was that if you cut the sphenopalatine ganglion, wait two weeks, and then repeat the experiments, you lose the effects of the GABA$_A$ receptor agonist. However, the plasma protein extravasation response does not differ. The loss of the GABA receptor agonist action led us to conclude that the receptor may well be on parasympathetic fibres.

Goadsby: It would not be surprising if something like the parasympathetics that were responsible for releasing NO, for example, made plasma extravasation worse.

Moskowitz: No, because parasympathectomy does not alter the response to trigeminal stimulation.

Ferrari: Did acute administration of valproic acid also block plasma extravasation?

Moskowitz: Yes, all these studies were done acutely and the effect lasted for about an hour. After chronic daily administration, the blockade lasted three to four hours. Valproate levels build up in tissues and perhaps this is the difference between the acute and prophylactic situation.

Schoenen: Is administration of valproic acid simultaneous with the ganglion stimulation?

Moskowitz: Valproate was given intraperitoneally 15 or 20 minutes before stimulation. Progesterone we gave a couple of hours before.

Schoenen: And pharmacologically is this sufficient to have GABA transaminase inhibition and increased GABA levels?

Goadsby: There are other things that valproate does: it acts on the voltage-dependent calcium channels in thalamus.

Moskowitz: The pharmacological evidence is quite strong that this is a GABA$_A$-mediated mechanism. The response is sensitive to the administration of progesterone metabolites, muscimol and bicuculline, but not GABA$_B$ receptor agonists and antagonists.

Ferrari: What is the role of the GABA receptor in any relationship between migraine and epilepsy?

Moskowitz: A receptor has its identity by virtue of where it is located and what it is coupled to, and so forth. Just because GABA happens to be an interesting chemical and receptor from the point of view of epilepsy does not necessarily tie the two together. The actions would seem, based on what we are looking at, to be quite independent. I would not use that evidence necessarily to link migraine and epilepsy.

Ferrari: You emphasized that the chloride ion is involved. Would that be another therapeutic approach?

Moskowitz: You mean drugs that increase or decrease chloride ion conductance. One problem with dealing with the GABA receptor is that the $GABA_A$ direct agonists, the muscimol-type compounds, have lots of side-effects. But that does not seem to be as much of a limitation with the allosteric modulators, mainly because they potentiate endogenous GABA rather than mimic the action of the endogenous ligand. There are more than 50 analogues of these steroids that are active at $GABA_A$ receptors. It might be possible to find a very potent benzodiazepine that could work in this way without causing hypnosis. Those might be preferred directions at present, rather than looking for a $GABA_A$ receptor agonist.

REFERENCES

Aloe, L., Alleva, E., Böhm, A. and Levi-Montalcini, R. (1986) Aggressive behaviour induces release of nerve growth factor from mouse salivary gland into the bloodstream. *Proceedings of the National Academy of Sciences USA*, **83**, 6184–6187.

Saudou, F., Amara, D.A., Dierich, A., LeMeur, M., Ramboz, S., Segu, L., Bukot, M.D. and Hen R. (1994) Enhanced aggressive behaviour in mice lacking 5-HT$_{1B}$ receptor. *Science*, **265**, 1875–1878.

13

The role of nitric oxide in migraine pain

Lars Lykke Thomsen and Jes Olesen

In 1980 Furchgott and Zawadzki reported that vasodilatation induced by acetylcholine depends on the presence of intact endothelium. The mediator of this endothelium-dependent vasodilatation was later identified as nitric oxide (NO), which had previously been considered to be merely an atmospheric pollutant (Palmer *et al.* 1987). Since then the biology of this small and short-lived messenger molecule has been increasingly and intensively investigated. Much is now known about the biology of NO and an increasing volume of evidence suggests that it plays a pivotal role in migraine pain (for reviews see Olesen *et al.* 1994, 1995, Thomsen *et al.* 1994a). Here we draw on our experiences with two experimental human headache models – intravenous infusion of glyceryl trinitrate (GTN, a donor of NO) and intravenous infusion of histamine (which probably activates endothelial NO formation) – to focus on nitric oxide mechanisms in migraine. We also provide evidence supporting the view that activation of the NO cascade of reactions is a common final pathway for headache induced by several other substances.

THE BIOLOGY OF NO

The highly reactive free radical NO is a lipophilic gas of formula $\cdot N = O$ (Kiechle and Malinski 1993). Its half-life is reported to be very short, in the range of 5–30s under bioassay conditions (Palmer *et al.* 1987, Kiechle

Migraine: Pharmacology and genetics
Edited by Merton Sandler, Michel Ferrari and Sara Harnett
Published in 1996 by Chapman & Hall
ISBN 1 86036 006 8

and Malinski 1993). NO is rapidly converted to nitrogen dioxide (NO_2) which again rapidly forms the more stable metabolites nitrite (NO_2^-) and nitrate (NO_3^-) (Wennmalm and Peterson 1991). NO is generated from the terminal guanidino nitrogen of L-arginine. The family of enzymes catalysing NO synthesis are known as NO synthases (NOS) (Knowles and Moncada 1994). NOS activity has been reported in many tissues, including endothelium, brain, peripheral nerves, vascular smooth muscle, myocardium, macrophages, neutrophils and microglia of several species (Kiechle and Malinski 1993). Purification and cloning of NOS has revealed the existence of at least three isoforms (Knowles and Moncada 1994). Two of these are constitutive and Ca^{++}/calmodulin dependent. One releases nitric oxide from endothelium (eNOS), the other from neurons (nNOS). This release is accelerated in response to stimulation of several specific membrane-bound receptors by glutamate, bradykinin, 5-hydroxytryptamine (5-HT), acetylcholine, histamine, endothelin-1, substance P (SP) and probably calcitonin gene-related peptide (CGRP) (Lüscher and Vanhoutte 1990, Garthwaite 1993, Gray and Marshall 1992, Toda 1990, Glusa and Richter 1993, De Nucci *et al.* 1988). Increased flow velocity and the subsequent increase of shear stress in endothelial cells may also stimulate eNOS (Lüscher and Vanhoutte 1990) (Figure 13.1). The third isoform of NO synthase is inducible and Ca^{++} independent (iNOS). iNOS generates nitric oxide for long periods and in large amounts in response to endotoxins and cytokines (Stuehr *et al.* 1991, Busse and Mülsch 1990, Wallace and Bisland 1994). Most physiological actions of NO are mediated via activation of soluble guanylate cyclase (sGC) and a consequent increase in cyclic guanosine monophosphate (cGMP) eventually leading to a decrease in intracellular Ca^{++} in target cells (Moncada *et al.* 1991, Mayer 1994) (Figure 13.1).

PHYSIOLOGY OF NO RELEVANT TO MIGRAINE

Nitric oxide has a large number of physiological effects throughout the body, several of which could be implicated in the pathophysiology of migraine. Thus, endothelium-dependent vasodilatation is of importance in cerebrovascular regulation, and neurogenic vasodilatation may be mediated via perivascular nerves (non-adrenergic non-cholinergic (NANC) nerves) which operate through nitric oxide. Furthermore, NO mediates neurotransmision in the central nervous system, which is important for pain perception (hyperalgesia). NO may contribute to sensory transmission in peripheral nerves. Also, NO contributes to the control of platelets and, when produced in large amounts, NO contributes to host defence reactions of importance in non-specific immunity and neurotoxicity (Moncada *et al.* 1991). Finally, NO may

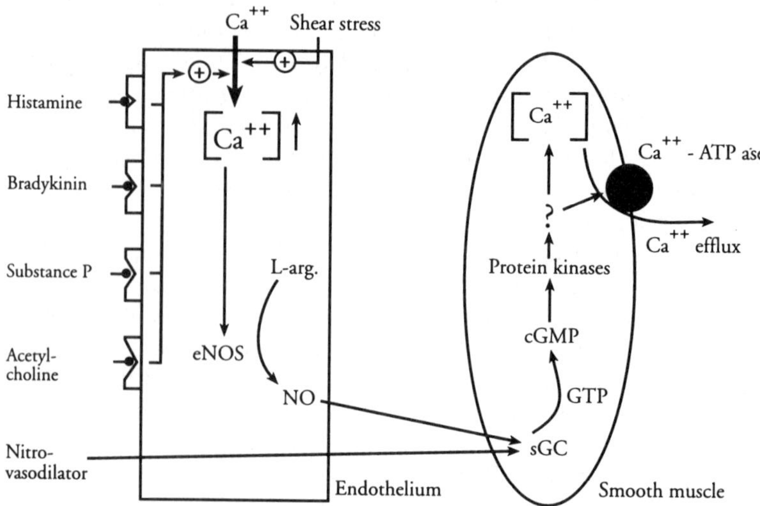

Figure 13.1 Molecular events in the nitric oxide pathway illustrated by endothelium-derived synthesis of nitric oxide (NO). Endothelium nitric oxide synthase (eNOS) is stimulated by an increase in intracellular calcium. NO diffuses from endothelial cells to smooth muscle cells and activates the soluble guanylate cyclase (sGC). This in turn leads to an increase in cyclic guanosine monophosphate (cGMP) and, via activation of protein kinases and subsequent poorly understood intermediary processes, stimulates the membrane bound Ca^{++}-ATPase. Ca^{++} diffuses out of the cell, eventually leading to smooth muscle relaxation and vasodilation. Nitrovasodilators act as NO donors and activate the same pathway.

release CGRP from perivascular nerve endings and may thus play a role in neurogenic inflammatory reactions (Wei *et al.* 1992).

EXPERIMENTAL HUMAN HEADACHE MODELS SUITABLE FOR THE STUDY OF NO MECHANISMS IN MIGRAINE

Histamine and glyceryl trinitrate (GTN) reliably and dose dependently produce headache in normal volunteers and migraine sufferers (Krabbe and Olesen 1980, Iversen *et al.* 1989a, Olesen *et al.* 1993). GTN itself has no known action in the human body but acts via liberation of NO and is thus generally regarded as a NO donor (Ignarro *et al.* 1981, Gruetter *et al.* 1981, Feelisch and Noack 1987). GTN is the most suitable substance for experimental studies of NO-induced headache as it is well tolerated and diffuses freely across membranes because of its lipid solubility. It may thus deliver NO to several tissues, including those protected by the blood–brain barrier. That GTN induces headache by liberating NO is supported by the following evidence: (a) GTN-induced headache in normal controls is very short lived and is unlikely to be caused by metabolites other than NO, since these have a longer half-life (Iversen *et al.* 1989a); (b) The long-acting nitrate 5-isosorbide-mononitrate (5-ISMN) induces a dose-dependent headache and arterial dilatation, but its metabolites apart from NO are different from those of GTN (Iversen *et al.* 1992); and (c) N-Acetylcysteine, which augments GTN effects in the heart by increasing the formation of NO or by enhancing the effect of NO itself, also augments the headache response to GTN and prolongs GTN-induced arterial dilatation of the superficial temporal artery but not of the radial arteries (Iversen 1992). Histamine also seems to induce headache via NO. In human cerebral blood vessels histamine stimulates an endothelial H_1 receptor which activates NOS (Toda 1990, Ottosen *et al.* 1991). Histamine thus stimulates the endogenous formation of NO whereas GTN delivers NO directly (Figure 13.1). The next question is: how relevant are these observations for migraine?

NO HYPERSENSITIVITY IN MIGRAINE

Previous studies have suggested that migraine patients experience a migraine-like headache in association with administration of GTN more often than non-migraineurs (Sicuteri *et al.* 1987). Controlled double-blind trials have confirmed that, with a delay of several hours (peak intensity 5.5 hours after infusion) migraineurs do develop a genuine migraine attack after GTN infusion (Olesen *et al.* 1993, Thomsen *et al.* 1994b) (Figure 13.2). This migraine headache is preceded by an immediate headache response during the infusion, resembling but not fulfilling International Headache Society (IHS) diagnostic criteria for migraine without aura (Headache Classification Committee 1988). This immediate response is seen in non-migraineurs, but is more severe in migraineurs (Olesen *et al.* 1993) (Figure 13.3). Thus, migraineurs are hypersensitive to GTN-induced headache and probably, therefore, to nitric oxide. An increased headache response could, however, reflect a greater general sensitivity to pain, or could be due to increased physiological sensitivity to nitric oxide. It is known that GTN dilates the middle cerebral artery via NO without affecting cerebral blood flow and thereby the arterioles (Dahl *et al.* 1989, Iversen *et al.* 1989b). Applying the ultrasound technique Transcranial Doppler (Thomsen and Iversen 1993), which provides an indirect measure of large intracranial artery diameters in situations of unchanged blood flow (Busija *et al.* 1981, Dahl *et al.* 1989, Iversen *et al.* 1989b, Friberg *et al.* 1991), we examined whether the increased sensitivity to the nitric oxide donor was reflected not only in increased headache in migraineurs but also in increased dilatation of the middle cerebral artery. Migraineurs were found to be more sensitive

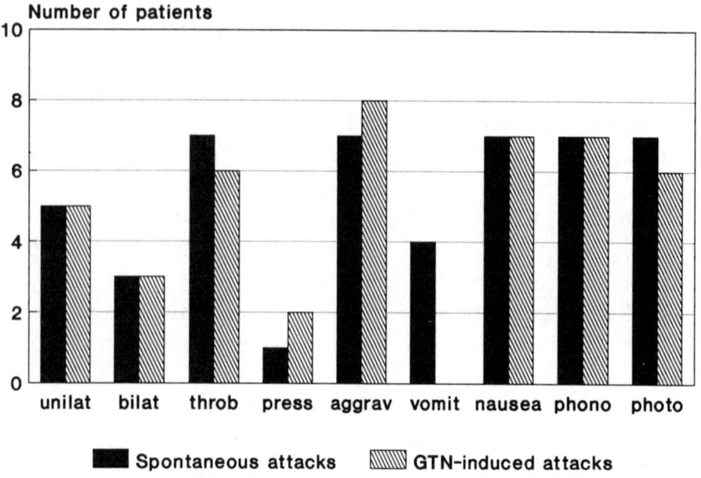

Figure 13.2 Clinical characteristics of glyceryl trinitrate (GTN) induced migraine. A comparison between spontaneous and GTN-induced migraine in eight out of ten migraine patients who developed migraine after GTN infusion (0.5 μg/kg/min for 20 min) is illustrated. The peak intensity of GTN-induced migraine occurred on average 5.5 hours after start of infusion. (Data from Thomsen *et al.* 1994b.) unilat, unilateral; bilat, bilateral; throb, throbbing; press, pressing; aggrav, aggravated by physical activity; phono, phonophobia; photo, photophobia.

in this respect as well (Figure 13.4). During a three hour observation period the time profile of the GTN-induced middle cerebral artery dilatation corresponded with the headache response (Thomsen *et al.* 1993, 1994b). Furthermore, a decreased collagen-induced platelet aggregation in combination with increased platelet arginine levels in migraineurs supports the view that migraineurs are supersensitive to physiological effects of NO (D'Andrea *et al.* 1994).

Migraineurs have been found to be hypersensitive to histamine in controlled trials (Krabbe and Olesen 1980, De-Marinis *et al.* 1990). The headache induced by histamine was almost completely blocked by the histamine H_1-blocker mepyramine whereas the H_2-blocker cimetidine only had a small effect (Krabbe and Olesen 1980). As mentioned above, activation of endothelial H_1 receptors induces the formation of nitric oxide (Toda 1990). Thus, the increased sensitivity to histamine in migraineurs may also be explained by hypersensitivity to activation of the NO pathway, and activation of this pathway is likely to be a final common pathway for the headache and arterial dilatation induced by

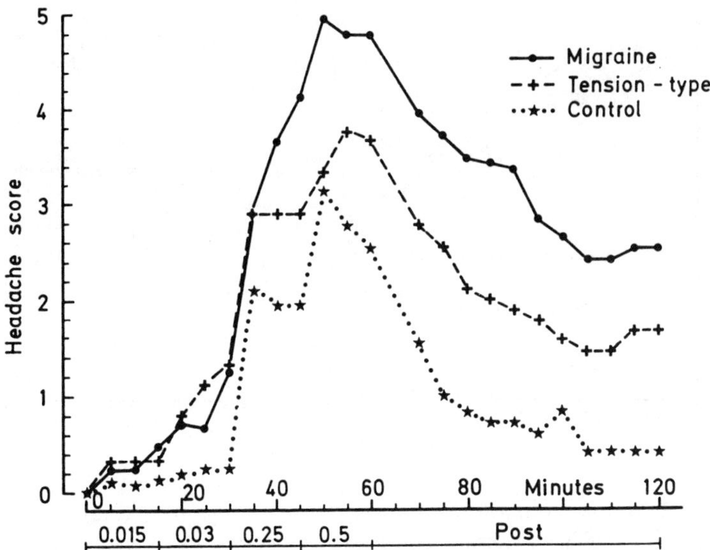

Figure 13.3 Headache intensity over time during four different doses (0.015, 0.03, 0.25, 0.5 μg/kg/min, each given for 15 min) of glyceryl trinitrate. Comparison of responses in migraineurs (n = 17), tension-type headache sufferers (n = 9) and healthy subjects (n = 17). During doses above 0.015 μg/kg/ min migraine patients experienced significantly more headache than controls ($p < 0.05$ Kruskal Wallis and multiple range test). (From Olesen *et al.* 1993, with permission.)

both histamine and GTN. Further evidence for the latter comes from the finding that GTN-induced headache could not be prevented by blocking histamine H_1 receptors, which indicates that the final common mechanism of histamine- and GTN-induced headache is not explained by histamine release after GTN infusion (Iversen and Olesen 1994).

NITRIC OXIDE: A FINAL COMMON PATHWAY FOR SEVERAL HEADACHE-INDUCING SUBSTANCES

Other substances that have been shown to reliably cause more headache than placebo in single-dose experiments, including reserpine, *m*-chlorophenylpiperazine (*m*-CPP) and, less convincingly, prostacyclin and hypoxia, may cause headache via NO (Olesen *et al.* 1995). The best known example of hypoxic headache is high-altitude headache. However, no formal study of the effects of hypoxia in migraine sufferers is available. Arregui *et al.* (1991) showed a greatly increased migraine prevalence in people living at high altitude. Hypoxia increases longevity

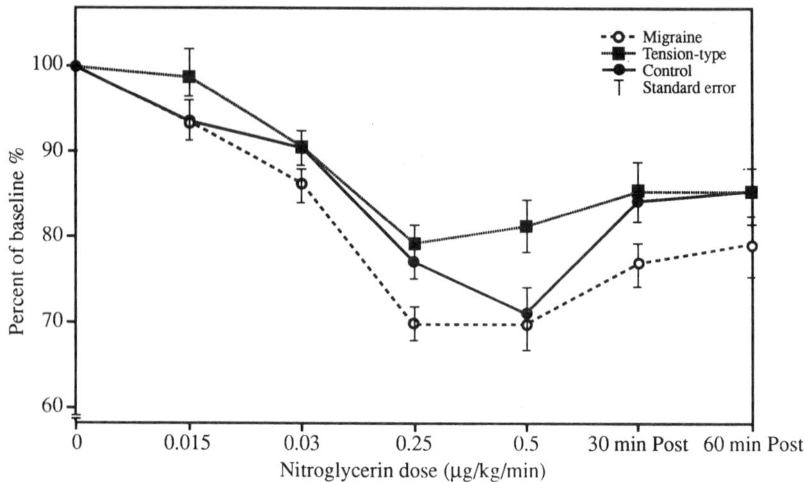

Figure 13.4 Middle cerebral artery responses during four different doses of glyceryl trinitrate (GTN). Comparison between responses in migraineurs ($n = 17$), tension-type headache sufferers ($n = 9$) and healthy subjects ($n = 17$). Migraineurs showed the most pronounced response ($p < 0.05$, ANOVA). A decrease in blood velocity indicates an increase in vessel area because cerebral blood flow is unchanged during GTN infusion. (From Olesen *et al.* 1994, with permission.)

of NO whereas pure oxygen acts as a NO scavenger, reducing the lifetime and thereby the effect of NO (Rengasamy and Johns 1991). Hypoxic vascular headache and hypoxia-induced migraine may thus be due to increased spontaneous NO concentration. Prostacyclin has been shown in one study to cause headache in migraineurs (Peatfield *et al.* 1981). Prostacyclin is a vasodilatator and may act directly on smooth muscle receptors, but in cerebral vessels protected by the blood–brain barrier is more likely to act via endothelial receptors by liberating NO (Lüscher and Vanhoutte 1990). In migraineurs reserpine has been shown to cause headache with some migrainous features (Lance 1991). Reserpine depletes not only platelets but also presynaptic nerve terminals of their content of monoamines. Substances released include 5-HT. The 5-HT$_{2C}$ (formerly 5-HT$_{1C}$) receptor has been suggested to play a crucial role in the initiation of migraine attacks (Fozard and Kalkman 1994). 5-HT caused an endothelium-dependent relaxing response in a number of vessels from different species, and this effect was mediated via the 5-HT$_{2C}$ receptor. The vascular response to 5-HT$_{2C}$ activation, at least in the pig, is primarily a consequence of the release of NO (Glusa and Richter 1993). *m*-CPP is a direct agonist at the 5-HT$_{2c}$ receptor and, therefore, is likely to cause vascular headache via NO synthesis (Fozard and Kalkman 1994). We conclude that NO is a likely common denominator for headaches induced by GTN, histamine, reserpine, *m*-CPP, prostacyclin and hypoxia (Olesen *et al.* 1995).

MECHANISMS OF NO-INDUCED MIGRAINE

Several neurotransmitters in brain tissue, periarterial cerebral nerves and blood stimulate the formation of NO in brain neurons and arterial endothelium and possibly also interact with NOS-containing nerve terminals (Lüscher and Vanhoutte 1990, Moncada *et al.* 1991, Garthwaite *et al.* 1988). Thus, fluctuations in neurotransmitter concentration in both brain and blood may trigger migraine headache in migraine patients because of their supersensitivity to nitric oxide. Formation of nitric oxide may also be elicited by pathological reactions such as: (a) spreading depression of Leão (Goadsby *et al.* 1992); (b) activation of the trigeminovascular system with liberation of, for example, substance P; and (c) fever and inflammation via interleukins and histamine, *etc.* (Olesen *et al.* 1994). At present it is not known in further detail how activation of the NO pathway causes migraine headache. Dilatation of large intra- and extracranial arteries may be involved because: (a) arterial dilatation is induced by NO liberated from endothelium and probably perivascular nerve endings (Moncada *et al.* 1991); (b) cephalic vaso-dilatation has been reported during spontaneous migraine headache (Iversen *et al.* 1990, Friberg *et al.* 1991, Thomsen *et al.* 1995); (c) mechanical dilatation of intracranial arteries causes referred pain in the areas where most patients feel their pain during migraine attacks (Nichols *et al.* 1990); and (d) agents such as ergotamine, dihydro-ergotamine (DHE) and sumatriptan which constrict arteries (but not arterioles) are effective in the treatment of the acute migraine attack. On the other hand, the moderate mechanical arterial dilatation reported during migraine attacks may not be enough to cause severe pain. Another possibility is central pain-modulating effects of nitric oxide. Direct activation of perivascular sensory nerve fibres and/or initiation of perivascular neurogenic inflammation (Moskowitz 1993) by nitric oxide are possible mechanisms. The direct noxious and cytotoxic effect of nitric oxide should also be considered. Whatever is true, it is striking that nitric oxide causes migraine with a delay of up to several hours (Thomsen *et al.* 1994b), a time course which mimics the slow development of migraine pain often seen during spontaneous migraine attacks. As mentioned, NO is an unstable free radical with a very short half-life. Other mediators or mechanisms therefore seem to be involved in the rather slow cascade of events set up by activation of the nitric oxide pathway and eventually leading to a migraine attack. The elucidation of these mechanisms and of steps further down the NO-activated cascade of reactions is a fascinating challenge likely to provide new therapeutic approaches to migraine.

Acknowledgements

We thank the University of Copenhagen and the Danish Migraine Society for financial support.

REFERENCES

Arregui, A., Carera, J., Leon-Velarde, F., Paredes, S., Viscarra, D. and Arbaiza, D. (1991) High prevalence of migraine in high-altitude population. *Neurology*, **41**, 1668–1669.

Busija, D.W., Heistad, D.D. and Marcus, M.L. (1981) Continuous measurements of cerebral blood flow in anesthetized cats and dogs. *American Journal of Physiology*, **241**, H228–H234.

Busse, R. and Mülsch, A. (1990) Induction of nitric oxide synthase by cytokines in vascular smooth muscle cells. *FEBS Letters*, **275**, 87–90.

Dahl, A., Russell, D., Nyberg-Hansen, R. and Rootwell, K. (1989) Effect of nitroglycerin on cerebral circulation measured by transcranial Doppler and SPECT. *Stroke*, **20**, 1733–1736.

D'Andrea, G., Cananzi, A.R., Perini, F., Alecci, F., Zamberlan, L., Hasselmark, L. and Welch, K.M.A. (1994) Decreased collagen-induced platelet aggregation and increased arginine levels in migraine: a possible link with the NO pathway. *Cephalalgia*, **14**, 352–357.

De-Marinis, M., Feliciani, M., Janiri, L., Cerbo, R. and Agnoli, A. (1990) Increased reactivity to a met-enkephalin analog in the control of autonomic responses in migraine patients. *Clinical Neuropharmacology*, **13**, 507–521.

De Nucci, G., Thomas, R., D'Orleans-Juste, P., Antunes, E., Walder, C., Warner, T.D. and Vane, J.R. (1988) Pressor effects of circulating endothelin are limited by its removal in the pulmonary circulation and by the release of prostacyclin and endothelium derived relaxing factor. *Proceedings of the National Academy of Sciences USA*, **85**, 9797–9800.

Feelisch, M. and Noack, E.A. (1987) Correlation between nitric oxide formation during degradation of organic nitrates and activation of guanylate cyclase. *European Journal of Pharmacology*, **139**, 19–30.

Fozard, J.R. and Kalkman, H.O. (1994) 5-Hydroxytryptamine (5-HT) and the initiation of migraine: new perspectives. *Naunyn-Schmiedeberg's Archives of Pharmacology*, **350**, 225–229.

Friberg, L., Olesen, J., Iversen, H.K. and Sperling, B. (1991) Migraine pain associated with middle cerebral artery dilatation: reversal by sumatriptan. *Lancet*, **338**, 13–17.

Furchgott, R.F. and Zawadzki, J.V. (1980) The obligatory role of endothelial cells in the relaxation of arterial smooth muscle by acetylcholine. *Nature*, **288**, 373–376.

Garthwaite, J. (1993) Nitric oxide signalling in the nervous system. *The Neurosciences*, **5**, 171–180.

Garthwaite, J., Charles, S.L. and Chess-Williams, R. (1988) Endothelium-derived relaxing factor release on activation of NMDA receptors suggests a role as intercellular messenger in the brain. *Nature*, **336**, 385–388.

Glusa, E. and Richter, M. (1993) Endothelium-dependent relaxation of porcine pulmonary arteries via 5-HT$_{1C}$-like receptors. *Naunyn-Schmiedeberg's Archives of Pharmacology*, **347**, 471–477.

Goadsby, P.J., Kaube, H. and Hoskin, K.L. (1992) Nitric oxide synthesis couples cerebral blood flow and metabolism. *Brain Research*, **595**, 167–170.

Gray, D.W. and Marshall, I. (1992) Human alpha-calcitonin gene-related peptide stimulates adenylate cyclase and guanylate cyclase and relaxes rat thoracic aorta by releasing nitric oxide. *British Journal of Pharmacology*, **107**, 691–696.

Gruetter, C.A., Kadowitz, P.J. and Ignarro, L.J. (1981) Methylene blue inhibits coronary arterial relaxation and guanylate cyclase activation by nitroglycerin, sodium nitrate and amyl nitrate. *Canadian Journal of Physiology and Pharmacology*, **59**, 150–156.

Headache Classification Committee of the International Headache Society (J. Olesen *et al.*) (1988) Classification and diagnostic criteria for headache disorders, cranial neuralgias and facial pain. *Cephalalgia*, **8** (Suppl. 7), 1–97.

Ignarro, L.J., Lipton, H., Edwards, J.C., Baricos, W.H., Hyman, A.L., Kadowitz, P.J. and Gruetter, C.A. (1981) Mechanisms of vascular smooth muscle relaxation by organic nitrates, nitrites, nitroprusside and nitric oxide: evidence for the involvement of S-nitrosothiols as active intermediates. *Journal of Pharmacology and Experimental Therapeutics*, **218**, 739–749.

Iversen, H.K. (1992) N-acetylcysteine enhances nitroglycerin-induced headache and cranial arterial responses. *Clinical Pharmacology and Therapeutics*, **52**, 125–133.

Iversen, H.K. and Olesen, J. (1994) Nitroglycerin-induced headache is not dependent on histamine release. Support for a direct nociceptive action of nitric oxide. *Cephalalgia*, **14**, 437–442.

Iversen, H.K., Olesen, J. and Tfelt-Hansen, P. (1989a) Intravenous nitroglycerin as an experimental model of vascular headache. Basic Characteristics. *Pain*, **38**, 17–24.

Iversen, H.K., Holm, S. and Friberg, L. (1989b) Intracranial hemodynamics during intravenous nitroglycerin infusion. *Cephalalgia*, **9** (Suppl. 10), 84–85.

Iversen, H.K., Nielsen, T.H., Olesen, J. and Tfelt-Hansen, P. (1990) Arterial responses during migraine headache. *Lancet*, **336**, 837–839.

Iversen, H.K., Nielsen, T.H., Garre, K., Tfelt-Hansen, P. and Olesen, J. (1992) Dose-dependent headache response and dilatation of limb and extracranial arteries after three doses of 5-isosorbide-mononitrate. *European Journal of Clinical Pharmacology*, **42**, 31–35.

Kiechle, F.L. and Malinski, T. (1993) Nitric oxide biochemistry, pathophysiology and detection. *American Journal of Clinical Pathology*, **100**, 567–575.

Knowles, R.G. and Moncada, S. (1994) Nitric oxide synthases in mammals. *Biochemical Journal*, **298**, 249–258.

Krabbe, A.E. and Olesen, J. (1980) Headache provocation by continuous intravenous infusion of histamine. Clinical results and receptor mechanisms. *Pain*, **8**, 253–259.

Lance, J.W. (1991) 5-Hydroxytryptamine and its role in migraine. *European Neurology*, **31**, 279–281.

Lüscher, T.F. and Vanhoutte, P.M. (1990) *The Endothelium: Modulator of Cardiovascular Functions*. CRC Press, Ann Abor, Boston.

Mayer, B. (1994) Regulation of nitric oxide synthase and soluble guanylyl cyclase. *Cell Biochemistry and Function*, **12**, 167–177.

Moncada, S., Palmer, R.M.J. and Higgs, E.A. (1991) Nitric oxide: physiology, pathophysiology and pharmacology. *Pharmacological Reviews*, **43**, 109–142.

Moskowitz, M.A. (1993) Neurogenic inflammation in the pathophysiology and treatment of migraine. *Neurology*, **43** (Suppl. 3), S16-S20.

Nichols, F.T. III, Mawad, M., Mohr, J.P., Stein, B., Hilal, S. and Michelsen, J. (1990) Focal headache during balloon inflation in the internal carotid and middle cerebral arteries. *Stroke*, **21**, 555–559.

Olesen, J., Iversen, H.K. and Thomsen, L.L. (1993) Nitric oxide supersensitivity. A possible molecular mechanism of migraine pain. *NeuroReport*, **4**, 1027–1030.

Olesen, J., Thomsen, L.L. and Iversen, H.K. (1994) Nitric oxide is a key molecule in migraine and other vascular headaches. *Trends in Pharmacological Sciences*, **15**, 149–153.

Olesen, J., Thomsen, L.L., Lassen, L.H. and Jansen-Olesen, I. (1995) The nitric oxide hypothesis of migraine and other vascular headaches. *Cephalalgia*, **15**, 94–100.

Ottosen, A.L.P., Jansen, I., Langemark, M., Olesen, J. and Edvinsson L. (1991) Histamine receptors in the isolated human middle meningeal artery. A comparison with cerebral and temporal arteries. *Cephalalgia*, **11**, 183–188.

Palmer, R.M.J., Ferrige, A.G. and Moncada, S. (1987) Nitric oxide release accounts for the biological activity of endothelium-derived relaxing factor. *Nature*, **327**, 524–526.

Peatfield, R.C., Gawel, M.J., and Clifford Rose, F. (1981) The effect of infused prostacyclin in migraine and cluster headache. *Headache*, **21**, 190–195.

Rengasamy, A. and Johns, R.A. (1991) Characterization of endothelium-derived relaxing factor/nitric oxide synthase from bovine cerebellum and mechanism of modulation by high and low oxygen tensions. *Journal of Pharmacology and Experimental Therapeutics*, **259**, 310–316.

Sicuteri, F., Del Bene, E., Poggioni, M. and Bonazzi, A. (1987) Unmasking latent dysnociception in healthy subjects. *Headache*, **27**, 180–185.

Stuehr, D.J., Cho H.J., Kwon N.S., Weise, M.F. Nathan, C.F. (1991) Purification and characterization of the cytokine-induced macrophage nitric oxide synthase: an FAD- and FMN-containing flavoprotein. *Proceedings of the National Academy of Sciences USA*, **88**, 7773–7777.

Thomsen, L.L. and Iversen, H.K. (1993) Experimental and biological variation of the three dimensional transcranial doppler measurements. *Journal of Applied Physiology*, **75**, 2805–2810.

Thomsen, L.L., Iversen, H.K., Brinck, T.A. and Olesen, J. (1993) Arterial supersensitivity to nitric oxide (nitroglycerin) in migraine sufferers. *Cephalalgia*, **13**, 395–399.

Thomsen, L.L., Iversen, H.K., Lassen, L.H. and Olesen, J. (1994a) The role of nitric oxide in migraine pain: therapeutic implications. *CNS Drugs*, **2**, 417–422.

Thomsen, L.L., Kruuse, C., Iversen, H.K. and Olesen, J. (1994b) A nitric oxide donor (nitroglycerin) triggers genuine migraine attacks. *European Journal of Neurology*, **1**, 73–80.

Thomsen, L.L., Iversen, H.K. and Olesen, J. (1995) Cerebral blood flow velocities are reduced during attacks of unilateral migraine without aura. *Cephalalgia*, **15**, 109–116.

Toda, N. (1990) Mechanism underlying responses to histamine of isolated monkey and human cerebral arteries. *American Journal of Physiology*, **258**, H311-H317.

Wallace, M.N. and Bisland, S.K. (1994) NADPH-diaphorase activity in activated astrocytes represents inducible nitric oxide synthase. *Neuroscience*, **59**, 905–919.

Wei, E.P., Moskowitz, M.A., Baccalini, P. and Kontos, H.A. (1992) Calcitonin gene related peptide mediates nitroglycerin and sodium nitroprusside induced vasodilation in feline cerebral arterioles. *Circulation Research*, **70**, 1313–1319.

Wennmalm, Å. and Peterson, A. (1991) Analysis of nitrite as a marker for endothelium-derived relaxing factor in biological fluids using electron paramagnetic resonance spectrometry. *Journal of Cardiovascular Pharmacology*, **17**, S34-S40.

DISCUSSION

Connor: Goadsby *et al.* (1990) reported that during a migraine headache there is an increase in calcitonin gene-related peptide (CGRP) within the external jugular vein. Is there an increase in CGRP during the late phase of the headache induced by nitroglycerin?

Thomsen: We are examining this. At the moment we are concentrating on the delayed headache response, but we do not have the data yet.

Moskowitz: Nitric oxide is involved in many different tissue reactions. What led you to focus on the coupling of nitric oxide and cyclic-GMP production, via guanylate cyclase activation?

Thomsen: It is known that nitric oxide-induced smooth muscle dilatation is mediated via this guanylate cyclase system. Both histamine and nitroglycerin are capable of inducing vasodilatation and migraine attacks. Histamine does not pass the blood–brain barrier, and seems to cause both vasodilatation and headache via H_1 receptor activation. H_1 receptors are known to be present particularly in intracranial endothelium and activation of these receptors causes activation of the NO–cGMP pathway.

Moskowitz: But why have you excluded other reaction products? You have not yet characterized the later headache which is so interesting and important.

Thomsen: I am simply saying that the initiation of the attack, at least the histamine-induced attack, seems to involve the endothelial H_1 receptor and subsequent activation of the nitric oxide–cGMP pathway. In the delayed headache response, many things could happen in between. It could be that the blood–brain barrier is broken, or it could be neurogenic inflammation mechanisms set off by nitric oxide.

Moskowitz: Charles Sherrington's definition of pain, accepted for almost 100 years, and perhaps even today, was the presence of real or threatened tissue injury. Since NO is thought to play a role as a cytotoxic agent, I wonder whether you might wish to consider mechanisms related to peroxynitrite anion and free radical formation which could then unify NO with the concept of real or threatened tissue injury.

Thomsen: I agree with you regarding the delayed headache response. We have to be very open-minded here, but I still think that there might be an association between the initiation of the induced attack and an involvement of vascular smooth muscle and this cGMP pathway.

Glover: Migraine attacks often end in diuresis and this might explain that if NO is acting via atriol natriuretic peptide receptors. I wonder if nitroglycerin causes diuresis.

Thomsen: We do not see excessive diuresis with nitroglycerin. Patients are able to lie still for three hours without asking to urinate.

Ferrari: Have you done experiments with patients on chronic pretreatment with migraine prophylactic drugs?

Thomsen: No, but we should.

Goadsby: Had any of your patients had aura previously, and do either of these stimuli ever cause aura?

Thomsen: We have not provoked anybody suffering from migraine with aura; they all suffered from migraine without aura.

Schoenen: Why do you link the first headache, which is apparently a vascular headache and is also provoked in normal subjects, to the delayed migraine attack?

Thomsen: From the histamine data, I would like to draw a link, but we don't know anything yet about the mechanisms of the delayed headache response. The characteristic factor must be what is set up by this triggering mechanism.

REFERENCE

Goadsby, P.J., Edvinsson, L. and Ekman, R. (1990) Vasoactive peptide release in the extracerebral circulation of humans during migraine headache. *Annals of Neurology*, **38**, 183-187.

14

5-Hydroxytryptamine and nitric oxide: the causal relationship between two endogenous precipitants of migraine

J.R. Fozard

INTRODUCTION

The most common factors claimed to precipitate migraine are stress in various forms, dietary considerations and, for women, hormonal events. However, few controlled trials have been carried out to verify such claims and the underlying mechanism(s) remain unexplained. In contrast, several drugs with well-defined pharmacological properties are able consistently to trigger (or alleviate) migraine. Analysis of these properties coupled with clinical biochemical evidence points strongly to a sudden release of 5-hydroxytryptamine (5-HT, serotonin) with subsequent activation of the 5-HT_{2B} receptor subtype as a key factor in the initiation of migraine. Moreover, the mechanims may involve the release of nitric oxide (NO) from the endothelial cells of the cerebral vasculature. This chapter reviews the evidence for this scenario. Since the basic theme has evolved over several years and been repeatedly reviewed (Fozard 1982, 1985, 1990, 1992, 1995, Fozard and Gray 1989, Kalkman 1994, Fozard and Kalkman 1994), emphasis will be placed on recent evidence implicating the 5-HT_{2B} receptor subtype and the

Migraine: Pharmacology and genetics
Edited by Merton Sandler, Michel Ferrari and Sara Harnett
Published in 1996 by Chapman & Hall
ISBN 1 86036 006 8

involvement of NO from the craniovascular endothelial cells in the initiation of migraine.

THE CASE FOR 5-HYDROXYTRYPTAMINE

Direct evidence that endogenous 5-HT is mobilized in migraine includes the observations that platelet 5-HT concentrations fall at the onset of an attack and that the urinary excretion of 5-hydroxyindoleacetic acid is increased in most patients. That an increase in 5-HT function rather than a deficit predisposes to migraine is indicated by the fact that attacks can be triggered by agents that release and/or block the uptake of 5-HT (reserpine, fenfluramine, zimelidine, viloxazine, femoxetine). In contrast, patients are generally protected in the depletion phase following a natural attack or administration of reserpine or uptake inhibitors and by prophylactic treatment by 5-HT receptor antagonists such as methysergide and pizotifen (see Fozard 1982, 1985, 1990).

THE CASE FOR INVOLVEMENT OF 5-HT$_{2B}$ RECEPTORS

In their original hypothesis, Fozard and Gray implicated the 5-HT$_{1C}$ receptor in the initiation of migraine (Fozard and Gray 1989). The evidence came from two sources. First, 1-(m-chlorophenyl)piperazine (m-CPP), a major metabolite of the antidepressant trazodone, induces migraine in humans (Brewerton *et al.* 1988); both the dose administered and the peak plasma concentrations are within the range of those which selectively activate 5-HT$_{1C}$ receptors (Fozard 1992). Second, several drugs effective at low doses in migraine prophylaxis (e.g. methysergide and pizotifen) have in common high affinity for, and antagonist effects at, 5-HT$_{1C}$ receptors (Fozard 1990, 1992). A revision of 5-HT receptor nomenclature (Hoyer *et al.* 1994) led to the reclassification of 5-HT$_{1C}$ receptors as 5-HT$_{2C}$ receptors and their inclusion, along with the 5-HT$_{2A}$ and 5-HT$_{2B}$ receptor subtypes, into the 5-HT$_2$ receptor family.

In a perceptive analysis, Kalkman (1994) pointed out that the 'pharmacological' arguments put forward to support 5-HT$_{2C}$ receptor involvement in the initiation of migraine hold equally well for the 5-HT$_{2B}$ receptor. Thus, m-CPP has equal or greater affinity for 5-HT$_{2B}$ receptors (Table 14.1) than for 5-HT$_{2C}$ receptors (Fozard 1992, Fozard and Kalkman 1994, Bonhaus *et al.* 1995) and is an agonist (Table 14.1). Further, the daily dose of eight drugs shown to have migraine prophylactic activity correlated highly significantly and marginally better with their antagonist potencies at the rat fundus 5-HT$_{2B}$ receptor than with their affinities for the 5-HT$_{2C}$ receptor (Kalkman 1994). Included in the analysis was propranolol which is one of the most consistently effective prophylactic agents in migraine (Weerasuriya *et al.*

Table 14.1 Activity of l-(*m*-chlorophenyl)piperazine

Cloned rat receptor pK_i	Cloned human receptor pK_i	Rat fundic strip pEC_{50}	Efficacy (% 5-HT)
7.6[a]	7.5[b]	8.1[a]	not given
		7.7[c]	38
		7.8[d]	40

Data from [a]Wainscott *et al.* (1993), [b]Bonhaus *et al.* (1995), [c]Baxter *et al.* (1994), [d]Cohen and Wittenauer (1986)

1982). At the doses used (120–240 mg/day) both peak (6×10^{-7} M) and trough (2×10^{-7} M) plasma concentrations (Walle *et al.* 1978) exceed those required to block 5-HT_{2B} and 5-HT_{2C} receptors (Kalkman 1994, Bodelsson *et al.* 1993). Overall, there is no good reason to favour a 5-HT_{2C} over a 5-HT_{2B} mechanism in the initiation of migraine. For reasons outlined below, the siting of the 5-HT_{2B} receptor on endothelial cells and its link to NO provides a plausible argument in favour of the 5-HT_{2B} site.

THE CASE FOR NITRIC OXIDE

The evidence for NO being involved in the triggering of migraine is summarized by Thomsen and Olesen (this volume). The key finding is that nitroglycerin, an NO donor, induces headache in migraine patients. Headache is slower in onset, more severe and of longer duration than that induced in control subjects and more often fulfils the diagnostic criteria for migraine. Broadly similar findings have been reported following infusion of histamine which induces severe headache by activating H_1 receptors (Krabbe and Olesen 1980). As argued in detail by Thomsen and Olesen, the most likely mechanism involved in histamine headache is stimulation of the endogenous formation of NO by activation of endothelial histamine H_1 receptors. NO has many pro-inflammatory and nociceptive properties which could contribute to the initiation and development of migraine headache: a variety of animal data suggests that NO can activate sensory nerve fibres, induce or augment oedema and modify the perception and processing of pain (reviewed in Fozard 1995). Of particular interest is the recent demonstration by Holthusen and Arndt (1994) that nitric oxide evokes pain in humans on intracutaneous injection.

THE LINK BETWEEN 5-HT AND NO

The human 5-HT_{2B} and 5-HT_{2C} receptors have been cloned (Kursar *et al.* 1994, Martin and Boess 1994, Schmuck *et al.* 1994, Bonhaus *et al.* 1995). Despite relatively low homology, the pharmacology and the signal transduction mechanisms of the two receptors are similar (Martin and Boess 1994, Bonhaus *et al.* 1995). Moreover, whilst Northern analysis and/or reverse transcription-polymerase chain reaction reveals a wide tissue distribution of mRNA for both 5-HT_{2B} and 5-HT_{2C} receptors (Bonhaus *et al.* 1995), little insight into their possible involvement in migraine can be gained from such data.

Significantly, however, functional studies reveal receptors with the pharmacological properties of 5-HT_{2B} receptors to be present on the endothelial cells of a wide variety of blood vessels and to mediate vasorelaxation when activated. In rat (Bodelsson *et al.* 1993, Ellis *et al.* 1995) and rabbit (Leff *et al.* 1987, Martin *et al.* 1993) jugular veins, pig vena cava (Sumner 1991) and pig pulmonary artery (Glusa and Richter 1993), 5-HT induces endothelium-dependent relaxant responses at low nM concentrations. Suppression of the responses by inhibitors of NO synthase (Sumner 1991, Glusa and Richter 1993) suggests the receptor stimulates the release of NO. Until recently, no suitable pharmacological tools were available (or recognized) to discriminate between 5-HT_{2B} and 5-HT_{2C} receptors and hence endothelium-mediated vasorelaxation could not be attributed unequivocally to the 5-HT_{2B} site. More recently, the use of both agonist (BW 723C86) and antagonist (yohimbine, SB 20646, SB 204741) ligands with potency and/or a degree of selectivity for 5-HT_{2B} receptors has established that endothelium-dependent relaxation of rat jugular vein is mediated by 5-HT_{2B} receptors (Ellis *et al.* 1995, Baxter *et al.* 1995). A further important point in this context is that the affinity of 5-HT for the 5-HT_{2B} receptor is, at close to 1 nM, some 100-fold higher than its affinity for 5-HT_{2A} or 5-HT_{2C} receptors (Bonhaus *et al.* 1995). The fact that endothelium-dependent relaxation to 5-HT in each of the vessels mentioned above occurs at low nM concentrations would be entirely consistent with their being 5-HT_{2B} receptor mediated.

Emerging *in vitro* and *in vivo* evidence suggests 5-HT_{2B} receptor-mediated endothelium-dependent vasorelaxation occurs in man. Martin (1994) quotes the unpublished finding of J. Angus that the use of BW 723C86 points to the presence of the 5-HT_{2B} receptor on the endothelium of arteries ($\sim$100 μm) taken from human buttock biopsies. Bruning *et al.* (1994) showed marked and sustained NO-dependent vasodilatation following infusion of 5-HT into the human forearm vascular bed. Although an extensive pharmacological evaluation of the response has not been carried out, 5-HT_{1A} receptors are not involved. It is of interest that the response could be blocked by tropisetron but not by other potent and highly selective 5-HT_3 antagonists such as ondansetron and granisetron (Bruning *et al.* 1992, 1993). It bears emphasis that tropisetron has been shown to be a surmountable antagonist of the endothelial 5-HT_{2B} receptor of rabbit jugular vein with a pK_B value of 6.45 (Martin *et al.* 1993). In support of these functional data, Ullmer *et al.* (1995) have recently demonstrated the presence of 5-HT$_{2B}$ receptor mRNA in primary human endothelial cells from pulmonary and coronary artery, umbilical vein and aorta: significantly, 5-HT$_{2C}$ receptor mRNA was not expressed in these cells.

Thus, in animal and human blood vessels, 5-HT shows activity analogous to that of histamine which in human cerebral arteries activates endothelium H$_1$ receptors to induce endothelial-dependent vasodilation mediated by NO (Ottoson *et al.* 1988, Toda 1990). As noted above, the latter mechanism was invoked by Olesen and his colleagues as the source of sufficient NO to produce migraine-like headaches following infusion of histamine in susceptible individuals. Similar reasoning applied in the context of the endothelial 5-HT$_{2B}$ receptor provides a plausible basis for a key role for a 5-HT–NO connection in the initiation of migraine.

A UNIFYING HYPOTHESIS

The data summarized above indicate that an important means by which migraine may be triggered is as a consequence of NO release by activation of 5-HT$_{2B}$ receptors present on the endothelial cells of key elements of the craniovascular bed. Activation may be induced pharmacologically with *m*-CPP, a compound with direct 5-HT$_{2B}$ agonist properties, or indirectly by 5-HT-releasing agents such as reserpine or fenfluramine. Blockade of 5-HT$_{2B}$ receptors can be achieved with methysergide, pizotifen and propranolol, the most consistently affective agents for the prophylactic treatment of migraine. The clinical response following treatment with these drugs implicates endogenous 5-HT as the trigger in the majority of cases of spontaneous migraine. The source of the 5-HT could be the blood platelet, but is more likely to reflect an increase in activity, in response to environmental precipitating factors including stress, of 5-HT-containing neurons, arising from nuclei in the brainstem, as well as peripheral sympathetic neurons which store and release both noradrenaline and 5-HT (for full discussion, see Fozard 1990). The released NO would, through its pro-inflammatory and nociceptive properties, provoke the sterile inflammatory response in the cerebral vasculature which is believed to be the key step in the development of migraine (see e.g. Fozard 1990, Moskowitz 1984, 1992).

REFERENCES

Baxter, G.S., Murphy, O.E. and Blackburn, T.P. (1994) Further characterisation of 5-hydroxytryptamine receptors (putative 5-HT$_{2B}$) in rat stomach fundus longitudinal muscle. *British Journal of Pharmacology*, **112**, 323–331.

Baxter, G.S., Ellis, E.S., Forbes, I.T., Jones, G.E., Kennett, G.A., Murphy, O.E. and Tilford, N. (1995) SB 204741: a potent and selective antagonist at 5-HT$_{2B}$ receptors. *British Journal of Pharmacology*, **114**, 157P.

Bonhaus, D.W., Bach, D., De Souza, A., Salazar, F.H.R., Matsuoka, B.D., Zuppan, P., Chan, H.W. and Eglen, R.M. (1995) The pharmacology and distribution of human 5-hydroxytryptamine$_{2B}$ (5-HT$_{2B}$) receptor gene products: comparison with 5-HT$_{2A}$ and 5-HT$_{2C}$ receptors. *British Journal of Pharmacology*, **115**, 622–628.

Bodelsson, M., Törnebrandt, K. and Arneklo-Nobin, B. (1993) Endothelial relaxing 5-hydroxytryptamine receptors in the rat jugular vein: similarity with the 5-hydroxytryptamine$_{1C}$ receptor. *Journal of Pharmacology and Experimental Therapeutics*, **264**, 709–716.

Brewerton, T.D., Murphy, D.L., Mueller, E.A. and Jimerson, D.C. (1988) Induction of migraine like headaches by the serotonin agonist m-chlorophenylpiperazine. *Clinical Pharmacology and Therapeutics*, **43**, 605–609.

Bruning, T.A., Chang, P.C., Blauw, G.J., Vermeij, P. and Van Zwieten, P.A. (1992) The 'nitric oxide-pathway' is involved in serotonin-mediated vaso-dilation in the human forearm: no additional evidence for the involvement of the 5-HT$_3$ receptor subtype. *Journal of Vascular Research*, **29**, 90.

Bruning, T.A., Chang, P.C., Blauw, G.J., Vermeij, P. and Van Zwieten, P.A. (1993) Serotonin-induced vasodilatation in the human forearm is mediated by the 'nitric oxide-pathway': no evidence for involvement of the 5-HT$_3$-receptor. *Journal of Cardiovascular Pharmacology*, **22**, 44–51.

Bruning, T.A., Van Zwieten, P.A., Blauw, G.J. and Chang, P.C. (1994) No functional involvement of 5-hydroxytryptamine$_{1A}$ receptors in nitric oxide-dependent dilatation caused by serotonin in the human forearm vascular bed. *Journal of Cardiovascular Pharmacology*, **24**, 454–461.

Cohen, M.L. and Wittenauer, L.A. (1986) Further evidence that the serotonin receptor in the rat stomach fundus is not 5-HT$_{1A}$ or 5-HT$_{1B}$. *Life Sciences*, **38**, 1–5.

Ellis, E.S., Byrne, C., Murphy, O.E., Tilford, N.S. and Baxter, G.S. (1995) Mediation by 5-hydroxytryptamine$_{2B}$ receptors of endothelium-dependent relaxation in rat jugular vein. *British Journal of Pharmacology*, **114**, 400–404.

Fozard, J.R. (1982) Serotonin, migraine and platelets. In: *Drugs and Platelets*, (eds P.A. Van Zwieten and E. Schönbaum), pp. 135–146. Gustav Fischer Verlag, Stuttgart.

Fozard, J.R. (1985) 5-Hydroxytryptamine in the pathophysiology of migraine. In: *Vascular Neuroeffector Mechanisms*, (eds J.A. Bevan, T. Godfraind, R.A. Maxwell, J.L. Stoclet and M. Worcel), pp. 321–328. Elsevier, Amsterdam.

Fozard, J.R. (1990) 5-HT in migraine: evidence from 5-HT receptor antagonists for a neuronal aetiology. In *Migraine: A Spectrum of Ideas*, (eds M. Sandler and G.M. Collins), pp. 128–146. Oxford University Press.

Fozard, J.R. (1992) 5-HT$_{1C}$ receptor agonism as an initiating event in migraine. In: *5-Hydroxytryptamine Mechanisms in Primary Headache*, (eds J. Olesen and P.R. Saxena), pp. 200–212. Raven Press, New York.

Fozard, J.R. (1995) The 5-hydroxytryptamine–nitric oxide connection: the key link in the initiation of migraine. *Archives Internationales de Pharmacodynamie et de Therapie*, **329**, 111–119.

Fozard, J.R. and Gray, J.A. (1989) 5-HT$_{1C}$ receptor activation: a key step in the initiation of migraine? *Trends in Pharmacological Science*, **10**, 307–309.

Fozard, J.R. and Kalkman, H.O. (1994) 5-Hydroxytryptamine (5-HT) and the initiation of migraine: new perspectives. *Naunyn-Schmiedeberg's Archives of Pharmacology*, **350**, 225–229.

Glusa, E. and Richter, M. (1993) Endothelium-dependent relaxation of porcine pulmonary arteries via $5-HT_{1C}$-like receptors. *Naunyn-Schmiedeberg's Archives of Pharmacology*, **347**, 471–477.

Holthusen, H. and Arndt, J.O. (1994) Nitric oxide evokes pain in humans on intracutaneous injection. *Neuroscience Letters*, **165**, 71–74.

Hoyer, D., Clarke, D.E., Fozard, J.R., Hartig, P.R., Martin, G.R., Mylecharane, E.J., Saxena, P.R. and Humphrey, P.P.A. (1994) International Union of Pharmacology classification of receptors for 5-hydroxytryptamine (Serotonin). *Pharmacological Reviews*, **46**, 157–203.

Kalkman, H.O. (1994) Is migraine prophylactic activity caused by $5-HT_{2B}$ or $5-HT_{2C}$ receptor blockade? *Life Sciences*, **54**, 641–644.

Krabbe, A.A. and Olesen, J. (1990) Headache provocation by continuous intravenous infusion of histamine. Clinical results and receptor mechanisms. *Pain*, **8**, 253–259.

Kursar, J.D., Nelson D.L., Wainscott, D.B., Cohen, M.L. and Baez, M. (1994) Molecular cloning, functional expression, and pharmacological characterization of a novel serotonin receptor ($5-hydroxytryptamine_{2B}$) from rat stomach fundus. *Molecular Pharmacology*, **92**, 549–557.

Leff, P., Martin, G.R. and Morse, J.M. (1987) Differential classification of vascular smooth muscle and endothelial cell 5-HT receptors by use of tryptamine analogues. *British Journal of Pharmacology*, **91**, 321–331.

Martin, G.R. (1994) Vascular receptors for 5-hydroxytryptamine: distribution, function and classification. *Pharmacology and Therapeutics*, **62**, 283–324.

Martin, G.R., Browning, C. and Giles, H. (1993) Further characterisation of an atypical 5-HT receptor mediating endothelium-dependent vasorelaxation. *British Journal of Pharmacology*, **110**, 137P.

Martin, I.L. and Boess, F.G. (1994) Molecular biology of 5-HT receptors. *Neuropharmacology*, **33**, 275–317.

Moskowitz, M.A. (1984) The neurobiology of vascular head pain. *Annals of Neurology*, **6**, 157–168.

Moskowitz, M.A. (1992) Neurogenic versus vascular mechanisms of sumatriptan and ergot alkaloids in migraine. *Trends in Pharmacological Sciences*, **13**, 307–311.

Ottosson, A., Jansen, I. and Edvinsson, L. (1988) Characterization of histamine receptors in isolated human cerebral arteries. *British Journal of Pharmacology*, **94**, 901–907.

Schmuck K., Ullmer, C., Engels, P. and Lübbert, H. (1994) Cloning and functional characterization of the human $5-HT_{2B}$ serotonin receptor. *FEBS Letters*, **324**, 85–90.

Sumner, M.J. (1991) Characterization of 5-HT receptor mediating endothelium-dependent relaxation in porcine vena cava. *British Journal of Pharmacology*, **102**, 938–942.

Thomsen, L.L. and Olesen, J. (1996) The role of nitric oxide in migraine pain. In: *Migraine: Pharmacology and Genetics*, (eds M. Sandler, M.D. Ferrari and S. Harnett, pp. 154–166. Chapman & Hall, London.

Toda, N. (1990) Mechanism underlying responses to histamine of isolated monkey and human cerebral arteries. *American Journal of Physiology*, **258**, H311–H317.

Ullmer, C., Schmuck, K., Kalkman, H.O. and Lübbert, H. (1995) Expression of serotonin receptor mRNAs in blood vessels. *FEBS Letters*, **370**, 215–221.

Wainscott, D.B., Cohen, M.L., Schenck, K.W., Audia, J.E., Nissen, J.S., Baez, M., Kursar, J.D., Lucaftes, V.L. and Nelson, D.L. (1993) Pharmacological characteristics of the newly cloned rat 5-hydroxytryptamine$_{2F}$ receptor. *Molecular Pharmacology*, **43**, 419–426.

Walle, T., Conradi, E.C., Walle, U.K., Fagan, T.C. and Gaffney, T.E. (1978) The predictable relationship between plasma levels and dose during chronic propranolol therapy. *Clinical Pharmacology and Therapeutics*, **24**, 668–677.

Weerasuriya, K., Patel, L. and Turner, P. (1982) β-adrenoceptor blockade and migraine. *Cephalalgia*, **2**, 33–45.

DISCUSSION

Goadsby: Does *m*-chlorophenylpiperazine (*m*-CPP) induce plasma extravasation?

Moskowitz: We tried that experiment once with Christian Waeber. There does not seem to be a major effect of *m*-CPP in our model.

Humphrey: 5-Hydroxytryptamine (5-HT) causes extravasation in rats, probably through this 5-HT$_2$ mechanism. It also has an anti-extravasation response mediated via 5-HT$_{1B}$ receptors, which is masked by the 5-HT$_2$ effect: the two actions cancel each other out. With α-methyl 5-HT, which is a selective 5-HT$_2$ receptor agonist, you only get extravasation. If *m*-CPP is not working here it may be because it is a partial agonist that produces varying effects at different sites. Perhaps that explains the long delay: *m*-CPP may initiate something that is insufficient in itself or takes a long time to establish. Whereas with reserpine we get massive release of 5-HT and onset of headache.

Fozard: There is a similar, rather long delay when headache is induced with a nitric oxide (NO) donor, so there is no need to postulate that there is anything strange or slow about a 5-HT receptor-mediated headache, assuming that it is going through the NO mechanism.

Humphrey: 5-HT, when released by reserpine or fenfluramine, seems to lead quickly to a headache, which is very different to the response to *m*-CPP.

Fozard: Yes, but we can live with that latency by invoking the NO link.

Humphrey: Are you saying that you do not want to involve NO in the headache-inducing effect of 5-HT?

Fozard: No. My feeling is that the data available do not allow us accurately to define true differences in onset times.

Humphrey: What extra action does 5-HT have that makes the headache come on much earlier?

Fozard: Looking at Dr Glover's data (Glover *et al.*, this volume), I have to accept that fenfluramine may trigger migraine through a different mechanism to *m*-CPP or that the data are such that we cannot make a quantitative comparison. Nevertheless, it still took two hours to develop a headache after fenfluramine. With a few more patients you might find you got closer to the onset time reported for *m*-CPP ($\geq$4 h).

Humphrey: I think that is wishful thinking, because reserpine is rapid in onset, just as Dr Glover showed for fenfluramine.

Fozard: All you can say is that the headache with *m*-CPP is not there at four hours and is substantial at eight hours. So it could be there at five hours.

Edvinsson: Does nitroglycerin, as a vasodilator, cause neurogenic inflammation?

Fozard: There is substantial evidence (see Fozard 1995) obtained using NO synthase inhibitors such as N^G-nitro-L-arginine methyl ester (L-NAME) or the substrate for NO synthase, L-arginine, that NO contributes to experimental inflammation or oedema, including neurogenic inflammation. Similar data have not been obtained with NO donors to my knowledge.

Edvinsson: Wouldn't it be easy to administer nitroglycerin as a vasodilator in this neurogenic model?

Moskowitz: The problem is that vasodilators usually lower blood pressure. If perfusion pressure drops, the assay can become invalid, so we avoided testing vasodilators. But the c-*fos* experiment is interesting: nitroglycerin will activate c-*fos*.

Fozard: Professor Moskowitz's experiment (Wei *et al.* 1992) in cat showing calcitonin gene-related peptide (CGRP) dependent vasodilator response to the NO donors may be relevant in that it suggests that you can activate sensory fibres to release CGRP. That may not give you oedema *per se*, but it is clear that the presence of CGRP will greatly enhance the oedema-forming properties of substance P or of any other oedema-forming inflammatory mediators (see Brain and Williams 1985).

Edvinsson: We could not show that infusion of nitroglycerin caused CGRP release in patients. They had the known nitroglycerin headache, but there was no CGRP release in this early headache. We have examined this in different animal models. Nitroglycerin worked as a vasodilator to the same degree in animals depleted of CGRP as in sensory intact animals. We have no evidence in support of nitroglycerin causing release of CGRP.

Fozard: There are now many papers that demonstrate that the release of CGRP from afferent nerve fibres can be facilitated by NO (Fozard 1995, Holzer *et al.* 1995).

Moskowitz: Our data are very clear. If you lesion the animal, thereby removing the CGRP fibres on one side of the head, and topically apply nitroglycerin or nitroprusside, the extent of the dilation is inhibited on the side of the denervation. Similarly, on the normal side, if you pretreat with a CGRP antagonist, the response to sodium nitroprusside is attentuated, suggesting that some of the action of nitroglycerin or nitroprusside is through CGRP release. Hermes Kontos and I did experiments independently. Peter Holzer, Susan Brain and others have been able to repeat this in other tissues. Not everyone agrees, however.

Fozard: Some of those experiments were done indirectly, not by measuring CGRP (see Hughes and Brain 1994). But you cannot argue with the data, which do not confirm Professor Moskowitz's work, but extend it to a variety of different models. The overall conclusion, that NO is involved in the release of CGRP from afferent neurons, is indisputable; it has been shown in several species and in two or three models.

Edvinsson: The evidence is indirect since the CGRP blocker, $CGRP_{8-37}$, has some activity of its own.

Fozard: Well, the results are published in quality journals and are generally accepted!

Lance: You are equating the $5\text{-}HT_{2B}$ and $5\text{-}HT_{2C}$ receptors. What is the difference between them?

Fozard: The receptors are structurally different but pharmacologically quite similar. It is not easy to tell the difference although the advent of new, selective ligands such as BW 723C86 and SB 204741 represents a considerable step forward in this respect.

Lance: And is the evidence for participation of nitric oxide simply endothelium-dependent relaxation? Is there no more direct evidence?

Fozard: No. But $5\text{-}HT_{2B}$ receptor-dependent vasorelaxation has been demonstrated in several tissues from a number of species and is suggested by an *in vivo* study in man (Bruning *et al.* 1994).

Schoenen: We have been looking for some time for a pharmacological property characterizing β-blockers which are active in migraine. You presented propranolol at a dose which is used in migraine therapy, but other β-blockers are active at much lower doses.

Peatfield: I was going to mention oxprenolol, which is believed to be inactive in migraine (Ekbom and Zetterman 1977).

Fozard: Another example of a β-blocker which is inactive in migraine is pindolol. However, the doses which have been given are relatively low, and it is unlikely that such doses would provide the concentrations needed to inhibit $5\text{-}HT_{2B}$ receptor-mediated, endothelium-dependent vasorelaxation (see Fozard and Kalkman 1994).

Peatfield: It would be interesting to study a wider range of β-blockers in that model.

Fozard: Yes. The problem would be, however, that you would have to relate your data to clinical observations with compounds that were not dosed as high as they should be to get the response. The beauty of propranolol is that it has always been overdosed relative to the β-blocking dose. Thus, one achieves plasma concentrations adequate to block 5-HT$_{2B}$ receptors and I suspect that accounts for the consistent prophylactic protection in migraine.

Ferrari: Do cyproheptadine, mianserin and tropisetron all have high affinity for the 5-HT$_{2B}$ receptor?

Fozard: Cyproheptadine and mianserin have affinities in the 10–50 nM range (Fozard and Kalkman 1994, Bonhaus *et al.* 1995). Tropisetron blocks the 5-HT$_{2B}$ receptor of the rabbit jugular vein with a pK_B of 6.45 (Martin *et al.* 1993), so it is not very potent.

Ferrari: None of these three compounds is effective in migraine prophylaxis.

Fozard: There **is** evidence that both cyproheptadine and mianserin are effective in migraine prophylaxis (see Fozard 1992), but I agree that further controlled studies with these drugs are needed. I was not suggesting tropisetron is effective in migraine. I was suggesting it may be effective in blocking endothelium-dependent vasodilation in man (Bruning *et al.* 1994) because it is a 5-HT$_{2B}$ receptor antagonist.

Humphrey: You went on to imply that 5-HT$_{2B}$ receptors were involved in the initiation of migraine attacks. That is why these questions are important.

Fozard: One should not forget that methysergide, pizotifen and propranolol are consistently effective prophylactic agents and have in common the capacity to block 5-HT$_{2B}$ receptors. Until drugs such as cyproheptadine and mianserin have been shown unequivocally not to be effective following appropriate dosing schedules, we should keep open minds on the hypothesis.

Goadsby: Would you aim a 5-HT$_{2B}$ drug into the brain or to act peripherally?

Fozard: That's a good question. My feeling is that brain penetration would not be necessary to achieve activity as a migraine prophylactic with a 5-HT$_{2B}$ receptor antagonist, because I think the relevant 5-HT$_{2B}$ receptors are those on the endothelial cells.

Hamel: Dr Fozard, you have been talking about models of vessels mainly in the periphery. Do you have any evidence in any species for a

5-HT receptor on cerebral vessels which induces relaxation through an endothelium-dependent mechanism?

Fozard: No.

Martin: We developed an agonist, BW 723C86, that is fairly selective for this 5-HT_{2B}-like endothelial receptor and have evidence for regional changes in cerebral blood flow with the agonist in rodents. It is indirect evidence, since there is no selective antagonist to check out the specificity of agonist effects, but the implication is that 5-HT_{2B} receptor activation will cause detectable dilatation.

Moskowitz: How do you know that it is not secondary to a metabolic action in the brain?

Martin: I cannot answer that. It is possible that vessel dilatation was secondary to some sort of local metabolic activation, but mRNA studies, as far as I am aware, suggest that the 5-HT_{2B} receptor is very sparsely distributed in the brain, so this would seem unlikely.

Fozard: Alberto Kaumann (personal communication) has seen vasodilatation in isolated human temporal arteries, but he has not yet analysed whether it is endothelium-dependent or which receptor site is involved. So you can see vasodilatation, but whether it is the same mechanism as I am proposing is not proven.

Goadsby: When Cudennec *et al.* (1993) looked at changes in cerebral blood flow in raphe activation, many of the areas with changed blood flow also had a parallel change in cerebral metabolic activity. If these drugs affect some area not otherwise specified by Dr Fozard, there could be a similar metabolic change and parallel changed blood flow.

REFERENCES

Bonhaus, D.W., Bach, D., De Souza, A., Salazar, F.H.R., Matsuoka, B.D., Zuppan, P., Chan, H.W. and Eglen, R.M. (1995) The pharmacology and distribution of human 5-hydroxytryptamine$_{2B}$ (5-HT_{2B}) receptor gene products: comparison with 5-HT_{2A} and 5-HT_{2C} receptors. *British Journal of Pharmacology*, **115**, 622–628.

Brain, S.D. and Williams, T.J. (1985) Inflammatory oedema induced by synergism between calcitonin gene-related peptide (CGRP) and mediators of increased vascular permeability. *British Journal of Pharmacology*, **86**, 855–860.

Bruning, T.A., Van Zwieten, P.A., Blauw, G.J. and Chang, P.C. (1994) No functional involvement of 5-hydroxytryptamine$_{1A}$ receptors in nitric oxide-dependent dilatation caused by serotonin in the human forearm vascular bed. *Journal of Cardiovascular Pharmacology*, **24**, 454–461.

Cudennec, A., Bonvento, G., Duverger, D., Lacombe, P., Seylaz, J. and MacKenzie, E.T. (1993) Effects of dorsal raphe nucleus stimulation on cerebral blood flow and metabolism coupling in the conscious rat. *Neuroscience*, **55**, 395–401.

Ekbom, K. and Zetterman, M. (1977) Oxprenolol in the treatment of migraine. *Acta Neurologica Scandinavica*, **56**, 181–184.

Fozard, J.R. (1992) 5-HT$_{1C}$ receptor agonism as an initiating event in migraine. In: *5-Hydroxytryptamine Mechanisms in Primary Headache*, (eds J. Olesen and P.R. Saxena), pp. 200–212. Raven Press, New York.

Fozard, J.R. (1995) The 5-hydroxytryptamine–nitric oxide connection: the key link in the initiation of migraine. *Archives Internationales de Pharmacodynamie et de Therapie*, **329**, 111–119.

Fozard, J.R. and Kalkman, H.O. (1994) 5-Hydroxytryptamine (5-HT) and the initiation of migraine: new perspectives. *Naunyn-Schmiedeberg's Archives of Pharmacology*, **350**, 225–229.

Glover, V., Ahmed, F., Hussein, N., Jarman, J. and Peatfield, R.C. (1996) Central 5-hydroxytryptamine supersensitivity in migraine. In: *Migraine: Pharmacology and Genetics*, (eds M. Sandler, M.D. Ferrari and S. Harnett), pp. 117–126. Chapman & Hall, London.

Holzer, P., Wachter, C., Heinemann, A., Jocic, M., Lippe, I.T. and Herbert, M.K. (1995) Sensory nerves, nitric oxide and NANC vasodilatation. *Archives Internationales Pharmacodynamie et de Therapie*, **329**, 67–79.

Hughes, S.R. and Brain, S.D. (1994) Nitric oxide-dependent release of vasodilator quantities of calcitonin gene-related peptide from capsaicin-sensitive nerves in rabbit skin. *British Journal of Pharmacology*, **111**, 425–430.

Martin, G.R., Browning, C. and Giles, H. (1993) Further characterisation of an atypical 5-HT receptor mediating endothelium-dependent vasorelaxation. *British Journal of Pharmacology*, **110**, 137P.

15

The possible role of neurotrophins in migraine

M. Sandler

With very few exceptions, the development of new drugs in the past fifty years has been in the hands of a small number of international pharmaceutical 'giants'. In the past decade, however, most particularly in the United States of America, a new type of corporate entity has emerged, the relatively tiny, entrepreneurial biotechnology company, whose appearance coincided with, and was designed to exploit, the molecular biology revolution. The complex and rapidly growing neuroscience arena has been specially prominent in these developments (Gershon 1994) and even within this research area the neurotrophins have occupied centre stage (Barinaga 1994a).

It is difficult to overstate the importance of the neurotrophins. Reviewing their evolutionary aspects, Barde (1994) has pointed out that they provide essential intercellular signals, preventing the elimination of many cells of the developing nervous system by apoptosis. However, whilst a substantial portion of the relevant literature has dwelt on the crucial role of these compounds in the developing nervous system in preventing the programmed cell death of certain neurons during development (e.g. Jacobson 1991, Raff *et al.* 1993), a continuous expression of brain-derived neurotrophic factor (BDNF) has been identified and followed into adult life, in the monkey brain at least (Huntley *et al.* 1992). Black (1993) concludes that trophic actions, influencing brain development, are critical throughout life, mediating learning, memory and regrowth after injury. In attempting to apply

Migraine: Pharmacology and genetics
Edited by Merton Sandler, Michel Ferrari and Sara Harnett
Published in 1996 by Chapman & Hall
ISBN 1 86036 006 8

their somewhat global concept of an 'amygdala kindling paradigm' to a specific subgroup of patients with migraine or affective illness who experience illness progression and drug tolerance, Post and Silberstein (1994) were the first to adumbrate the possibility of a neurotrophin connection with this group of illnesses.

THE CAST LIST

We now know that a large, complex and heterogeneous assembly of neurotrophic factors provides trophic support for neurons of the central and peripheral nervous system (see Loughlin and Fallon 1993). As is well known, nerve growth factor (NGF) was the first representative of the group to be identified and represents the start of the now classical target-derived growth factor concept, whereby innervated tissues produce a signal to innervating neurons for the selective limitation of neuronal death occurring during development (e.g. Purves 1986, Oppenheim 1991). Thus, many neurons put out axons but only those which reach their proper target, to be nourished by just sufficient NGF, continue to survive. In the peripheral nervous system, NGF plays a crucial role in keeping alive developing dorsal root ganglia and sympathetic neurons (Johnson and Gorin 1980, Levi-Montalcini 1987). After its production by target cells, NGF is bound to its specific receptor, internalized by the neuron, and undergoes retrograde neuronal transport to the cell body, where it acts via the cotransported receptor molecule (Levi-Montalcini 1987, Thoenen *et al.* 1987). Although Gnahn *et al.* (1983), and many others subsequently, identified an important central role for NGF in neostriatal and basal forebrain cholinergic neurons, recently Holtzman *et al.* (1995) have been able to demonstrate NGF action in nine further brain neuronal populations, so that new functions for this agent seem likely to emerge. I shall suggest in this chapter that NGF may play a role in the sequence of events leading to migraine headache (Sandler 1995), but even so, it seems necessary not to study this agent in isolation but to view it against a complex backcloth of other neurotrophins.

Over the past dozen years, NGF, the first representative of this group, has multiplied into a neurotrophin family by the emergence of the related factors, BDNF, neurotrophin-3 (NT-3) and neurotrophin-4/5 (NT-4/5) (see Loughlin and Fallon 1993). Recently, neurotrophin-6 (NT-6) has been detected in an African species of teleost fish (Götz *et al.* 1994); it appears to possess a similar but weaker spectrum of action to that of NGF. The neurotrophins possess their own specific set of tyrosine kinase receptors (see Parada *et al.* 1992), the products of the proto-oncogenes, *trk* A, by which NGF acts, *trk* B, the receptor system for both BDNF and NT-4/5, and *trk* C, specific for NT-3. There also exists a low affinity receptor common to all these neurotrophins but, although much has been written about it, its precise function is obscure.

BDNF became of particular interest to the Parkinson's disease research community with the demonstration that it provides neurotrophic support to dopaminergic neurons of the substantia nigra in tissue culture (Hyman *et al.* 1991). However, a new trophic factor has emerged which appears to be more highly specific for cells of this kind, glial cell-derived neurotrophic factor (GDNF) (Lin *et al.* 1993), a hot candidate for the treatment of Parkinson's disease (Barinaga 1995)! Even so, its action turns out to be less specific than had originally been claimed. It also appears to be the most potent motoneuron trophic factor discovered to date (Yan *et al.* 1995). Other main groupings of trophic factors, which have, in fact, major actions outside the nervous system, include the neurocytokines, particularly ciliary neurotrophic factor (CNTF) (Lo 1993), the fibroblast growth factors (FGF), especially basic FGF (bFGF) (Matsuyama *et al.* 1992), the transforming growth factors (TGF), particularly the TGF-β family (Chalazonitis *et al.* 1992), the epidermal growth factors (EGF) (Abe and Saito 1992), platelet-derived growth factor (PDGF) (Nikkhah *et al.* 1993), and midkine and pleiotrophin (Yasuhara *et al.* 1993). In fact, it has gradually become obvious, with our increasingly detailed knowledge of neurotrophin interactions, that the original 'classical' target-derived growth factor concept of action must be modified (Korsching 1993). Interactions are less specific and more complex than had been assumed, with a considerable overlap in biological activities. Signalling is not limited to the retrograde messenger mode but may include local trophic interactions, autocrine signalling and anterograde trophic signals.

Many agents are known to enhance the action of NGF (Carswell 1993), including tumour necrosis factor α (TNF-α) (Hattori *et al.* 1993) and certain TGF-β isoforms, which regulate the expression of NGF and NT-3 mRNA (Buchman *et al.* 1994). Tuttle and Creedon (1993) have shown that PDGF-BB increases NGF synthesis in vascular smooth muscle fortyfold, whilst TGF-β increases it tenfold: acting together, however, they promote a massive increase, one hundred and ninety three times greater than baseline. Exogenous compounds exist, too, which potentiate NGF, e.g. fellutamide A, a tripeptide derivative of *Penicillium fellutanum*, a potent enhancer of NGF synthesis and secretion, at least *in vitro* (Yamaguchi *et al.* 1993), or the immunosuppressant, FK506 (Lyons *et al.* 1994). Other agents are known which mimic the actions of NGF, such as certain guanidine compounds related to isaxonine (Lehmann *et al.* 1993) and another antibiotic, BU-4314 from a *Microtetraspora* sp. (Toda *et al.* 1993). Compounds like these, which cross the blood–brain barrier, may intensify the action of the endogenous neurotrophin. Whether they are present in certain foodstuffs, particularly those such as red wine, which may play a role in the initiation of migraine headache (Sandler *et al.* 1995), is unknown, but the possibility is obviously of interest in the light of the NGF hypothesis of migraine headache discussed below.

NGF and BDNF synthesis appear to be interconnected in the rat hippocampus (Knipper *et al.* 1994). Kokaia *et al.* (1993a) have also noted this association in hippocampal as well as in cortical neurons, together with co-expression of their respective receptors, *trk* A and *trk* B. Seizures resulted in increased levels of both in these 'double-labelled' cells. Such parallel increases in NGF and *trk* A have been observed by Goodness *et al.* (1994) in transgenic mice, accompanied by an unexpected increase in *trk* C (not *trk* B).

SPREADING DEPRESSION, SEIZURES AND KINDLING

Despite doubts in some quarters, we now seem to be reaching a consensus that the migraine aura can be equated with spreading depression (e.g. Welch *et al.* 1993). The biochemical sequelae of this phenomenon have been subjected to closer examination. Thus, Herrera *et al.* (1993) found that the production of spreading depression by the application of KCl to the rat cerebral cortex results in transient up-regulation of the immediate early gene, c-*fos*, which reaches its peak at 6 h. This was followed by an increase in NGF mRNA, reaching its highest concentration, in the entorhinal cortex, at 12 h, with a concentration fifty times greater than baseline. Although there also seemed to be an increase in NGF-like protein, maximal at 24 h, the antibody used for its assay may not have been entirely specific. In similar experimental circumstances, Kokaia *et al.* (1993b) identified a rapid induction of BDNF mRNA in rat cerebral cortex following spreading depression, with a peak at 2 h, a finding mirrored by Kawahara *et al.* (1994) who found spreading depression to up-regulate BDNF similarly. Whilst Kokaia *et al.* (1993b) were unable to detect any change in NGF mRNA concentration, it is not clear from their paper whether they followed up the KCl-treated animals for a sufficient length of time to monitor such an effect.

NGF and BDNF are the only two neurotrophic factors so far to have been scrutinized, even if partially, in this 'experimental migraine' context but further relevant evidence may be provided by examining the biochemical consequences of other types of excess electrical activity in the brain. The prime example, perhaps, is that of electroconvulsive shock which brings about a substantial increase in brain NGF and BDNF concentrations (Gall 1992a,b, Lindvall *et al.* 1994, Nibuya *et al.* 1994), even if stimulation activity is minimal (Follesa *et al.* 1994). Kindling-induced seizures will, likewise, generate increased NGF and BDNF concentrations in adult rat brain (Bengzon *et al.* 1992, Kokaia *et al.* 1994,

Sato *et al.* 1994). Electroconvulsive shock is, of course, widely employed in man for the treatment of depressive illness and another approach to this disorder, at one time widely in vogue, was the induction of hypoglycaemia: it is now known that hypoglycaemic coma causes a rise in brain neurotrophic factors (Lindvall *et al.* 1992, Kokaia *et al.* 1994).

How are we to interpret these rises in NGF and BDNF concentrations in response to electrical events? We must probably assume, as a working hypothesis, that they are compensatory and neuroprotective. Frim *et al.* (1993), for example, demonstrated a protective effect of engineered NGF-secreting fibroblasts against excitotoxic lesions in rat striatum and Emerich *et al.* (1994) have reported similar data. Further observations are obviously required.

Do people who suffer from migraine headache, despite its obvious clinical drawbacks, derive any selective advantage from it? There is insufficient evidence to say but I shall attempt to put forward a case, in a following section, incriminating NGF as a plausible candidate for the putative nociceptive substance liberated during migraine attacks even though it may provide longer-term benefit. Intracerebroventricular NGF, NT-3 and NT-4/5, but not BDNF, cause increased acquisition and retention of spatial memory in aged rats (Fischer *et al.* 1994). Compensatory overproduction in man of NGF, at least, might thus lead to pain in certain sensitive, i.e. migraine-predisposed, subjects (see below), despite trophic benefit. BDNF may have its own relatively specific role to play and this aspect of the problem will be discussed more fully in the section below dealing with the possible relationship between migraine and depressive illness.

ROLE OF c-*FOS*

The role of c-*fos* in the spreading depression model came to the attention of migraine researchers first in the experiments of Herrera *et al.* (1993) (mentioned above), preceding the appearance of NGF. Kawahara *et al.* (1994) also noted intense c-*fos* activity in ipsilateral cortical neurons and bilateral dentate gyri, 3 h after KCl, as did Hoffman *et al.* (1994) in 2 h samples, followed at 10 h by the appearance of glial fibrillary acidic protein (GFAP). The protein product of c-*fos* is also known to show itself in male rat brain following intraventricular NGF injection (Peng *et al.* 1993): Ginty *et al.* (1994) have shown that NGF activates a *Ras*-dependent protein kinase that stimulates c-*fos* transcription via phosphorylation of CREB (cyclic AMP response element binding protein), i.e. the mechanism by which the NGF signal is transduced to the nucleus to induce gene expression. CREB may function in the nucleus as a general mediator of growth factor responses. Moskowitz *et al.* (1993) have demonstrated that cortical spreading depression provokes the expression of c-*fos* protein-like immunoreactivity within the trigeminal nucleus caudalis (in addition to the cortex) via trigeminovascular mechanisms. Both chronic surgical transection of meningeal afferents and sumatriptan reduce this effect.

Our knowledge of these aura-initiated biochemical events is superficial and it is probably safest not to draw too many conclusions from the scanty evidence that we possess. Even so, the migraine aura seems to be emerging as merely another triggering event for a migraine headache, to take its place with other triggering events which initiate migraine without aura (Sandler 1995). If this interpretation is correct, then the difference between migraine-disposed and non-migraine disposed subjects lies in the sensitivity of the former to triggering events of a number of different kinds.

POSSIBLE ROLE OF bFGF

Apart from NGF and BDNF, a trophic factor with an important neuroprotective role in the brain is bFGF. Its intraventricular injection has been shown to protect against ischaemic brain damage (Berlove *et al.* 1991, Yamada *et al.* 1991). Moreover, mice transgenic for bovine bFGF show increased resistance to ischaemic brain damage (MacMillan *et al.* 1993). Paradoxically, however, Rosenblatt *et al.* (1994) were able to demonstrate that bFGF causes dilatation of rat pial arterioles. Thus, if the vascular hypothesis of the disease be favoured, it is possible that migraine headache stems from vasodilatation brought about by hypersensitivity to bFGF, secreted as a protective mechanism against potential brain ischaemic damage from spreading depression (Sandler 1995).

Kawahara *et al.* (1994) showed that the induction of spreading depression in rats protects CA1 pyramidal neurons from cerebral ischaemia following cardiac arrest, whatever the mechanism. It is known that brief, nonlethal periods of cerebral ischaemia protect against subsequent otherwise lethal injury (Simon *et al.* 1994). Electrical stimulation of the cerebellar fastigial nucleus of the rat for 1 h protects the brain from ischaemic infarction. These changes are not due to alterations in cerebral blood flow or metabolism: their mechanism may involve rapid transcription of protective genes (Reis *et al.* 1994).

NGF AND HYPERALGESIA

NGF administration, both to neonatal and mature rats, causes profound behavioural hyperalgesia (Lewin *et al.* 1993) and this phenomenon also occurs in mice (Lewin and Mendell 1993). In addition, transgenic mice over-expressing NGF in their skin manifest gross hyperalgesia (Lewin and Mendell 1993). In man, intravenously administered recombinant human NGF results in muscle pain while subcutaneous administration leads to hyperalgesia at the injection site, persisting for up to eight weeks (Petty *et al.* 1994). Intracerebroventricular NGF has been associated with severe abdominal pain in three Alzheimer patients (B. Winblad, personal communication, 1994), details of only one of whom have been published (Olson *et al.* 1992). Is it possible that the headache phase of migraine derives from this agent? It must be remembered that the time-course of the rise and fall in NGF level recorded by Herrera *et al.* (1993) in rats is likely to be too prolonged to fit into the human clinical migraine pattern. Even so, it is tempting to speculate that NGF (or some similar factor) might be the putative nociceptive substance of Moskowitz and Macfarlane (1993), released from the neocortex into the interstitial space in response to unknown ionic mechanisms associated with the aura. In this context, we should note that an important aspect of normal glial function is its ability to mop up excess chemicals, such as potassium and glutamate, spilling over from synapses (Travis 1994). Perhaps migraine, under certain circumstances, might stem from some deficit of glial function.

We must not blind ourselves to the fact that pain responses of the kind produced by NGF are not completely specific: administration of certain cytokines, for example, may also result in hyperalgesia (Watkins *et al.* 1994). CNTF, apparently quite toxic to man (Barinaga 1994a), appears to number the ability to generate pain among its disadvantages (Lindsay 1995). BDNF, on the contrary, tends to produce a long-lasting analgesia (Siuciak *et al.* 1994a). Despite our ignorance about the possible nociceptive ability of other trophic factors, NGF stands out as an interesting candidate for further study in this context. One important line of investigation seems apposite: using an animal model of experimental inflammation, Woolf *et al.* (1994) demonstrated local sensory hypersensitivity and increased substance P and calcitonin gene-related peptide (CGRP) in primary sensory neurons innervating inflamed tissue itself. The behavioural sensitivity and hyperalgesia could be neutralized by anti-NGF serum, preventing the increase in substance P and CGRP but not affecting swelling and erythema.

MIGRAINE AND DEPRESSION

There is no longer any doubt that a strong relationship exists between migraine and depressive illness (Breslau and Davis 1993, Glover *et al.* 1993, Merikangas *et al.* 1993). Despite intensive clinical and experimental effort over many years, the pathogenesis of depression, like that of migraine, remains unknown. Much of the focus of investigation has been on monoamine economy and, indeed, it seems likely that such compounds play a major role in the development of this illness. And yet, the most important argument undermining the key role of monoamines in its development stems from the timing of the clinical response to antidepressant drug therapy. Although these drugs do increase brain monoamine levels when administered acutely, chronic dosage is required in order to achieve clinical benefit, with a response lag of up to several weeks. Thus, some type of long-term adaptation is probable, involving regulation of intracellular sites and gene expression.

It seems not unlikely that neurotrophins, which are known to regulate neuronal growth and plasticity under certain circumstances, play a major part in the development of this illness, with a deficit leading to abnormal neuronal death (Margolis *et al.* 1994). As mentioned earlier, the neurotrophins are of overriding importance in preventing the programmed cell death of certain neurons during development (Jacobson 1991, Raff *et al.* 1993); their role in the adult is more problematic. BDNF, however, is exceptional in that its continued expression has been identified and followed into adult life in monkey brain (Huntley *et al.* 1992), whilst adult rat spinal and brainstem neurons retain *trk* B mRNA and thus their responsiveness to BDNF (Yan *et al.* 1994). It thus seems likely that, in man, some populations of responsive cells require trophic support from this and other neurotrophins for survival and maintenance of function.

Whether abnormal neuronal death occurs in depressive illness is still unclear although cell loss has been claimed in some forms of bipolar affective disorder (Beckmann and Jakob 1991). However, evidence has begun to mount that treatment procedures that are effective in this illness have in common their ability to give rise to a facilitated production of neurotrophins. Perhaps the prime example is that of electroconvulsive therapy, reviewed earlier, which brings about a substantial increase in brain NGF and BDNF levels, whilst even lesser amounts of electrical over-activity, including Leão's spreading depression, as discussed, will heighten the presence of these factors, as will hypoglycaemic coma. Even the finding that protracted exercise in rats provokes an increase in BDNF gene expression (Neeper *et al.* 1995), tends to support anecdotal accounts of lightening of affect in man after prolonged exertion. Of outstanding potential importance, however, in this connection, are the preliminary observations of Duman *et al.* (1994) who found that 21-day administration of tranylcypromine, desipramine or sertraline also causes an increase of BDNF in the frontal cortex. Whether the ability of desipramine pretreatment to prevent the death of PC12 cells by apoptosis following 6-hydroxydopamine exposure (Walkinshaw and Waters 1994) is relevant in this context is unknown (it may, equally, be due just to the blockade of 6-hydroxydopamine uptake by these cells). It is of particular interest, therefore, that infusion of BDNF into the midbrain had an antidepressant action in two rat models of depression (Siuciak *et al.* 1994b). And in view of the known central antinociceptive action of BDNF, mentioned earlier (Siuciak *et al.* 1994a), the use of monoamine oxidase inhibitors (Anthony and Lance 1969, Sandyk and Iacono 1987) or tricyclic antidepressants (Couch *et al.* 1976) in migraine and in other pain syndromes takes on a new complexion.

All these data provide a *prima facie* case for neurotrophic factor implication in the response to antidepressant treatment and, conversely, indicate that depressive illness represents a state of neurotrophin deficiency. To what extent immobilization stress in the rat approximates to a depressive state is unknown but this animal model is characterized by a reduction in BDNF mRNA in the hippocampus and throughout the limbic system (Smith 1994). Perhaps the well documented hypersensitivity to pain in depressive illness (Blumer and Heilbronn 1982) corresponds with a BDNF deficiency state. And with the known interrelationship between migraine and depressive illness, it seems possible that the organism attempts to compensate for a depressive state by facilitated production of BDNF; but because both BDNF and NGF are expressed in the same hippocampal and cortical neurons, so that seizures cause the release of both (Kokaia *et al.* 1993a), it seems perfectly likely that spreading depression or other triggering mechanism will also liberate NGF as well as BDNF. If, as suggested earlier, migrainous subjects are distinguished by particular sensitivity to NGF, then a headache episode will ensue.

TESTING THE HYPOTHESES

Many of the data on neurotrophin economy recorded in the literature have been based on mRNA measurements. Assay procedures for the active proteins themselves have been more difficult, relying on immunological measurements. Thus, although serum levels of NGF are on record (e.g. Haddad *et al.* 1994), we have so far been unable to replicate these findings. The problem may be compounded by the fact that NGF forms a complex, in serum, with α_2-macroglobulin, from which it is necessary to liberate it before any measurement can be made (Murase *et al.* 1992, Liebl and Koo 1993). NGF, and bFGF too, have been identified in the cerebrospinal fluid of brain-injured human patients (Patterson *et al.* 1993), so that, in conditions such as migraine, where an excess production has been predicated, serial collections of this material across an attack may be worth evaluation.

Although truncated forms of *trk* B are likely to be of major clinical importance (Beck *et al.* 1993), reference has also been made in the literature to a truncated NGF receptor which, it has been claimed, appears in the urine in patients with diabetic neuropathy (Hruska *et al.*

1993). If this finding can be replicated, it might be interesting to look for material of this kind across a migraine attack.

The hypothesis that hypersensitivity to NGF exists in a migrainous population might conveniently be tested by skin testing, in patients and control subjects, with low concentrations of this compound, in a similar manner to that employed by Petty *et al.* (1994), noting any differences in response. This approach might also be useful in detecting whether depressed patients display greater sensitivity to NGF than controls.

It might also be feasible to devise a therapeutic test for NGF hyper-production employing anti-NGF serum (e.g. Woolf *et al.* 1994) or using the staurosporine-related protein kinase inhibiting antibiotic, K-252b (Nakanishi *et al.* 1986), although this compound does not readily penetrate the cell membrane (Nakanishi *et al.* 1991). K-252b is a selective and nontoxic inhibitor of NGF action on cultured brain neurons (Knüsel and Hefti 1991, 1992) and biochemical variations on its structure might well lead to a therapeutically useful product. Anti-NGF compounds also appear to be on the way (Barinaga 1994b) and may prove to be useful for therapeutic testing.

Investigation of BDNF production might be more straightforward, in that Yamamoto and Gurney (1990) have noted that human platelets contain this agent, a finding which has been confirmed elsewhere (unpublished). Whether platelet values reflect central BDNF concentrations is a problem which obviously must be investigated.

In summary, therefore, evidence is presented pointing to a possible involvement of the neurotrophins in migraine. Nerve growth factor (NGF) in particular, with its known ability to provoke pain, may well be a prime target for study in this condition. A high correlation is known to exist between migraine and depressive illness. The possibility of depression representing a brain-derived neurotrophic factor (BDNF) deficiency state has been evaluated in this context.

REFERENCES

Abe, K. and Saito, H. (1992) Protective effect of epidermal growth factor on glutamate neurotoxicity in cultured cerebellar neurons. *Neuroscience Research*, **14**, 117–123.

Anthony, M. and Lance, J.W. (1969) Monoamine oxidase inhibition in the treatment of migraine. *Archives of Neurology*, **21**, 263–268.

Barde, Y.A. (1994) Neurotrophic factors: an evolutionary perspective. *Journal of Neurobiology*, **25**, 1329–1333.

Barinaga, M. (1994a) Neurotrophic factors enter the clinic. *Science*, **264**, 772–774.

Barinaga, M. (1994b) Watching the brain remake itself. *Science*, **266**, 1475–1476.

Barinaga, M. (1995). Researchers broaden the attack on Parkinson's disease. *Science*, **267**, 455–456.

Beck, K.D., Lamballe, F., Klein, R., Barbacid, M., Schauwecker, P.E., McNeill, T.H., Finch, C.E., Hefti, F. and Day, J.R. (1993) Induction of noncatalytic trk B neurotrophin receptors during axonal sprouting in the adult hippocampus. *Journal of Neuroscience*, **13**, 4001–4014.

Beckmann, H. and Jakob, H. (1991) Prenatal disturbances of nerve cell migration in the entorhinal region: a common vulnerability factor in functional psychoses? *Journal of Neural Transmission*, **84**, 155–164.

Bengzon, J., Söderström, S., Kokaia, Z., Kokaia, M., Ernfors, P., Persson, H., Ebendal, T. and Lindvall, O. (1992) Widespread increase of nerve growth factor protein in the rat forebrain after kindling-induced seizures. *Brain Research*, **587**, 338–342.

Berlove, D.J., Caday, C.G., Moskowitz, M.A. and Finklestein, S.P. (1991) Basic fibroblast growth factor (bFGF) protects against ischemic neuronal death in vivo. *Society of Neuroscience Abstracts*, **17**, 1267.

Black, I.B. (1993) Environmental regulation of brain trophic interactions. *International Journal of Developmental Neuroscience*, **11**, 403–410.

Blumer, D. and Heilbronn, M. (1982) Chronic pain as a variant of depressive disease. *Journal of Nervous and Mental Diseases*, **7**, 381–393.

Breslau, N. and Davis, G.C. (1993) Migraine, physical health and psychiatric disorder: a prospective epidemiologic study in young adults. *Journal of Psychiatric Research*, **27**, 211–221.

Buchman, V.L., Sporn, M. and Davies, A.M. (1994) Role of transforming growth factor-beta isoforms in regulating the expression of nerve growth factor and neurotrophin-3 mRNA levels in embryonic cutaneous cells at different stages of development. *Development*, **120**, 1621–1629.

Carswell, S. (1993) The potential for treating neurodegenerative disorders with NGF-inducing compounds. *Experimental Neurology*, **124**, 36–42.

Chalazonitis, A., Kalberg, J., Twardzik, D.R., Morrison, R.S. and Kessler. JA. (1992) Transforming growth factor β has neurotrophic actions on sensory neurons in vitro and is synergistic with nerve growth factor. *Developmental Biology*, **152**, 121–132.

Couch, J.R., Ziegler, D.K. and Hassanein, R. (1976) Amitriptyline in the prophylaxis of migraine. *Neurology*, **26**, 121–127.

Duman, R.S., Nibuya, M., Rydelek-Fitzgerald, L. and Morinobu, S. (1994) Regulation of neurotrophins by antidepressant treatments. *Abstracts of the American College of Neuropsychopharmacology*, p. 76.

Emerich, D.F., Hammang, J.P., Baetge, E.E. and Winn, S.R. (1994) Implantation of polymer-encapsulated human nerve growth factor-secreting fibroblasts attenuates the behavioral and neuropathological consequences of quinolinic acid injections into rodent striatum. *Experimental Neurology*, **130**, 141–150.

Fischer, W., Sirevaag, A., Wiegand, S.J., Lindsay. R.M. and Björklund, A. (1994) Reversal of spatial memory impairments in aged rats by nerve growth factor and neurotrophins 3 and 4/5 but not by brain-derived neurotrophic factor. *Proceedings of the National Academy of Science USA*, **91**, 8607–8611.

Follesa, P., Gale, K. and Mocchetti, I. (1994) Regional and temporal pattern of expression of nerve growth factor and basic fibroblast growth factor mRNA in rat brain following electroconvulsive shock. *Experimental Neurology*, **127**, 37–44.

Frim, D.M., Short, M.P., Rosenberg, W.S., Simpson, J., Breakefield, X.O. and Isacson, O. (1993) Local protective effects of nerve growth factor-secreting fibroblasts against excitotoxic lesions in the rat striatum. *Journal of Neurosurgery*, **78**, 267–273.

Gall, C.M. (1992a) Regulation of brain neurotrophin expression by physiological activity. *Trends in Pharmacological Science*, **13**, 401–403.

Gall, C.M. (1992b) Seizure-induced changes in neurotrophin expression: implications for epilepsy. *Experimental Neurology*, **124**, 150–166.

Gershon, D. (1994) Changing times for neuroscientists. *Nature*, **372**, 203–204.

Ginty, D.D., Bonni, A. and Greenberg, M.E. (1994) Nerve growth factor activates a Ras-dependent protein kinase that stimulates c-*fos* transcription via phosphorylation of CREB. *Cell*, **77**, 713–725.

Glover, V., Jarman, J. and Sandler, M. (1993) Migraine and depression: biological aspects. *Journal of Psychiatric Research*, **27**, 223–231.

Gnahn, H., Hefti, F., Heumann, R., Schwab, M.E. and Thoenen, H. (1983) NGF-mediated increase of choline acetyltransferase (ChAT) in the neonatal rat forebrain: evidence for a physiological role of NGF in the brain. *Developmental Brain Research*, **9**, 42–52.

Goodness, T.P., Albers, K.M., Davis, F.F. and Davis, B.M. (1994) Neurotrophin receptor expression in trigeminal ganglia of mice overexpressing NGF in skin. *Society for Neuroscience Abstracts*, **20**, 39.

Götz, R., Köster, R., Winkler, C., Raulf, F., Lottspelch, F., Schartl, M. and Thoenen, H. (1994) Neurotrophin-6 is a new member of the nerve growth factor family. *Nature*, **372**, 266–269.

Haddad, J., Vilge, V., Juif, J.G., Maitre, M., Donato L., Messer, J. and Mark, J. (1994) β-Nerve growth factor levels in newborn cord sera. *Pediatric Research*, **35**, 637–639.

Hattori, A., Tanaka, E., Murase, K., Ishida, N., Chatani, Y., Tsujimoto, M., Hayashi, K. and Kohno, M. (1993) Tumour necrosis factor stimulates the synthesis and secretion of biologically active nerve growth factor in non-neuronal cells. *Journal of Biological Chemistry*, **268**, 2577–2582.

Herrera, D.G., Maysinger, D., Gadient, R., Boeckh, C., Otten, U. and Cuello, A.C. (1993) Spreading depression induces c-*fos*-like immunoreactivity and NGF mRNA in the rat cerebral cortex. *Brain Research*, **602**, 99–103.

Hoffman, T.L., Macklin, W.B., Lust, W.D., Solman, W.R. and Ratcheson, R.A. (1994) Changes in gene expression following multiple spreading depressions. *Society for Neuroscience Abstracts*, **20**, 1480.

Holtzman, D.M., Kilbridge, J., Li, Y., Cunningham Jr, E.T., Lenn, N.J., Clary, D.O., Reichardt, L.F. and Mobley, W.C. (1995) TrkA expression in the CNS: evidence for the existence of several novel NGF-responsive CNS neurons. *Journal of Neuroscience*, **15**, 1567–1576.

Hruska, R.E., Chertack, M.M. and Kravis, D. (1993) Elevation of nerve growth factor receptor-truncated in the urine of patients with diabetic neuropathy. *Annals of the New York Academy of Science*, **679**, 299–305.

Huntley, G.W., Benson, D.L., Jones, E.G. and Isackson, P.J. (1992) Developmental expression of brain derived neurotrophic factor mRNA by neurons of fetal and adult monkey prefrontal cortex. *Developmental Brain Research*, **70**, 53–63.

Hyman, C., Hofer, M., Barde, Y-A., Juhasz, M., Yancopoulos, G.C., Squinto, S.P. and Lindsay, R.M. (1991) BDNF is a neurotrophic factor for dopaminergic neurons of the substantia nigra. *Nature*, **350**, 230–223.

Jacobson, M. (1991) Neuronal death and neurotrophic factors. In: *Developmental Neurobiology*, 3rd Edn, pp. 311–58. Plenum Press, New York.

Johnson, E.M. and Gorin, P.G. (1980) Dorsal root ganglion neurons are destroyed by exposure *in utero* to maternal antibody to nerve growth factor. *Science*, **210**, 916–918.

Kawahara, N., Reutzler, C.A., Wiegand, S.J., Croll, S. and Klatzo, I. (1994)

Induction of protective mechanisms in cerebral ischemia. *Society for Neuroscience Abstracts*, **20**, 1480.

Knipper, M., Berzaghi, M., Blöchl, A., Breer, H., Thoenen, H. and Lindholm, D. (1994) Positive feedback between acetylcholine and the neurotrophins nerve growth factor and brain-derived neurotrophic factor in the rat hippocampus. *European Journal of Neuroscience*, **6**, 668–671.

Knüsel, B. and Hefti, F. (1991) K-252b is a selective and nontoxic inhibitor of nerve growth factor action on cultured brain neurons. *Journal of Neurochemistry*, **57**, 955–962.

Knüsel, B. and Hefti, F. (1992) K-252 compounds: modulators of neurotrophin signal transduction. *Journal of Neurochemistry*, **59**, 1987–1996.

Kokaia, Z., Bengzon, J., Metsis, M., Kokaia, M., Persson, H. and Lindvall, O. (1993a) Coexpression of neurotrophins and their receptors in neurons of the central nervous system. *Proceedings of the National Academy of Science USA*, **90**, 6711–6715.

Kokaia, Z., Gido, G., Ringstedt, T., Bengzon, J., Kokaia, M., Siesjo, B.K., Persson, H. and Lindvall, O. (1993b) Rapid increase of BDNF mRNA levels in cortical neurons following spreading depression: regulation by glutamatergic mechanisms independent of seizure activity. *Molecular Brain Research*, **19**, 277–286.

Kokaia, Z., Metsis, M., Kokaia, M., Bengzon, J., Elmer, E., Smith, M-J., Timmusk, T., Siesjo, B.K., Persson, H. and Lindvall, O. (1994) Brain insults in rats induce increased expression of the BDNF gene through differential use of multiple promoters. *European Journal of Neuroscience*, **6**, 587–596.

Korsching, S. (1993) The neurotrophic factor concept: a reexamination. *Journal of Neuroscience*, **13**, 2739–2748.

Lehmann, S., Quirosa-Guillou, C., Becherer, U., Thal, C. and Zanetta, J-P. (1993) Neurite outgrowth of neurons of rat dorsal root ganglia induced by new neurotrophic substances with guanidine group. *Neuroscience Letters*, **152**, 57–60.

Levi-Montalcini, R. (1987) The nerve growth factor 35 years later. *Science*, *237*, 1154–1162.

Lewin, G.R. and Mendell, L.M. (1993) Nerve growth factor and nociception. *Trends in Neurological Science*, **16**, 353–359.

Lewin, G.R., Ritter, A.M. and Mendel, L.M. (1993) Nerve growth factor-induced hyperalgesia in the neonatal and adult rat. *Journal of Neuroscience*, **13**, 2136–2148.

Liebl, D.J. and Koo, P.H. (1993) Comparative binding of neurotrophins (NT-3, CNTF and NGF) and various cytokines to α_2-macroglobulin. *Biochemical and Biophysical Research Communications*, **193**, 1255–1261.

Lin, F.H., Doherty, D.H., Lile, J.D., Bektesh, S. and Collins, F. (1993) GDNF: a glial cell line-derived neurotrophic factor for midbrain dopaminergic neurons. *Science*, **260**, 1130–1132.

Lindsay, R.M. (1995) Neuron saving schemes. *Nature*, **373**, 289–373.

Lindvall, O., Emfors, P., Bengzon, J., Kokaia, Z., Smith, M-L., Siesjo, B.K. and Persson, H. (1992) Differential regulation of mRNAs for nerve growth factor, brain derived neurotrophic factor, and neurotrophin 3 in the adult rat brain following cerebral ischemia and hypoglycemic coma. *Proceedings of the National Academy of Science USA*, **89**, 648–652.

Lindvall, O., Kokaia, Z., Bengzon J., Elmér, E. and Kokaia, M. (1994) Neurotrophins and brain insults. *Trends in Neurological Sciences*, **17**, 490–496.

Lo, D.C. (1993) A central role for ciliary neurotrophic factor? *Proceedings of the National Academy of Science USA*, **90**, 2557–2558.

Loughlin, S.E. and Fallon, J.H. (eds) (1993) *Neurotrophic Factors*, Academic Press, San Diego.

Lyons, W.E., George, E.B., Dawson, T.M., Steiner, J.P. and Snyder, S.H. (1994) Immunosuppressant FK506 promotes neurite outgrowth in cultures of PC12 cells and sensory ganglia. *Proceedings of the National Academy of Science USA*, **91**, 3191–3195.

MacMillan, V., Judge, D., Wiseman, A., Settles, D., Swain, J. and Davis, J. (1993) Mice expressing a bovine basic fibroblast growth factor transgene in the brain show increased resistance to hypoxemic-ischemic cerebral damage. *Stroke*, **24**, 1735–1739.

Margolis, R.L., Chuang, D-M. and Post, R.M. (1994) Programmed cell death: implications for neuropsychiatric disorders. *Biological Psychiatry*, **35**, 946–956.

Matsuyama, A., Iwata, H., Okumura, N., Yoshida, S., Imaizumi, K., Lee, Y., Shiraishi, S. and Shiosaka, S. (1992) Localization of basic fibroblast growth factor-like immunoreactivity in the rat brain. *Brain Research*, **587**, 49–65.

Merikangas, K.R., Merikangas, J.R. and Angst, J. (1993) Headache syndromes and psychiatric disorders: association and familial transmission. *Journal of Psychiatric Research*, **27**, 197–210.

Moskowitz, M. and Macfarlane, R. (1993) Neurovascular and molecular mechanisms in migraine headaches. *Cerebrovascular Brain Metabolic Review*, **5**, 159–177.

Moskowitz, M.A., Nozaki, K. and Kraig, R.P. (1993) Neocortical spreading depression provokes the expression of *C-fos* protein-like immunoreactivity within trigeminal nucleus caudalis via trigeminovascular mechanisms. *Journal of Neuroscience*, **13**, 1167–1177.

Murase, K., Takeuchi, R., Iwata, E., Furukawa, Y., Furukawa, S. and Hayashi, K. (1992) Development changes in nerve growth factor level in rat serum. *Journal of Neuroscience Research*, **33**, 282–288.

Nagashima, K., Nakanishi, S. and Matsuda, Y. (1991) Inhibition of nerve growth factor-induced neurite outgrowth of PC12 cells by a protein kinase inhibitor which does not permeate the cell membrane. *FEBS Letters*, **293**, 119–123.

Nakanishi, S., Matsuda, Y., Iwahashi, K. and Kase, H. (1986) K-252b, c and d, potent inhibitors of protein kinase C from microbial origin. *Journal of Antibiotics*, **39**, 1066–1071.

Neeper, S.A., Gomez-Pinilla, F., Chol, J. and Cotman, C. (1995) Exercise and brain neurotrophins. *Nature*, **373**, 109.

Nibuya, M., Rudelek-Fitzgerald, L., Morinobu, S., Russell, D.S., Nestler, E.J. and Duman, R.S. (1994) Induction of BDNF and trkB by electroconvulsive seizure (ECS): regional regulation and role of CREB. *Society for Neuroscience Abstracts*, **20**, 1312.

Nikkhah, G., Odin, P., Smits, A., Tingström, A., Othberg, A., Brundin, P., Funa, K. and Lindvall, O. (1993) Platelet-derived growth factor promotes survival of rat and human mesencephalic dopaminergic neurons in culture. *Experimental Brain Research*, **92**, 516–523.

Olson, L., Nordberg, A., von Holst, H., Bäckman, L., Ebendal, T., Alafuzoff, I., Amberla, K., Hartvig, P., Herlitz, A., Lilja, A., Lundqvist, H., Långström, B., Meyerson, B., Persson, A., Viitanen, M., Winblad, B. and Seiger, A. (1992) Nerve growth factor affects C-nicotine binding, blood flow, EEG, and verbal episodic memory in an Alzheimer patient (Case Report). *Journal of Neural Transmission*, **4**, 79–95.

Oppenheim, R.W. (1991) Cell death during development of the nervous system. *Annual Review of Neuroscience*, **14**, 453–501.

Parada, L.F., Tsoulfas, S., Tessarollo, L., Blair, J., Reid, S.W. and Soppet, D. (1992). The trk family of tyrosine kinases: receptors for NGF-related neurotrophins. *Cold Spring Harbor Symposium*, **57**, 45–52.

Patterson, S.L., Grady., M.S. and Bothwell, M. (1993) Nerve growth factor and a fibroblast growth factor-like neurotrophic activity in cerebrospinal fluid of brain injured human patients. *Brain Research*, **605**, 43–49.

Peng, Z-C., Chen, S., Fusco, M., Vantini, G. and Bentivoglio, M. (1993) Fos induction by nerve growth factor in the adult rat brain. *Brain Research*, **632**, 57–67.

Petty, B.G., Cornblath, D.R., Adornato, B.T., Chaudhry, V., Flexner, C., Wachsman, M., Sinicropi, D., Burton, L.E. and Peroutka, S.J. (1994) The effect of systemically administered recombinant human nerve growth factor in healthy human subjects. *Annals of Neurology*, **36**, 244–246.

Post, R.M. and Silberstein, S.D. (1994) Shared mechanisms in affective illness, epilepsy, and migraine. *Neurology*, **44**, (Suppl. 7), S37–S47.

Purves, D. (1986) The trophic theory of neural connections. *Trends in Neuroscience*, **9**, 486–489.

Raff, M.C., Barres, B.A., Burne, J.F., Coles, H.S., Ishizaki, Y. and Jacobson, M.D. (1993) Programmed cell death and the control of cell survival: lessons from the nervous system. *Science*, **262**, 695–700.

Reis, D.J., Golanov, E.V., Yamamoto, S., Kobylarz, K. and Prabhakar, V. (1994) Conditioned neuroprotection from ischemic infarction elicited by electrical stimulation of the cerebellar fastigial nucleus (FN) in rat. *Society for Neuroscience Abstracts*, **20**, 1480.

Rosenblatt, S., Irikura, K., Caday, C.G., Finklestein, S.P. and Moskowitz, M.A. (1994) Basic fibroblast growth factor dilates rat pial arterioles. *Journal of Cerebral Blood Flow and Metabolism*, **14**, 70–74.

Sandler, M. (1995) Migraine to the year 2000. *Cephalalgia*, **15**, 259–264.

Sandler, M., Li, N-Y., Jarrett, N. and Glover, V. (1995) Dietary migraine: recent progress in the red (and white) wine story. *Cephalalgia*, **15**, 101–103.

Sandyk, R. and Iacono, R.P. (1987) Phenelzine in migraine headaches. *Journal of Neuroscience*, **35**, 243.

Sato, K., Kashibara, K., Morimoto, K., Otsuki, K., Fujiwara, Y., Akiyama, K., Hayahara, T. and Kuroda, S. (1994) Regional increase in brain-derived neurotrophic factor and nerve growth factor mRNA, but not in acidic and basic fibroblast growth factor mRNA in kindling. *Society for Neuroscience Abstracts*, **20**, 1312.

Simon, R.P., Chen, J., Lan, J.O., Zhu, L., Swanson, R.A. and Graham, S.H. (1994) Characterization of induced ischemic tolerance in focal cerebral ischemia in rats. *Society for Neuroscience Abstracts*, **20**, 1480.

Siuciak, J.A., Altar, C.A., Wiegand, S.J. and Lindsay, R.M. (1994a) Antinociceptive effect of brain-derived neurotrophic factor and neurotrophin-3. *Brain Research*, **633**, 326–330.

Siuciak, J.A., Lewis, D., Wiegand, S.J. and Lindsay, R.M. (1994b) Brain derived neurotrophic factor (BDNF) produces an anti-depressant like effect in two animal models of depression. *Society for Neuroscience Abstracts*, **20**, 1106.

Smith, M.A. (1994) Neurotrophins, stress and drugs. Stress alters the expression of neurotrophic factors in the rat brain. *Abstracts of the American College of Neuropsychopharmacology*, p. 76.

Thoenen, H., Bandtlow, C. and Heumann, R. (1987) The physiological function of nerve growth factor in the central nervous system: comparison with the periphery. *Reviews of Physiology, Biochemistry and Pharmacology*, **109**, 145–178.

Toda, S., Yamamoto, S., Tenmyo, O., Tsuno, T., Hasegawa, T., Rosser, M., Oka, M., Sawada, Y., Konishi, M. and Oki, T. (1993) A new neuritogenetic compound BU-4514N produced by *Microtetraspora* sp. *Journal of Antibiotics*, **46**, 875–883.

Travis, J. (1994) Glia: the brain's other cells. *Science*, **266**, 970–972.

Tuttle, J.B. and Creedon, D.J. (1993) Pharmacology of nerve growth factor output by target cells. *Annals of the New York Academy of Science*, **692**, 273–276.

Walkinshaw, G. and Waters, C.M. (1994) Neurotoxin-induced cell death in neuronal PC12 cells is mediated by induction of apoptosis. *Neuroscience*, **63**, 975–987.

Watkins, L.R., Wiertelak, E.P., Goehler, L.E., Smith, K.P., Martin, D. and Maier, S.F. (1994) Characterization of cytokine-induced hyperalgesia. *Brain Research*, **654**, 15–26.

Welch, K.M.A., Barkley, G.L., Tepley, N. and Ramadan, N.M. (1993) Central neurogenic mechanisms of migraine. *Neurology*, **43**, S21–S25.

Woolf, C.J., Safieh-Garabedian, B., Ma, Q.-P, Crilly, P. and Winters J. (1994) Nerve growth factor contributes to the generation of inflammatory sensory hypersensitivity. *Neuroscience*, **62**, 327–331.

Yamada, K., Kinoshita, A., Kohmura, E., Sakaguchi, T., Taguchi, J. and Kataoka K. (1991) Basic fibroblast growth factor prevents thalamic degeneration after cortical infarction. *Journal of Cerebral Blood Flow and Metabolism*, **11**, 472–478.

Yamaguchi, K, Tsuji, T., Wakuri, S., Yazawa, K., Kondo, K., Shigemori, H. and Kobayashi, J. (1993) Stimulation of nerve growth factor synthesis and secretion by fellutamide A in vitro. *Bioscience Biotechnology and Biochemistry*, **57**, 195–199.

Yamamoto, H. and Gurney, M.E. (1990) Human platelets contain brain-derived neurotrophic factor. *Journal of Neuroscience*, **10**, 3469–3478.

Yan, Q., Matheson, C. and Lopez, O.T. (1995) *In vivo* neurotrophic effects of GDNF on neonatal and adult facial motor neurons. *Nature*, **373**, 341–344.

Yan, Q., Matheson, C., Lopez, O.T. and Miller, J.A. (1994) The biological responses of axotomized adult motoneurons to brain-derived neurotrophic factor. *Journal of Neuroscience*, **14**, 5281–5291.

Yasuhara, O., Muramatsu, H., Kim, S.U., Muramatsu, T., Maruta, H. and McGeer, P.L. (1993) Midkine, a novel neurotrophic factor, is present in senile plaques of Alzheimer disease. *Biochemical and Biophysical Research Communication*, **192**, 246–251.

DISCUSSION

Fozard: Do we understand what is happening at the neuronal level when nerve growth factor (NGF) produces hyperalgesia?

Sandler: No, I do not think it has been investigated.

Fozard: Woolf *et al.* (1994) found that the release of the sensory transmitters was normal, so at least it seems that it is not interfering with the release of those transmitters but perhaps sensitizing the neurons to the effects of such transmitters.

Sandler: Yes, after local anti-NGF serum administration the inflammatory process seemed to be unaltered and neuropeptide concentrations were unchanged, but the animal did not have any pain.

Schoenen: NGF has been shown to be trophic for dorsal root ganglion neurons and to inhibit transganglionic degeneration in the spinal cord dorsal horn after sciatic nerve section.

Sandler: Yes. The dorsal root ganglion is a great target!

Schoenen: Would migraine be the first disorder where an excess of one of these factors is suspected? Until now hypotheses have mainly involved deficient activity of these neurotrophic factors, for example in Alzheimer's and Parkinson's disease or neuropathies.

Sandler: If it were true, then it might be.

Schoenen: Would your hypothesis involve an excessive release or production at a given time, or some long-standing excessive production or activity?

Sandler: You are right to pin me down! One possible mechanism might be hypersensitivity to a normal production of nerve growth factor, perhaps after spreading depression, which is probably what many of us think the migraine aura has turned out to be (Lauritzen 1994). Or it may be that any of the triggering phenomena initiate a secondary release of NGF.

Schoenen: What about the relationship with the neurotransmitters, for example, 5-hydroxytryptamine? You alluded to acetylcholine systems which are known to be centrally controlled: NGF is trophic for these cholinergic systems.

Sandler: Brain-derived neurotrophic factor (BDNF) to some extent controls the dopaminergic system (Hyman *et al.* 1991), but also other factors, in particular the glial-derived neurotrophic factor, have a powerful effect on dopaminergic system growth (Lin *et al.* 1993). I would stress that there are so many of these factors acting together, some in a sort of see-saw relationship, that the problem is difficult to elucidate (for review, see Korsching 1993).

Connor: Presumably the anti-nerve growth factor serums or anti-*trk* A serums could have quite detrimental effects within the CNS.

Sandler: Yes. It depends where they home in. We will have to approach this very carefully.

Humphrey: It is difficult to see how you can get an idea for an analgesic drug here because of the physiological importance of growth factors. An anti-growth factor serum or a tyrosine kinase receptor blocker could be fairly disastrous clinically.

Sandler: We assume that these proteins do not cross the blood–brain barrier. NGF certainly does not cross the blood–brain barrier. To get

NGF into the brain, to try to treat Alzheimer's disease, for example, you can give it intraventricularly (Olson *et al.* 1992) or you can conjugate it to a transferrin receptor antibody to facilitate its passage (Friden *et al.* 1993).

Humphrey: But in a scenario involving damage leading to algesia, the growth factor would be expected to be important for essential repair.

Sandler: Well, what would no growth factor do in an inflammatory situation? We have no information. Many things come to the fore during the inflammatory process.

Moskowitz: How do you address the relatively long time for NGF induction with respect to headache and migraine? It seems that the induction of pain takes time.

Sandler: It may be that small amounts are produced well before the peak production that we measured. Perhaps some individuals are sensitive to these small amounts. I have not really addressed myself to the question in man.

Peatfield: Is there a valid distinction between the functions of nerve growth factors in the development of the nervous system, and the function of the growth factors in the fully grown nervous system where they might act in a hormone-like way, or by influencing nerve terminals?

Sandler: Yes. The only proven continuous activity in the adult seems to be connected with BDNF (Huntley *et al.* 1992, Acheson *et al.* 1995). This might be relevant to the depression story.

Peatfield: We do need to explore that and perhaps not pay quite so much attention to some of the original discoveries, which seem to be related to the development of the nervous system, and why a proportion of cells disintegrate during development.

Sandler: There isn't much information in adult man. NGF stimulates expression of 5-HT$_3$ receptors (Isenberg *et al.* 1993). One wonders about its possible action on other ion channel receptors.

Peatfield: What happens if you raise antibody to NGF and infuse it into adult animals, assuming it has access to all the sites of action of NGF?

Sandler: The protein would not have that access.

Peatfield: I recognize that problem, but I wonder whether this kind of approach might shed any light on what NGF does in an adult animal.

Fozard: There appear to be several receptor sites for neurotrophins. There might, therefore, be some opportunity for selective blockade of, say, the receptors producing hyperalgesia.

REFERENCES

Acheson, A., Conover, J.C., Fandl, J.P., DeChiara, T.M., Russell, M., Thadani, A., Squinto, S.P., Yancopoulos, G.D. and Lindsay, R.M. (1995) A BDNF autocrine loop in adult sensory neurons prevents cell death. *Nature*, **374**, 450–453.

Friden, P.M., Walus, L.R., Watson, P., Doctrow, S.R., Kozarich, J.W., Bäckman, L., Bergman, H., Hoffer, B., Bloom, F. and Granholm, A.-C. (1993) Blood–brain barrier penetration and in vivo activity of an NGF conjugate. *Science*, **259**, 373–377.

Huntley, G.W., Benson, D.L., Jones, E.G. and Isackson, P.J. (1992) Developmental expression of brain derived neurotrophic factor mRNA by neurons of fetal and adult monkey prefrontal cortex. *Developmental Brain Research*, **70**, 53–63.

Hyman, C., Hofer, M., Barde, Y.-A., Juhasz, M., Yancopoulos, G.C., Squinto, S.P. and Lindsay, R.M. (1991) BDNF is a neurotrophic factor for dopaminergic neurons of the substantia nigra. *Nature*, **350**, 230–232.

Isenberg, K.E., Ukhun, I.A., Holstad, S.G., Jafri, S., Uchida, U., Zorumski, C.F. and Yang, J. (1993) Partial cDNA cloning and NGF regulation of a rat 5-HT$_3$ receptor subunit. *NeuroReport*, **5**, 121–124.

Korsching, S. (1993) The neurotrophic factor concept: a re-examination. *Journal of Neuroscience*, **13**, 2739–2748.

Lauritzen, M. (1994) Pathophysiology of the migraine aura. *Brain*, **117**, 199–210.

Lin, F.H., Doherty, D.H., Lile, J.D., Bektesh, S. and Collins, F. (1993) GDNF: a glial cell line-derived neurotrophic factor for midbrain dopaminergic neurons. *Science*, **260**, 1130–1132.

Olson, L., Nordberg, A., von Holst, H., Bäckman, L., Ebendal, T., Alafuzoff, I., Amberia, K., Hartvig, P., Herlitz, A., Lilja, A., Lundqvist, H., Längström, B., Meyerson, B., Persson, A., Viitanen, M., Winblad, B. and Seiger, A. (1992) Nerve growth factor affects C-nicotine binding, blood flow, EEG, and verbal episodic memory in an Alzheimer patient (Case Report). *Journal of Neural Transmission*, **4**, 79–95.

Woolf, C.J., Safieh-Garabedian, B., Ma, Q-P., Crilly, P. and Winters, J. (1994) Nerve growth factor contributes to the generation of inflammatory sensory hypersensitivity. *Neuroscience*, **62**, 327–331.

16

The role of perivascular peptides in migraine

Lars Edvinsson

INTRODUCTION

The early classical studies by Ray and Wolff (1940) showed that large cerebral arteries at the base of the brain and meningeal (dural) arteries and sinusoids were sensitive to noxious stimuli. This directed interest to the wall of the intracranial vessels. Radner (1947), when performing the first series of selective vertebral angiography, observed that all his patients complained of acute headache when he injected the contrast media. This was later confirmed by Hauge (1954) in an extensive study where visual phenomena with resemblance to migraine headache and with some associated facial symptoms were described (see also Sjaastad and Saunte 1983). The effect of contrast media on brain vessels was much later suggested to be the result of vasodilatation due to the increase in local osmolarity (Edvinsson *et al.* 1987a, Jansen *et al.* 1987): the effect remained after removal of the endothelium. The currently used contrast media are iso-osmolar and therefore have less direct vascular effects.

Alcohol and some vasodilators such as nitroglycerin and histamine can induce bilateral pulsating headache which is rarely accompanied by nausea, photo- and phonophobia in healthy subjects (Lance 1993, Iversen *et al.* 1989). However, migraine-like episodes can be triggered in migraine sufferers (Olesen *et al.* 1993; Thomsen *et al.* 1993). On the other hand, vasoconstrictors such as the ergots, 5-hydroxytryptamine and

Migraine: Pharmacology and genetics
Edited by Merton Sandler, Michel Ferrari and Sara Harnett
Published in 1996 by Chapman & Hall
ISBN 1 86036 006 8

noradrenaline can abort the attack, probably through vasoconstriction of the larger arteries at the base of the brain given their relative inability to cross the blood–brain barrier (Lance 1993).

PERIVASCULAR NERVES

This obviously opens the following questions for the vessel wall: Are there sensors? How is the information propagated? Is there a neuro-anatomical link to explain referred pain? Are there connections to the brainstem and central neuronal components of the pain system?

The first detailed study of the innervation of the human cerebral circulation focused on the 'classical' autonomic transmitters noradrenaline (NA) and acetylcholine (ACh) (Edvinsson *et al.* 1976). By 1664 Thomas Willis had already described nerve fibres on the anterior and the posterior cerebral arteries. With modern histochemical techniques their origin, distribution, neurotransmitter content and ultrastructural criteria are still being described by work on laboratory animals (Edvinsson *et al.* 1993). In brief, the perivascular nerves can be classified into three systems.

The **sympathetic system** arises in hypothalamic neurons passing to the intermediolateral cell column of the spinal cord and synapsing before proceeding out to the superior cervical ganglion. Here they again synapse and give rise to the fibres that innervate the vessels. This system is marked by the transmitters noradrenaline, neuropeptide Y (NPY) (Edvinsson *et al.* 1983) and possibly adenosine triphosphate (ATP). It is fundamentally a vasoconstrictor pathway (Edvinsson *et al.* 1993). The **parasympathetic system** arises from cell bodies in the superior salivatory nucleus passing out with fibres of the facial nerve (VII cranial nerve) and synapsing in the sphenopalatine and otic ganglia (Gibbins *et al.* 1984, Suzuki *et al.* 1988). In some species there are additional microganglia on the internal carotid artery. This system is marked by the neurotransmitters acetylcholine, vasoactive intestinal polypeptide (VIP) (Larsson *et al.* 1976), and peptide histidine isoleucine (PHI) and methionine (PHM) (Edvinsson and McCulloch 1985). In addition, pituitary adenylate cyclase-activating peptide (PACAP) (Uddman *et al.* 1993a), helospectin (Uddman *et al.* 1993b) and nitric oxide synthase (NOS) activity (Nozaki *et al.* 1993) have been found in the parasympathetic nerves. Physiologically, the system is vasodilatory (Edvinsson *et al.* 1985). Lastly, there is sensory innervation of cranial vessels and dura mater from the **trigeminal system**. The cell bodies are bipolar and located in the trigeminal ganglion. They make functional first-order connections with neurons in the trigeminal nucleus caudalis and in its related extension down to the C2 level (see Goadsby and Zagami 1991). This system is marked by calcitonin gene-related peptide

(CGRP) (Uddman *et al.* 1985), substance P (SP) (Edvinsson *et al.* 1981) and neurokinin A (NKA) (Edvinsson *et al.* 1988). A minor population of NOS-positive and a relatively large population of PACAP-positive cell bodies are seen. It is an essentially vasodilatory system as well as having a primary involvement in sensory functions (Edvinsson *et al.* 1986).

PEPTIDERGIC MECHANISMS IN MAN

Innervation

Different human cerebral vessels have been examined using either autopsy specimens of large cerebral arteries or cortical vessels obtained during neurosurgical tumour resections (Edvinsson *et al.* 1987b, 1994, Edvinsson and Ekman 1984, Jansen *et al.* 1992, 1986, Allen *et al.* 1984). All major arteries belonging to the circle of Willis (post-mortem tissue) are supplied with a very dense innervation. This is readily illustrated using immunofluorescence: numerous NPY immunoreactive fibres can be seen. There is a close similarity in the innervation patterns for NPY and tyrosine hydroxylase (TH), a noradrenaline synthesis enzyme. The supply of CGRP/SP as well as that of VIP is sparse.

A markedly different degree of density is seen in whole-mount preparations of fresh human cortical arteries and veins obtained during neurosurgical tumour resections. The density of NPY and TH immuno-reactivity is quite marked. There is a close similarity in the distribution of NPY and TH immunoreactive fibres, supporting their putative sympathetic origin. Also, the human cortical veins are supplied by a moderate number of NPY and TH immunoreactive fibres. In contrast, only few scattered fibres were seen to contain VIP, CGRP or SP immunoreactivity (Edvinsson *et al.* 1994).

Quantitative studies

HPLC extracts of the human cerebral arteries have revealed that NPY, VIP and CGRP immunoreactivity each elute in one major component with the same elution volume as the synthetic human NPY, VIP, and human α-CGRP, respectively (Edvinsson *et al.* 1987b, 1994, Jansen *et al.* 1992). SP elutes as two peaks, one major peak with the same retention volume as SP, and in a second peak with the same elution volume as oxidized SP (Jansen *et al.* 1992). Quantitative measurements in the human middle cerebral artery revealed the following concentrations (pmol/g $\pm$ SEM); NPY, 3.0 $\pm$ 2.4; VIP, 2.3 $\pm$ 0.7; CGRP, 3.9 $\pm$ 1.1; and SP, 2.3 $\pm$ 0.8. There was no significant difference in the different peptide concentrations. However, in one quantitative study (Edvinsson *et al.* 1987) it was observed that there is a continuous decline in the concentrations of all the perivascular peptides from the newborn to the elderly.

Vasomotor responses

Administration of NPY elicits a concentration-dependent contraction of human cerebral arteries (Edvinsson *et al.* 1987b). The responses induced by NPY are somewhat stronger than those induced by NA, and the potency significantly higher for NPY than for NA. The contractile response to NA is antagonized in a competitive fashion by the α_1-adrenoceptor antagonist prazosin. The NPY-induced contractions are instead mediated via the Y_1 subtype of NPY receptors since Pro^{34} -NPY and NPY are equipotent while NPY_{13-36} has only weak effects on human brain vessels (Edvinsson *et al.* 1991). The NPY contractions are blocked in a competitive manner by the new NPY antagonist BIBP3226.

In precontracted vessel segments, ACh, VIP and PHM cause dilatation (Edvinsson *et al.* 1987, Jansen *et al.* 1992). The relative potency for relaxation in the cerebral arteries is VIP > PHM > ACh. There are significant differences in potency between VIP and PHM-27, and between VIP and ACh: the amount of relaxation varies between 76 and 87%. The ACh relaxation occurs via a muscarinic receptor and involves the release of nitric oxide from the endothelium while VIP causes activation of adenylyl cyclase.

CGRP, SP and NKA act as strong vasodilators. The order of potency is CGRP > SP > NKA. CGRP induces relaxation with the highest I_{max} (91%) compared to SP (70%) and NKA (80%). The existence of specific peptide receptors is supported by agonist and antagonist studies. In particular, selective NK-1 antagonists may block the SP-induced relaxation in a competitive manner. These responses cause relaxation via release of nitric oxide from the endothelial cells. The CGRP receptor activation involves stimulation of adenylyl cyclase and appears, by and large, to be independent of the endothelium.

HUMAN IN VIVO DATA

Human data will be considered under the three major headache categories that have been studied, migraine with and without aura and cluster headache. It is important to note, in order to link the basic science to the clinical data, some observations of direct trigeminal ganglion stimulation in man.

Trigeminal ganglion stimulation

The trigeminal system provides the only known pain-sensitive innervation of the cranial vasculature by virtue of the central convergence of trigeminal and upper cervical pain inputs. This takes place at the second-order neurons. When these pathways are activated in animals there is no resting tone on regional cerebral blood flow (rCBF) or regional glucose use (Edvinsson *et al.* 1986). Trigeminal ganglion stimulation increases both bulk extracerebral (Goadsby *et al.* 1986) and regional cerebral blood flow, specifically in the frontal and parietal cortex (Goadsby and Duckworth 1987). The effect upon extracerebral blood flow is mediated through strong reflex connections with the facial nerve dilator system, which relays some 80% of the dilatation in some species, while the remaining 20% is mediated antidromically (Lambert *et al.* 1984).

In man, Tran-Dinh and colleagues (1992) observed that thermal stimulation of the trigeminal ganglion resulted in a bilateral cortical blood flow increase, slightly more ipsilateral, thus supporting the available animal data (Goadsby and Duckworth 1987).

Trigeminal ganglion stimulation results in local cranial release of both CGRP and SP in the cat, both acting as markers of trigeminal activation (Goadsby *et al.* 1988). Patients under treatment for trigeminal neuralgia by thermocoagulation of the ganglion were noted to flush ipsilateral to the side of stimulation. As this flush occurred, blood samples were taken from the external jugular vein (EJV) and compared with samples taken immediately before coagulation. There was a marked increase in both CGRP and SP in the patients who flushed compared to the control precoagulation levels (Goadsby *et al.* 1988).

Migraine with aura

Prodromal

Early studies of this condition were confined to either peripheral venous blood or cerebrospinal fluid (CSF). In peripheral blood, VIP and SP levels were not altered during the headache (Blegvad *et al.* 1986). Furthermore, the often described symptoms of altered bladder habit, or hunger, have led to the suggestion that this may reflect a hypothalamic disturbance and therefore be a manifestation of an essentially central nervous system disorder. However, analysis of vasopressin levels during headache (unchanged) has not supported this hypothesis (Blegvad *et al.* 1986). In an attempt to examine brain function more directly, the levels of various agents in CSF have been determined. Morphine-like substances have been reported to be reduced during migraine (Anselmi *et al.* 1980), although no change in β-endorphin or ACTH was detected (Bach *et al.* 1985). Interestingly, plasma and platelet met-enkephalin levels were moderately increased during headache (Ferrari *et al.* 1987, Mosnaim *et al.* 1985).

Aura

In a series of studies Olesen *et al.* (1981, 1990) showed a pattern of 'spreading oligaemia' or 'spreading hypoperfusion'. This was, however, only apparent in patients with migraine with aura. The hypoperfusion is ipsilateral to the headache pain and contralateral to the symptoms of aura. Woods *et al.* (1994) demonstrated support for the spreading nature of hypoperfusion in one subject with a spontaneous migraine. They performed blood flow measurements with positron emission tomography (PET) and oxygen-15-labelled water and noted, in addition, that the headache was associated with bilateral hypoperfusion that started in the occipital lobes and spread anteriorly into the temporal and parietal lobes ipsilaterally. It is interesting to note that the involvement spread across the cortical surface at a relatively constant rate, sparing the cerebellum, the basal ganglia and the thalamus. During this course it ultimately spanned the vascular distribution territories of four major cerebral arteries. These studies lend much support to the hypothesis of spreading depression in migraine (Lauritzen 1994).

Experimental studies in cat (and unpublished in monkey) with induced spreading depression revealed the expected flow changes but no neuropeptide release (Piper *et al.* 1993). One study in man came to the same conclusion when sampling central venous blood (Friberg *et al.* 1994). Thus, the vasoconstriction of cortical arterioles may result in dilatation of the large arteries at the base of the brain in order to maintain relatively constant cerebral blood flow. Depending on region, extent and situation of the aura, minor or larger areas of the cortex may be affected.

Headache

The results of trigeminal ganglion stimulation in man led us to examine the levels of various neuropeptides in man during migraine. Blood samples were drawn from the external jugular vein during headache. We assessed patients using markers for the sympathetic (NPY), parasympathetic (VIP), and trigeminovascular systems (CGRP, SP). There were no changes in the peripheral blood levels of the peptides studied or in NPY, VIP, or SP in the EJV blood. However, there was a marked increase in CGRP in external jugular venous blood: from control levels of 40 pmol/l to 91 ± 11 pmol/l during the migraine headache (Goadsby *et al.* 1990). Two patients with some symptoms similar to those seen in cluster headache, e.g. nasal congestion and rhinorrhea, had increases in VIP, but this was not significant for the whole group. We have confirmed these observations in a further series of patients who had blood sampled during headache and then after administration of sumatriptan. Remarkably, the CGRP levels returned to control after administration of sumatriptan with successful amelioration of the headache (Goadsby and Edvinsson 1991, 1993a). The changes in VIP suggest that some reflex parasympathetically mediated event is also taking place, but this requires further characterization (Zagami and Lambert 1990, Lambert *et al.* 1988).

Migraine without aura

A similar picture to that seen for migraine with aura emerges for migraine without aura. Plasma levels of SP and VIP are normal both during an attack and interictally (Blegvad *et al.* 1986). Again, as with migraine with aura, plasma vasopressin levels were unchanged during headache (Blegvad *et al.* 1986). Conflicting data emerged concerning the opioids: in two studies met-enkephalin and β-endorphin were shown to be marginally elevated (Ferrari *et al.* 1987, Mosnaim *et al.* 1985), while in other studies no change was found, specifically for β-endorphin and ACTH (Bach *et al.* 1985). Studies of the cerebrospinal fluid demonstrated that there is no change in either SP or somatostatin during headache (Vecchiet *et al.* 1987).

Again, we examined patients with migraine without aura during headache by sampling blood from the EJV. As with migraine with aura, substantial increases in CGRP levels were found in the external jugular venous blood. There were no changes in SP, VIP or NPY in jugular or in peripheral blood (Goadsby *et al.* 1990). Nicolodi and Del Bianco (1990) sampled saliva and analysed peptides in association with migraine without aura. They saw increases in both SP and CGRP along with a reduction in VIP during headache (Nicolodi and Del Bianco 1990). The difference in the changes seen with these techniques probably represents the different field of sampling. While the cerebral circulation has a preferentially CGRP-rich trigeminal innervation (O'Connor and van der Kooy 1988) the innervation of the salivary glands is not as well characterized.

Cluster headache

Cluster headache is a rare severe disorder with a poorly understood pathophysiology. Although it would seem to be an ideal condition to examine, in that it is a well-described clear-cut clinical syndrome in which a number of attacks can be studied, analysis of neuropeptide release has not been particularly helpful. Plasma levels of SP and somatostatin show only very modest change (Sicuteri *et al.* 1985), while met-enkephalin and β-endorphin levels appear consistently elevated during headache (Appenzeller *et al.* 1981, Hardebo *et al.* 1985).

Cerebrospinal fluid changes are similar with only changes in met-enkephalin being noted reliably (Hardebo and Ekman 1986). Interestingly, both substance P and VIP levels were elevated in the saliva during headache. This may well indicate activation of the central and peripheral arms of the trigeminovascular reflex (Goadsby and Lance 1988), but further studies are needed to clarify the relationship between salivary peptide changes and headache.

In a recent study, patients with episodic cluster headache fulfilling the criteria of the International Headache Society (Headache Classification Committee 1988) were examined during an acute spontaneous attack of headache to determine the local cranial release of neuropeptides (Goadsby and Edvinsson 1993b, 1994). Blood was sampled from the EJV ipsilateral to the pain before and after treatment of the attack. Samples were assayed for CGRP, VIP, SP and NPY. The attacks were treated with either oxygen inhalation, sumatriptan or an opiate. Thirteen patients were studied. All had well-established typical attacks of cluster headache when blood was sampled. During the attacks, external jugular vein blood concentrations of CGRP and VIP were raised while there was no change in NPY or SP. CGRP concentrations rose to 110 ± 7 pmol/l (control, <40), while VIP levels rose to 20 ± 3 pmol/l (control, <7). Treatment with oxygen or sumatriptan (subcutaneous) reduced the CGRP level to normal, while opiate administration did not alter the peptide levels. These data demonstrate for the first time *in vivo* human evidence for activation of the trigeminovascular system and the cranial parasympathetic nervous system in an acute attack of cluster headache. All subjects had release of VIP. This is in concert with the facial symptoms that are well known to the symptomatology of this rare disorder. Furthermore, it was shown that both oxygen and sumatriptan, while aborting the attacks, terminate activity in the trigeminovascular system. This agrees well with the results of Fanciullacci *et al.* (1995) demonstrating release of CGRP in nitroglycerin-elicited attacks of cluster headache.

Thus, CGRP, which marks the trigeminovascular system, and VIP, which marks parasympathetic activity, are both elevated in the cranial venous blood of patients with an acute spontaneous attack of cluster headache. The termination of the attack with either sumatriptan or oxygen causes normalization of the CGRP levels, reflecting cessation of activity in the trigeminovascular system, whereas pain relief along with an opiate agonist apparently terminates the attack but does not immediately cause trigeminovascular activity to cease. The finding of both CGRP and VIP in the cranial venous blood suggests that there is activation of a brainstem reflex, the afferent arc of which is the trigeminal nerve and the efferent the cranial parasympathetic outflow from the VIIth nerve. This investigation of cluster headache allows us to examine some important aspects of the neural innervation of the cranial circulation. Such studies provide general physiological information applicable to our understanding of vascular headaches such as migraine.

SUBARACHNOID HAEMORRHAGE AND NEUROPEPTIDES

A possible involvement of perivascular vasodilatory neuropeptides in subarachnoid haemorrhage (SAH) has been evaluated in man by measuring the levels of CGRP, SP and VIP in the cranial venous outflow and in CSF in thirty-four patients admitted to hospital after an acute SAH (Juul *et al.* 1990, 1995). After surgery with aneurysm clipping and nimodipine treatment, blood samples were taken from the external jugular vein or CSF and analysed for neuropeptide levels during the postoperative course. The degree of vasoconstriction in the patients was monitored with Doppler ultrasound recordings bilaterally from the middle cerebral (MCA) and internal carotid (ICA) arteries following the EJV blood sampling every second day. The mean value of all CGRP measurements in EJV during the entire course of SAH revealed a significantly higher level compared to the control. The highest CGRP levels were found in patients with the highest velocity index values (vasospasm). The relationship $V_{mean\ MCA}/V_{mean\ ICA}$ was used as an index of vasoconstriction. In patients with MCA aneurysms ($n = 10$), a significant correlation (r $= 0.65$, $p < 0.05$) was found between the vasospasm index and the CGRP levels. There were no changes observed in the SP and VIP levels. Alterations in cerebrovascular tone induced by changing arterial CO_2 tension or lowering of blood pressure (ketanserin infusion test) did not alter the levels of the perivascular peptides in the EJV. Inhalation of CO_2, hyperventilation (lowering of CO_2), or lowering of the blood pressure with ketanserin infusion resulted in the expected changes in cerebral blood flow as published separately (Olsen *et al.* 1992), but there were no significant changes in the EJV levels of CGRP, SP or NPY. The levels of VIP remained low. In addition, CGRP, SP, VIP and NPY were analysed in CSF in the postoperative course after subarachnoid haemorrhage in 14 patients. The CSF VIP was lower in SAH than in controls. In individual patients with marked vasoconstriction increased concentrations of CGRP (up to 14 pmol/l) and NPY (up to 232 pmol/l) were observed. Thus, the alterations seen in this study of neuropeptide profile following SAH, or as previously reported in migraine (Goadsby and Edvinsson 1993a, Goadsby *et al.* 1990) are not due simply to changes *per se* in cerebral blood flow or in cerebrovascular tone. This is supported by the study of CSF neuropeptides in SAH patients: the highest levels of CGRP were found in subjects with marked vasospasm.

These results demonstrate that in a strict and clear-cut intracranial arterial constrictory disorder the trigeminovascular reflex (McCulloch *et al.* 1986) is active to counterbalance vasospasm by release of the vasodilator CGRP. This is verified both by measurements in the jugular vein outflow and by CGRP increase in the CSF. The degree of vasospasm correlates well with CGRP levels in EJV blood and CSF. This lends support to our data on neuropeptide release in migraine and cluster headache.

CONCLUSIONS

The study of neuropeptide levels in migraine and cluster headache is now providing the link between the clinic and research work that is so crucial if the basic pathophysiology of the problem is to be determined. In both migraine with and without aura there are marked changes in cranial levels of CGRP indicating activation of the trigeminal system. These levels are rendered normal by the new and highly effective antimigraine agents sumatriptan and zolmitriptan, coincident with the relief of the headache (Goadsby and Edvinsson 1994). Similarly, CGRP is released with trigeminal activation in studies on animals and, at least for the rat, the changes are also inhibited by sumatriptan. These data substantiate the usefulness of the animal models employed. Work is underway to explore the neural innervation of the cerebral and extracerebral vessels which, along with pharmacological studies of the transmitters involved, should permit both a better understanding of the pathogenesis of migraine and more effective treatment.

Acknowledgements

This study was supported by the Swedish Medical Research Council (project no. 5958), and by the Faculty of Medicine, Lund University.

REFERENCES

Allen, J.M., Todd, N., Crockard, H.A., Schon, F., Yeats, J.C. and Bloom, S.R. (1984) Presence of neuropeptide Y in human circle of Willis and its possible role in cerebral vasospasm. *Lancet*, **ii**, 550–552.

Anselmi, B., Baldi, E., Casacci, F. and Salmon, S. (1980) Endogenous opioids in cerebrospinal fluid and blood in idiopathic headache sufferers. *Headache*, **20**, 294–299.

Appenzeller, O., Atkinson, R.A. and Standefer, J.C. (1981) Serum β-endorphin in cluster headache and common migraine. In: *Progress in Migraine Research*, (eds F. Clifford Rose and K. Zilkha), pp.106–109. Pitman, Bath.

Bach, F.W., Jensen, K., Blegvad, N., Fenger, M., Jordal, R. and Olesen, J. (1985) β-Endorphin and ACTH in plasma during attacks of common and classic migraine. *Cephalalgia*, **5**, 177–182.

Blegvad, N., Jensen, K., Fahrenkrug, J., Schaffalitzky de Muckadell, O.B. and

Olesen, J. (1986) Plasma VIP and substance P during migraine attack. *Cephalalgia*, **5** (Suppl. 2), 252–253.

Edvinsson, L. and Ekman, R. (1984) Distribution and dilatory effect of vasoactive intestinal polypeptide (VIP) in human cerebral arteries. *Peptides*, **5**, 329–331.

Edvinsson, L. and McCulloch, J. (1985) Distribution and vasomotor effects of peptide HI (PHI) in feline cerebral blood vessels in vitro and in situ. *Regulatory Peptides*, **10**, 345–356.

Edvinsson, L., Owman, C. and Sjöberg, N-O. (1976) Autonomic nerves, mast cells, and amine receptors in human brain vessels. A histochemical and pharmacological study. *Brain Research*, **115**, 337–393.

Edvinsson, L., McCulloch, J. and Uddman, R. (1981) Substance P: immunohisto-chemical localization and effect upon cat pial arteries in vitro and in situ. *Journal of Physiology*, **325**, 251–258.

Edvinsson, L., Emson, P., McCulloch, J., Tatemoto, K. and Uddman, R. (1983) Neuropeptide Y: cerebrovascular innervation and vasomotor effects in the cat. *Neuroscience Letters*, **43**, 79–84.

Edvinsson, L., Fredholm, B.B., Hamel, E., Jansen, I. and Verrecchia, C. (1985) Perivascular peptides relax cerebral arteries concomitant with stimulation of cyclic adenosine monophosphate accumulation or release of an endothelium-derived relaxing factor in the cat. *Neuroscience Letters*, **58**, 213–217.

Edvinsson, L., McCulloch, J., Kingman, T.A. and Uddman, R. (1986) On the functional role of the trigemino-cerebrovascular system in the regulation of cerebral circulation. In: *Neural Regulation of the Cerebral Circulation*, (eds C. Owman and J.E. Hardebo), pp. 4007–4018. Elsevier, Amsterdam.

Edvinsson, L., Golman, K. and Jansen, I. (1987a) Site of action of contrast media on cerebral vessels. *Cephalalgia*, **7**, 83–85.

Edvinsson, L., Ekman, R., Jansen, I., Ottosson, A. and Uddman, R. (1987b) Peptide containing nerve fibres in human cerebral arteries: immunocyto-chemistry, radioimmunoassay and in vitro pharmacology. *Annals of Neurology*, **21**, 431–437.

Edvinsson, L., Brodin, E., Jansen, I. and Uddman, R. (1988) Neurokinin A in cerebral vessels: characterization, localization and effects in vitro. *Regulatory Peptides*, **20**, 181–197.

Edvinsson, L., Adamsson, M. and Jansen, I. (1991) Characterization of neuropeptide Y (NPY) responses in human and rodent brain vessels with the selective NPY receptor agonist (Pro 34) NPY and the antagonist D-myo-inositol-1, 2, 6-triphosphate (PP 56). *Journal of Cerebral Blood Flow and Metabolism*, **11** (Suppl. 2), 275.

Edvinsson, L., MacKenzie, E.T. and McCulloch, J. (1993) *Cerebral Blood Flow and Metabolism*, Raven Press, New York. pp.1–683.

Edvinsson, L., Jansen, I., Cunha e Sa, M. and Gulbenkian, S. (1994) Demonstration of neuropeptide containing nerves and vasomotor responses to perivascular peptides in human cerebral arteries. *Cephalalgia*, **4**, 88–96.

Fanciullacci, M., Alessandri, M., Figini, M., Geppetti, P. and Michelacci, S. (1995) Increases in plasma calcitonin gene-related peptide from extracerebral circulation during nitroglycerin-induced cluster headache attack. *Pain*, **60**, 119–123.

Ferrari, M.D., Frolich, M., Odkink, J., Tapparelli, C., Portielje, J.E.A. and Bruyn, G.W. (1987) Methionine-enkephalin and serotonin in migraine and tension headache. In: *Advances in Headache Research*, (ed. F. Clifford Rose), pp.227–234. John Libbey, London.

Friberg, L., Olesen, J., Skyhøj Olsen, T., Karle, A., Ekman, R. and Fahrenkrug, J. (1994) Absence of vasoactive peptide release from brain to cerebral circulation during onset of migraine with aura. *Cephalalgia*, **14**, 47–54.

Gibbins, I.L., Brayden, J.E. and Bevan, J.A. (1984) Perivascular nerves with immunoreactive vasoactive intestinal polypeptide in cephalic arteries of the cat: distribution, possible origins and functional implications. *Neuroscience*, **13**, 127–134.

Goadsby, P.J. and Duckworth, J.W. (1987) Effect of stimulations of trigeminal ganglion on regional cerebral blood flow in cats. *American Journal of Physiology*, **253**, R270–R274.

Goadsby, P.J. and Edvinsson, L. (1991) Sumatriptan reverses the changes in calcitonin gene-related peptide seen in the headache phase of migraine. *Cephalalgia*, (Suppl. 11), 3–4.

Goadsby, P.J. and Edvinsson, L. (1993a) The trigeminovascular system and migraine: studies characterizing cerebrovascular and neuropeptide changes seen in humans and cats. *Annals of Neurology*, **33**, 48–56.

Goadsby, P.J. and Edvinsson, L. (1993b) Evidence of trigeminovascular activation in man during acute cluster headache. *Cephalalgia*, **13**, 30

Goadsby, P.J. and Edvinsson, L. (1994) Human in vivo evidence for trigemino-vascular activation in cluster headache. Neuropeptide changes and effects of acute attack therapies. *Brain*, **117**, 427–434.

Goadsby, P.J. and Lance, J.W. (1988) Brainstem effects on intra- and extracerebral circulations. Relation to migraine and cluster headache. In: *Basic Mechanisms of Headache*, (eds J. Olesen and L. Edvinsson), pp. 413–427. Elsevier, Amsterdam.

Goadsby, P.J., Lambert, G.A. and Lance, J.W. (1986) Stimulation of the trigeminal ganglion increases flow in the extracerebral but not the cerebral circulation of the monkey. *Brain Research*, **381**, 63–67.

Goadsby, P.J. and Zagami, A.S. (1991) Stimulation of the superior sagittal sinus increases metabolic activity and blood flow in certain regions of the brainstem and upper cervical spinal cord of the cat. *Brain*, **114**, 1001–1004.

Goadsby, P.J., Edvinsson, L. and Ekman, R. (1988) Release of vasoactive peptides in the extracerebral circulation of humans and the cat during activation of the trigeminovascular system. *Annals of Neurology*, **23**, 193–196.

Goadsby, P.J., Edvinsson, L. and Ekman, R. (1990) Vasoactive peptide release in the extracerebral circulation of humans during migraine headache. *Annals of Neurology*, **28**, 183–187.

Hardebo, J.E., and Ekman, R. (1986) Substance P and opioids in cluster headache. In: *Trends in Cluster Headache*, (eds F. Sicuteri, L. Vecchiet and M. Fanciullaci), pp. 145–158. Elsevier, Amsterdam.

Hardebo, J.E., Ekman, R., Eriksson, M., Holgersson, S. and Rydberg, B. (1985) CSF opioid levels in cluster headache. Effects of acupuncture. In: *Migraine: Clinical and Research Advances*, (ed. F. Clifford Rose), pp. 79–85. Karger, Basel.

Hauge, T. (1954) Catheter vertebral angiography. *Acta Radiologica*, (Suppl. 109).

Headache Classification Committee of the International Headache Society (J. Olesen *et al.*) (1988) Classification and diagnostic criteria for headache disorders, cranial neuralgias and facial pain. *Cephalalgia*, **8**, (Suppl. 7), 1–97.

Iversen, H.K., Olesen, J. and Tfelt-Hansen, P. (1989) Intravenous nitroglycerin as an experimental model of vascular headache. Basic characteristics. *Pain*, **38**, 17–24.

Jansen, I., Uddman, R., Hocherman, M., Ekman, R., Jensen, K. and Olesen, J. *et al.* (1986) Localization and effects of neuropeptide Y, vasoactive intestinal polypeptide, substance P and calcitonin gene-related peptide in human temporal arteries. *Annals of Neurology*, **20**, 496–501.

Jansen, I., Golman, K. and Edvinsson, L. (1987) Mechanisms of action of contrast media on cranial vessels. Comparison of diatrizoate, ioxaglate, iohexol mannitol and NaCl on rabbit basilar and ear arteries. *Investigative Radiology*, **22**, 814–821.

Jansen, I., Uddman, R., Ekman, R., Olesen, J., Ottosson, A. and Edvinsson, L. (1992) Distribution and effects of neuropeptide Y, vasoactive intestinal peptide, substance P and calcitonin gene-related peptide in human middle meningeal arteries: comparison with cerebral and temporal arteries. *Peptides*, **13**, 527–536.

Juul, R., Edvinsson, L., Gisvold, S.E., Ekman, R., Brubakk, A.O. and Fredriksen, T.A. (1990) Calcitonin gene-related peptide-LI in subarachnoid haemorrhage in man. Signs of activation of the trigemino-cerebrovascular system? *British Journal of Neurosurgery*, **4**, 171–180.

Juul, R., Hara, H., Gisvold, S.E., Brubakk, A.O., Fredriksen, T.A., Waldemar, G., Schmidt, J.F., Ekman, R. and Edvinsson, L. (1995) Alterations in perivascular dilatory neuropeptides (CGRP, SP, VIP) in the external jugular vein and in the cerebrospinal fluid following subarachnoid haemorrhage in man. *Acta Neurochirurgica*, **132**, 32–41.

Lambert, G.A., Bogduk, N., Goadsby, P.J., Duckworth, J.W. and Lance, J.W. (1984) Decreased carotid arterial resistance in cats in response to trigeminal stimulation. *Journal of Neurosurgery*, **61**, 307–315.

Lambert, G.A., Goadsby, P.J., Zagami, A.S. and Duckworth, J.W. (1988) Comparative effects of stimulation of the trigeminal ganglion and the superior sagittal sinus on cerebral blood flow and evoked potentials in the cat. *Brain Research*, **453**, 143–149.

Lance, J.W. (1993) The pathogenesis of migraine. In: *The Mechanism and Management of Headache*, 5th edn, pp. 111–121. Butterworth Heinemann, London.

Larsson, L.I., Edvinsson, L., Fahrenkrug, J., Håkanson, R., Owman, C., Schaffalitzky de Muckadel, O.B. *et al.* (1976) Immunohistochemical localization of a vasodilatory polypeptide (VIP) in cerebrovascular nerves. *Brain Research*, **113**, 400–404.

Lauritzen, M. (1994) Pathophysiology of migraine aura: the spreading depression theory. *Brain*, **117**, 199–210.

McCulloch, J., Uddman, R., Kingman, T.A. and Edvinsson, L. (1986) Calcitonin gene-related peptide. Functional role in cerebrovascular regulation. *Proceedings of the National Academy of Science USA*, **83**, 5731–5735.

Mosnaim, A.D., Wolf, M.E., Chevesich, J., Callaghan, O.H. and Diamond, S. (1985) Plasma methionine enkephalin levels. A biological marker for migraine? *Headache*, **25**, 259–261.

Nicolodi, M. and Del Bianco, E. (1990) Sensory neuropeptides (substance P, calcitonin gene-related peptide) and vasoactive intestinal polypeptide in human saliva: their pattern in migraine and cluster headache. *Cephalalgia*, **10**, 39–50.

Nozaki, K., Markowitz, M.A., Maynard, K.I., Koketsu, N., Dawson, T.M., Bredt, D.S. *et al.* (1993) Possible origins and distribution of immunoreactive nitric oxide synthase-containing nerve fibres in cerebral arteries. *Journal of Cerebral Blood Flow and Metabolism*, **13**, 70–79.

O'Connor, T.P. and van der Kooy, D. (1988) Enrichment of a vasoactive neuropeptide (calcitonin gene-related peptide) in the trigeminal sensory projection to the intracranial arteries. *Journal of Neurosciences*, **8**, 2468–2476.

Olesen, J., Larsen, B. and Lauritzen, M. (1981) Focal hyperemia followed by spreading oligemia and impaired activation of rCBF in classic migraine. *Annals of Neurology*, **9**, 344–352.

Olesen, J., Friberg, L. and Skyhøj Olsen, T. (1990) Timing and topography of cerebral blood flow, aura, and headache during migraine attacks. *Annals of Neurology*, **28**, 791–798.

Olesen, J., Iversen, H.K. and Thomsen, L.L. (1993) Nitric oxide supersensitivity. A possible molecular mechanisms of migraine pain. *NeuroReport*, **4**, 1027–1030.

Olsen, K.S., Videbaek, C., Schmidt, J.F. and Paulson, O.B. (1992) The effect of ketanserin on cerebral blood flow and cerebrovascular CO_2 reactivity in healthy volunteers. *Acta Neurochirurgica*, **119**, 7–11.

Piper, R.D., Edvinsson, L., Ekman, R. and Lambert, G.A. (1993) Cortical spreading depression does not result in the release of calcitonin gene-related peptide into the external jugular vein of the cat: relevance to human migraine. *Cephalalgia*, **13**, 180–183.

Radner, S. (1947) Intracranial angiography via the vertebral artery. *Acta Radiologica*, **28**, 838–843.

Ray, B.S. and Wolff, H.G. (1940) Experimental studies on headaches, pain sensitive structures of the head and their significance in headaches. *Archives of Surgery*, **41**, 813–856.

Sicuteri, F., Fanciullacci, M., Geppetti, P., Renzi, D. and Spillantini, M.G. (1985) Substance P mechanisms in cluster headache: evaluation in plasma and cerebrospinal fluid. *Cephalalgia*, **5**, 143–149.

Sjaastad, O. and Saunte, C. (1983) Unilaterality of headache. Hauge's studies revisited. *Cephalalgia*, **3**, 201–205.

Suzuki, N., Hardebo, J.E. and Owman, C. (1988) Origins and pathways of cerebrovascular vasoactive intestinal polypeptide-positive nerves in rat. *Journal of Cerebral Blood Flow Metabolism*, **8**, 697–712.

Thomsen, L.L., Iversen, H.K., Brinck, T.A. and Olesen, J. (1993) Arterial supersensitivity to nitric oxide in migraine sufferers. *Cephalalgia*, **13**, 395–399.

Tran-Dinh, Y.R., Thurel, C., Cunin, G., Serrie, A. and Seylaz, J. (1992) Cerebral vasodilation after the thermocoagulation of the trigeminal ganglion in humans. *Neurosurgery*, **31**, 658–662.

Uddman, R., Edvinsson, L., Ekman, R., McCulloch, J. and Kingman, T.A. (1985) Innervation of feline cerebral vasculature by nerve fibres containing calcitonin gene-related peptide: trigeminal origin and co-existence with substance P. *Neuroscience Letters*, **62**, 131–136.

Uddman, R., Goadsby, P.J., Jansen, I. and Edvinsson, L. (1993a) PACAP, a VIP-like peptide, immunohistochemical localization and effect upon cat pial arteries and on cerebral blood flow. *Journal of Cerebral Blood Flow and Metabolism*, **13**, 291–297.

Uddman, R., Goadsby, P.J., Jansen, I. and Edvinsson, L. (1993b) Helospectin-like peptides: immunohistochemical localization and effects on cat pial arteries and on cerebral blood flow. *Journal of Cerebral Blood Flow and Metabolism*, **13**, (Suppl. 1), S206.

Vecchiet, L., Geppetti, P., Marchionni, A., Spillantini, M.G., Fanciullacci, M. and Sicuteri, F. (1987) Cerebrospinal fluid (methionin[5])-enkephalin, substance P and somatostatin-like immunoreactivities in painful and pain-less human diseases. In: *Trends in Cluster Headache*, (eds F. Sicuteri, L. Vecchiet and M. Fanciullacci), pp. 135–143. Exerpta Medica, Amsterdam.

Willis, T. (1664) *Cerebri Anatome*. Martin and Allestry, London.

Woods, R.P., Iacoboni, M. and Mazziotta, J.C. (1994) Bilateral spreading cerebral hypoperfusion during spontaneous migraine headache. *New England Journal of Medicine*, **31**, 689–692.

Zagami, A.S. and Lambert, G.A. (1990) Stimulation of cranial vessels excites nociceptive neurones in several thalamic nuclei of the cat. *Experimental Brain Research*, **81**, 552–566.

DISCUSSION

Ferrari: What happens to neuropeptide Y (NPY) after sumatriptan?

Edvinsson: We found no difference between NPY levels in controls and during migraine headache. When patients were given sumatriptan the concentrations of NPY increased markedly in all cases (Goadsby *et al.* 1990). We tried to see if this was a general biological phenomenon but could not replicate it in the cat.

Ferrari: Did it occur in both cluster headache and migraine?

Edvinsson: We saw no change in NPY values during cluster headache attacks. We did not analyse NPY in cluster headache after sumatriptan.

Branchek: I would assume that if the NPY receptors are on the presynaptic trigeminal terminals then NPY would reinforce the sumatriptan stimulus to prevent further transmitter release. I don't know why the sumatriptan is causing the release of NPY or what the source of NPY is, but mechanistically an excess could help in the migraine.

Lance: You suggest that the release of calcitonin gene-related peptide (CGRP) is in reaction to a vascular spasm, to relax the vessel, rather than acting primarily as a vasodilator. Where does the CGRP come from, given that you have shown that CGRP-containing fibres are sparse in the cerebral cortex?

Edvinsson: That is a good question. The CGRP that can be released comes from peripheral terminals of the trigeminal ganglion. We cannot say that it is released only from arteries in the brain. The signal we see could come from other cephalic arteries as well.

Lance: Is the sparse distribution you have shown present in the vessels plunging into the cerebral cortex, not in the pial vessels on the surface?

Edvinsson: There are few CGRP-positive fibres in the pial vessels on the cortex surface and in man probably none in intracortical vessels. The large circle of Willis arteries at the base of the brain have a fairly rich innervation by CGRP-positive fibres. In animals the innervation seems to be more extended: we see these fibres more often in cortex arteries. But in man we were surprised not to find many of them on the cortical surface.

Hamel: Did you see them in the circle of Willis and the middle cerebral artery in man? You are saying that in fresh small pial vessels from cortical biopsies you see very few fibres, but when you get large vessels at the base of the brain from post-mortem tissues, then you see CGRP fibres.

Edvinsson: Yes. Our impression is that histochemistry underestimates the extent. Quantitative analysis has to some extent confirmed this.

Thomsen: What is the significance for the question of where CGRP is released of the negative findings in the internal jugular vein during migraine with aura attacks (Friberg *et al.* 1994)?

Edvinsson: Only a few cases were studied. Friberg *et al.* measured many things in the internal jugular vein, among them CGRP and substance P. I think further studies are needed.

Ferrari: You found that cortical spreading depression was not able to activate sensory fibres. How does that fit with Professor Moskowitz's observations that cortical spreading depression does activate the trigeminal system?

Edvinsson: We induced cortical spreading depression in the cat and the monkey and measured neuropeptides in the jugular vein. The results were clear-cut: there was no change during induced spreading depression (Piper *et al.* 1993). There is first a vasodilatory phase and then depression of the blood flow. The vasodilatory phase can be reduced in the presence of $CGRP_{8-37}$, the CGRP receptor antagonist. In Professor Moskowitz's work, excessive stimulation (up to nine spreading depressions) appears necessary for c-*fos* activation. Perhaps the difference lies in the use of only one spreading depression in our studies.

Moskowitz: To resolve this Professor Edvinsson's experiment could be done with sufficient intensity to activate c-*fos*, looking at that time to see if there is any release of CGRP in the jugular vein.

Edvinsson: I agree. We would be happy to examine samples obtained during such circumstances. Have you induced just one spreading depression and seen no c-*fos* activation?

Moskowitz: No, we have not done that. Based on what we know about humans, we cannot say anything yet about the number and duration of spreads and the effects on blood flow. It is an open issue that needs to be addressed.

However, the critical issue here is not the number of spreads. The critical issue is how much of the noxious chemical accumulates into the perivascular and extracellular space. In some people, or in some animals, one spread might be sufficient. In rodents we used one spreading depression every nine minutes.

Edvinsson: The other interesting aspect is Dr Diener's data in migraine without aura (Diener and May, this volume). There was no spreading across the cortex, but activation of nuclei in the brainstem. Perhaps there could be a connection from this area to the blood vessels. The headache and the spreading depression might be two separate phenomena.

Sandler: Am I right in thinking that neither CGRP nor substance P produce pain in their own right?

Edvinsson: Administration of CGRP does not produce pain, but the patients become very red from cutaneous vasodilatation.

Moskowitz: The inference from Professor Edvinsson's data is that activation of the trigeminal system occurred with the vasoconstrictor, noradrenaline. With respect to the hypothesis that dilation is causing pain and that constriction is relieving pain, these results would appear to be contradictory. If activation of the trigeminal system causes pain, how does one reconcile the hypothesis that vasoconstriction relieves pain based on these data?

Humphrey: There is a big difference between changes in normal vessel calibre associated with normal changes in arterial flow and the vascular changes envisaged in migraine. The simple concept of vasodilatation causing pain is not tenable: you can sit in a bath and not get a headache. It is distension of the blood vessel wall with increases in transmural pressure that causes pain.

Moskowitz: That is because the connective tissue is injured and pain is a response to tissue injury. That is not what happens in humans under conditions of migraine.

Humphrey: We can argue about this, but the pain only occurs while the vessels are distended. When the distension is reduced, the pain goes away. You are not looking at damage there.

Moskowitz: Yes, but how do you reconcile this notion of constriction activating a system which is associated with the production of pain?

Humphrey: This looks like a protective mechanism. People have speculated that a CGRP antagonist might be useful in migraine. Might it be very deleterious to have a blocker of the vasodilatatory action of CGRP? Is it functioning physiologically to protect the brain blood flow?

Edvinsson: I agree that it would be logical to examine the effect of a CGRP blocker on acute migraine attacks. However, as yet there is no clinically useful blocker.

Fozard: Is the very potent relaxant response to CGRP on the human cerebral vessels endothelium-dependent?

Edvinsson: There are suggestions that in some other regions, in some species but not in man, part of the response to CGRP can be endothelium dependent. In our experiments in the guinea-pig, cat and human brain vessels, it appears not to be dependent to a significant degree. After N^G-nitro-L-arginine methyl ester (L-NAME) or N^G-monomethyl-L-arginine (L-NMMA), or removal of the endothelium, we saw no modulation of the CGRP response: for the substance P response the endothelium is essential. We found a nice parallel relation between dilator response of CGRP and cAMP generation.

Sandler: CGRP produces oedema. I wonder if the observation by Goltman (1935–36) of the brain bulging out of a defect in the skull could be due to CGRP release?

Moskowitz: Brain changes which occur so dramatically over short periods of time are probably due to an increase in brain volume (i.e. an increase in the venous compartment) rather than primarily oedema of the brain itself.

Schoenen: What is the direct evidence that CGRP release is due to the calibre change of the vessel and not to some metabolic change in the tissue? For the subarachnoid haemorrhage, you showed that there is a relation between vessel calibre and the release of CGRP, but there is also a relationship between the amount of blood in the meninges and the vasospasm. Professor Moskowitz has used experimental blood injections into rat meninges and showed activation of the trigeminovascular system. Could the blood directly excite trigeminal fibres and produce the release of CGRP?

Edvinsson: In the cat model we took a few microlitres of blood and injected it in the vascular wall. That caused a pronounced, almost complete, constriction of the pial arterioles. The amount of constriction was the same in trigeminal lesioned animals and in controls, but the time for the vessel to normalize was significantly prolonged in the lesioned group. That is direct evidence that blood components can cause contraction of the vessel. The trigeminovascular reflex is activated secondarily to release the stored neuropeptides.

Schoenen: This does not directly prove that the reflex release of CGRP is due to the calibre change of the vessel.

Edvinsson: We used a number of different contractile stimuli: barium chloride, alkaline pH, prostaglandin F$_{2\alpha}$ and noradrenaline. They all resulted in the same activation. We also examined dilatation by acidic CSF and did not see any change of the dilatory response following trigeminal lesioning.

Ferrari: If you apply other vasoconstrictors, not blood, do you see the same increase in CGRP? For instance, if you were to apply sumatriptan would you see CGRP increase?

Edvinsson: It is an interesting idea that sumatriptan might *per se* activate the trigeminovascular system. As stated above, circumstantial evidence may indicate this. However, we have not measured CGRP release at the same time in the cat.

Fozard: Four or five vasoconstrictor stimuli all resulted in CGRP release. Was the CGRP release with different vasoconstrictors the same, possibly as a reflection of metabolic factors? Were the vasoconstrictor responses to the various stimuli identical?

Edvinsson: No, they were different. We could have varied the doses given. Barium chloride and blood caused almost complete contraction of the blood vessel. The other agents resulted in contraction of between 20% and 30%, so there were two different levels of constrictor activity.

Fozard: Did the ones that caused a high level of constriction give the greatest release of CGRP?

Edvinsson: We did not measure CGRP release in this model. I do not think there is a marked difference.

Moskowitz: In a rabbit subarachnoid haemorrhage model, we found tremendous release of tachykinins from primary afferent fibres innervating blood vessels and an increase in preprotachykinin mRNA turnover within the trigeminal ganglion (Linnik *et al.* 1989). I am convinced that blood application, or for that matter any headache stimulus (and subarachnoid haemorrhage is certainly one of them) will activate and release peptides from perivascular afferents.

Lance: Is it correct that in the trigeminally lesioned animals, the application of any vasoconstrictor has a potentiated effect?

Edvinsson: Not for NPY. Although the response to NPY is as strong as those of the other constrictors, it takes a long time for it disappear from the receptors. Its disappearance with or without the trigeminal lesion is the same, probably due to its longer association with the receptor.

Lance: But other vasoconstrictor actions are potentiated because the trigeminal section has abolished the CGRP content of the nerve. What happens if you apply vasodilators?

Edvinsson: We have only looked at the effect of low pH in mock CSF. The response was not altered. It would be interesting to test a number of other vasodilators, such as nitroglycerin.

Lance: De Marinis *et al.* (1984) showed that after thermocoagulation of the trigeminal ganglion the flushing reaction to intravenous histamine was diminished on the trigeminally sectioned side. Presumably trigeminal lesions have some effect on vasodilatator as well as constrictor systems.

Edvinsson: We should differentiate between intra- and extracranial tissues, because studies with neuroanatomy and True Blue retrograde tracing tend to show that although the cerebral circulation is preferentially rich in CGRP fibres as compared to substance P, other cranial structures have more substance P.

Martin: Professor Moskowitz has commented that if vasoconstriction elicits CGRP release, indicating activation of trigeminal sensory neurons, constriction *per se* should be proalgesic. Isn't it probable that CGRP release occurs by virtue of local axon reflex?

Moskowitz: I was trying to be provocative! My point is that an analysis based on vessel calibre alone is not a productive way to view migraine or its treatment mechanism.

Humphrey: That was the point of asking whether it was physiological or not, because if it is a normal mechanism at a local level, it is there for a good reason, in a protective role rather than activation of the trigeminal nerve and algesia *per se*.

Moskowitz: To the best of our knowledge, the trigeminal nerve itself does not participate to any significant extent in normal vascular physiology. It is not a tonically firing system. It is intended to sense real or threatened tissue injury, such as in the presence of large amounts of noradrenaline, blood, ischaemia-reperfusion, bacterial meningitis or severe hypertension beyond the limits of autoregulation. Large differences in blood flow develop in response to the above conditions. After unilateral trigeminalectomy, differences in flow develop between the two sides which can be equated with peptide release. The trigemino-vascular system is not involved in autoregulation or the hypercapnia response. It is a back-up system to modulate flow under intense pathophysiological conditions (Moskowitz and Macfarlane 1993).

Martin: If substance P is co-stored, and presumably co-released with CGRP, why doesn't substance P increase or why can't you measure it increasing?

Edvinsson: When we stimulate the trigeminal ganglia in cat or in man we can readily measure both peptides. Under these conditions there is initially more substance P than CGRP in the jugular venous blood. The low levels of substance P do not change during migraine or cluster headache attacks.

Moskowitz: Could this relate to the half-life of substance P and CGRP?

Goadsby: It is either that or it is selectivity of innervation. If you stimulate the trigeminal ganglion you turn on every sensory afferent in the head, from stroking on the face to intracranial pain. I would suggest that pain from migraine or cluster headache is more specific, so it is not surprising that the fibres which are activated are more selective than the non-specific results of trigeminal ganglion stimulation.

Martin: I thought the issue was that substance P and CGRP are co-stored in the same terminals.

Goadsby: But they are not co-stored in the same terminals. The cerebrovascular innervation from the trigeminal system preferentially has CGRP (O'Connor and van der Kooy 1988).

Moskowitz: I disagree with that. About 35% of the ganglion cells contain CGRP and about 15% contain substance P, and among those substance P-containing cells there is a significant overlap of CGRP.

Connor: The half-life of substance P in plasma is a lot less than that of CGRP, so it is possible that some metabolic differences can account for the fact that you see CGRP levels increase but you can't detect substance P. We cannot discount that as one reason for the difference.

Edvinsson: Tracing experiments have shown that one-third of the trigeminal cells contain CGRP and then one-third of those cells contain substance P. We can easily measure the SP/CGRP release during trigeminal stimulation and also the baseline levels. During headache attacks we record similar baseline levels of SP but marked increases in CGRP. Support for our data has come from Fanciullacci *et al.* (1995) in cluster headache patients and from Nicolodi and Del Bianco (1990) who observed SP release in nasal secretion and in saliva. So I do not think that metabolism of substance P is the explanation.

Connor: Nasal secretions and saliva might be different from plasma.

Edvinsson: That is true. The innervation pattern is different: there is more substance P innervation in the face than in the cerebral circulation. Therefore substance P can be more easily detected. We analysed SP in the jugular vein plasma but not in the cubital fossa. I could see your argument if we were only sampling in the cubital fossa since substance P would have to circulate in the entire system before we could measure it. Sampling in the jugular vein offers measurement a very short distance from where we believe the peptide is released. The half-life would have to be only a few seconds to be a significant factor.

Connor: There might be a very localized release. Just by measuring samples from the jugular vein, you may not detect very small localized changes, which in combination with the fact that substance P can be broken down so rapidly may explain the negative findings.

Edvinsson: We can never disregard the possibility of small changes, of course, but I would be surprised. If the ratio of three CGRP to one substance P is reasonable there could be a little substance P being released which we cannot detect.

Moskowitz: When you investigate plasma from the internal *vs* the external jugular vein, what structures are you draining in these respective pools of blood?

Edvinsson: That is a good question which I am not able to answer. This is partly why we did the subarachnoid haemorrhage project: to have clearly localized vasoconstriction where we could correlate this by transcranial doppler, and also the possibility of measuring peptides both in CSF and in the external jugular vein.

Moskowitz: At some point we need to know whether the peptide levels in blood reflect events occurring in a certain compartment or a specific tissue. That is very important.

Goadsby: Quite clearly, by taking blood from the neck you are observing levels from the head. The first thing we wanted to do was move from the periphery to the head. The internal jugular vein drains the large sinus directly, but it is not practical to study that in patients. The external jugular vein drains the head, and the largest part would be all the extracranial tissues and some intracranial components.

Moskowitz: Do we know whether the anterior one-third of the sagittal sinus drains into the external jugular vein?

Goadsby: From angiography, that part of the jugular drains down into the external system. It is not possible to be more precise, because the distribution of that has not been well studied. You make a good point: if you make an observation, then you like to know where it arose from. I don't think the data implied necessarily an exclusively dural or exclusively brain or exclusively extra-brain origin for the change in the levels. It would probably be better to be able to do selective sampling, but I don't think it is possible.

Moskowitz: Let us say, for example, that one-tenth of the drainage into the external jugular vein is coming from the sagittal sinus. And let us say that CGRP levels were increased 20-fold in sagittal sinus above baseline, and there was also a five-fold increase for substance P. With 10-fold dilution, the 20-fold increase becomes a two-fold CGRP increase, and a five-fold SP increase would be at baseline in the external jugular blood.

Goadsby: I don't think the data have ever suggested absolutely that there is no involvement of substance P, but it is for substance P to make the grade yet. The data do clearly suggest that there is an involvement of CGRP.

Humphrey: The weight of the argument seems to be moving in favour of the locus of the pathophysiological changes being at the level of blood vessels that are predominantly innervated by CGRP- rather than substance P-containing fibres. Therefore, Professor Edvinsson, studies such as yours should be able to tell us whether human dural vessels, meningeal vessels or the large arteries have such an innervation and hence are implicated.

Edvinsson: With immunoelectron microscopy we can see NPY- and VIP-containing vesicles in the nerve terminals close to the smooth muscle.

The substance P- and CGRP-containing vesicles in the temporal artery are located further out in the adventitia, indicative of a more sensory role in the vessel wall. The supply of all these fibres is fairly rich.

Humphrey: But that is not a major vascular bed in which we should be interested, although in some migraineurs it might be implicated. The meningeal vasculature is the interesting area: it would be exciting if the innervation there was predominantly CGRP.

Edvinsson: We have not yet finished our work on the human meningeal artery but in the preliminary work only a few SP/CGRP fibres have been seen.

REFERENCES

De Marinis, M., Martucci, N., Gagliadi, F.M., Feliciani, M. and Agnoli, A. (1984) Trigeminal control of cranio-facial vasomotor response: 1: histamine test in patients with unilateral Gasserian ganglion lesions. *Cephalalgia*, **4**, 243–251.

Diener, H.C. and May, A. (1996) Positron emission tomography studies in acute migraine attacks. In: *Migraine: Pharmacology and Genetics* (eds M. Sandler, M.D. Ferrari and S. Harnett), pp. 109–116. Chapman & Hall, London.

Fanciullacci, M., Alessandri, M., Figini, M., Geppetti, P. and Michelacci, S. (1995) Increases in plasma calcitonin gene-related peptide from extracerebral circulation during nitroglycerin-induced cluster headache attack. *Pain*, **60**, 119–123.

Friberg, L., Olesen, J., Olsen, T.S., Karle, A., Ekman, R. and Fahrenkrug, J. (1994) Absence of vasoactive peptide release from brain to cerebral circulation during onset of migraine with aura. *Cephalalgia*, **14**, 47–54.

Goadsby, P.J., Edvinsson, L. and Ekman, R. (1990) Vasoactive peptide release in the extracerebral circulation of humans during migraine headache. *Annals of Neurology*, **28**, 183–187.

Goltman, A.M. (1935–36) The mechanism of migraine. *Journal of Allergy*, **7**, 351–355.

Linnik, M.D., Sakas, D.E., Uhl, G.R. and Moskowitz, M.A. (1989) Subarachnoid blood and headache: altered trigeminal tachykinin gene expression. *Annals of Neurology*, **25**, 179–184.

Moskowitz, M.A. and Macfarlane, R. (1993) Neurovascular and molecular mechanism in migraine headaches. *Cerebral and Brain Metabolism Reviews*, **5** (3), 159–177.

Nicolodi, M. and Del Bianco, E. (1990) Sensory neuropeptides (substance P, calcitonin gene-related peptide) and vasoactive intestinal polypeptide in human saliva: their pattern in migraine and cluster headache. *Cephalalgia*, **10**, 39–50.

O'Connor, T.P. and van der Kooy, D. (1988) Enrichment of a vasoactive neuropeptide (calcitonin gene-related peptide) in trigeminal sensory projection to the intracranial arteries. *Journal of Neuroscience*, **8**, 2468–2476.

Piper, R.D., Edvinsson, L., Ekman, R. and Lambert, G.A. (1993) Cortical spreading depression does not result in the release of calcitonin gene related peptide into the external jugular vein of the cat: relevance to human migraine. *Cephalalgia*, **13**, 180–183.

17

Somatostatin receptor activation and analgesia

Patrick P.A. Humphrey

INTRODUCTION

About a decade after its discovery the tetradecapeptide mediator, somatostatin, was found to have analgesic effects in patients with cluster headache (Sicuteri *et al.* 1984a). Perhaps surprisingly, in view of its short half-life in plasma, other analgesic actions of somatostatin have since been described in various clinical conditions, including intractable pain associated with cancer (Sicuteri *et al.* 1984a, Mollenholt *et al.* 1994, Taura *et al.* 1994). The more metabolically stable octapeptide analogue of somatostatin, octreotide, has also been shown to have analgesic effects but the clinical efficacy observed with both peptides appears specific to some individuals and some types of pain (Penn *et al.* 1992, Gullo and Barbara 1991, Schmidt *et al.* 1993). This raises questions about the potential mechanism or mechanisms involved and whether better therapeutic agents can be designed. These issues have not been properly explored, largely because of the lack of knowledge about somatostatin receptor pharmacology. However, research interest has been re-awakened by the cloning of five distinct somatostatin receptor genes (see Hoyer *et al.* 1995). These have been named chronologically from sst_1 to sst_5. Pharmacologically these recombinant receptors can be classified into two groups, the so-called $SRIF_1$ group (sst_2, sst_3 and sst_5), at which octreotide has relatively high affinity, and the $SRIF_2$ group (sst_1 and sst_4) for which octreotide has little or no affinity (Hoyer *et al.* 1994).

Migraine: Pharmacology and genetics
Edited by Merton Sandler, Michel Ferrari and Sara Harnett
Published in 1996 by Chapman & Hall
ISBN 1 86036 006 8

On a cautionary note, there is evidence that octreotide has much lower affinity for the human sst_5 receptor compared to the rodent equivalent, making its selectivity in man even more marked (O'Carroll *et al.* 1994). It remains to be seen whether this is an advantage, or possibly a disadvantage, in the absence of much data about which receptor types mediate which of the many actions of somatostatin. In addition, there is evidence that octreotide may behave as a partial agonist in some situations, which could limit its clinical efficacy (Feniuk *et al.* 1993).

POSSIBLE ANALGESIC MECHANISMS

Somatostatin produces a variety of effects which could result in analgesia (Table 17.1). Since vascular headaches such as migraine or cluster headache can be treated acutely with vasoconstrictor agents such as the ergots or sumatriptan (Humphrey and Goadsby 1994), the vascular effects of somatostatin could theoretically be relevant to the treatment of head pain. It has been shown experimentally in the clinic that somatostatin will constrict the human hand vein but there are few reports of its effects on cranial blood vessels (Panconesi *et al.* 1987, Long *et al.* 1992, Shirahase *et al.* 1993). One report indicates that canine isolated basilar arteries will contract to somatostatin and that this contractile action is endothelium-dependent, involving the release of thromboxane A_2 (Shirahase *et al.* 1993). Somatostatin has also been reported to constrict rat pial vessels *in vivo* when applied topically (Long *et al.* 1992). However, we have been unable to show any contractile effects of somatostatin on dog or rat isolated cerebral vessels (unpublished observations). We have found, however, that the human isolated saphenous vein, is contracted by somatostatin. This effect was not endothelium-dependent and appears to involve a direct action on the smooth muscle, mediated via an sst_2 receptor type (Dimech *et al.* 1995). The contractile effects of somatostatin were tachyphylactic in the human saphenous vein, which might explain the paucity of reports of its vasoconstrictor effects and suggests that this action may not be clinically relevant.

If somatostatin receptor activation leads to analgesia, it is likely to result from a direct neuronal inhibitory action. It is evident that mRNA for all five somatostatin receptor types occurs throughout the central nervous system (Bruno *et al.* 1993). There is also evidence from functional studies for somatostatin receptors on peripheral nerve terminals, which mediate inhibition of the release of various neurotransmitters including acetylcholine and ATP (Feniuk *et al.* 1993, Feniuk and Humphrey 1994). Clearly somatostatin might have localized analgesic effects at some sites by a local inhibitory action on sensory nerve terminals, analogous with the proposed mechanism of action for the

Table 17.1 Possible mechanisms involved in analgesic actions of somatostatin

Mechanism	*Location*	*References*
Vasoconstriction	Some cranial arteries and peripheral veins	Panconesi *et al.* (1987), Shirahase *et al.* (1993), Long *et al.* (1992), Dimech *et al.* (1995)
Inhibition of release of hormone or enzymes	E.g. growth hormone, gastrointestinal hormones and enzymes	Brazeau *et al.* (1973), Lewin (1992)
Neuronal inhibition	Both peripheral and central neurons	Feniuk *et al.* (1993), Feniuk and Humphrey (1994), Gazelius *et al.* (1981), Randic and Miletic (1978), Sandkühler *et al.* (1990), Chapman and Dickenson (1992), Gothert (1980)
Increased neurotransmitter release	Brain 5-hydroxytryptamine, noradrenaline, acetylcholine, GABA and dopamine	Tanaka and Tsujimoto (1981), Tsujimoto and Tanaka (1981), Araujo *et al.* (1990), Meyer *et al.* (1989), Chesselet and Reisine (1983)
Neurodegeneration	Central neuronal damage occurs at high local concentrations and may not be receptor mediated	Long (1988), Mollenholt *et al.* (1988, 1990), Long *et al.* (1992)

antimigraine drug, sumatriptan, on perivascular sensory nerves of intracranial vessels (Humphrey and Goadsby 1994). In this respect, there is evidence that somatostatin can abolish the release of substance P from dental pulp neurons in the anaesthetized cat (Gazelius *et al.* 1981). In the Moskowitz trigeminovascular model in the rat, octreotide inhibits plasma protein extravasation in the dura, suggestive of inhibition of neuropeptide release from sensory nerves, but the doses necessary were surprisingly high (up to 1 mg/kg intravenously; see Figure 1 in Matsubara *et al.* 1992).

There is evidence for an inhibitory action of locally administered somatostatin on nociceptive stimuli in the dorsal horn of the spinal cord (Randic and Miletic 1978, Sandkühler *et al.* 1990). A neuronal hyper-polarizing action of somatostatin has also been described in a rat isolated spinal cord preparation but the concentrations required were in the micromolar range (Murase *et al.* 1982). In the brain somatostatin appears to have predominantly excitatory rather than inhibitory actions. Indeed, several studies have shown somatostatin to cause (rather than inhibit) release of other neurotransmitters from central neurons (Table 17.1). This is consistent with reports of depolarizing effects of somatostatin in brain neurons from both cortex and hippocampus (Dodd and Kelly 1978, Delfs and Dichter 1983). On the basis of these studies, it seems likely that the analgesic effects of somatostatin are likely to occur at the level of the spinal cord (Chapman and Dickenson 1992). In this respect, *in situ* hybridization studies suggest that the most prominent somatostatin receptor within the dorsal horn is the sst_3 receptor, at which octreotide has much lower affinity than for the sst_2 receptor (Hoyer *et al.* 1995, Señaris *et al.* 1995). However, a recent study (Helmchen *et al.* 1995) has provided evidence that somatostatin produces inhibition within the dorsal horn by activating descending inhibitory fibres at the level of the medullary nucleus raphe magnus and the periaqueductal grey (Figure 17.1).

Studies to investigate the analgesic potential of somatostatin receptor activation have frequently used epidural administration. There is some controversy about the potential neurotoxic effects of somatostatin and octreotide when administered in this way but examination of clinical autopsy tissue from patients who have died from cancer has provided no evidence for spinal neurotoxicity (Mollenholt *et al.* 1988, 1990, 1994). In laboratory studies in rats, octreotide has been shown to produce marked reductions in spinal blood flow and evidence of neuro-degeneration (Long *et al.* 1992). In contrast, no such changes have been observed in similar studies in the guinea-pig (Mollenholt *et al.* 1992). Nevertheless, it is evident that extremely high concentrations (up to 1 mg/ml) are being used for epidural administration and at these concentrations similar neurotoxic effects have been observed experi-

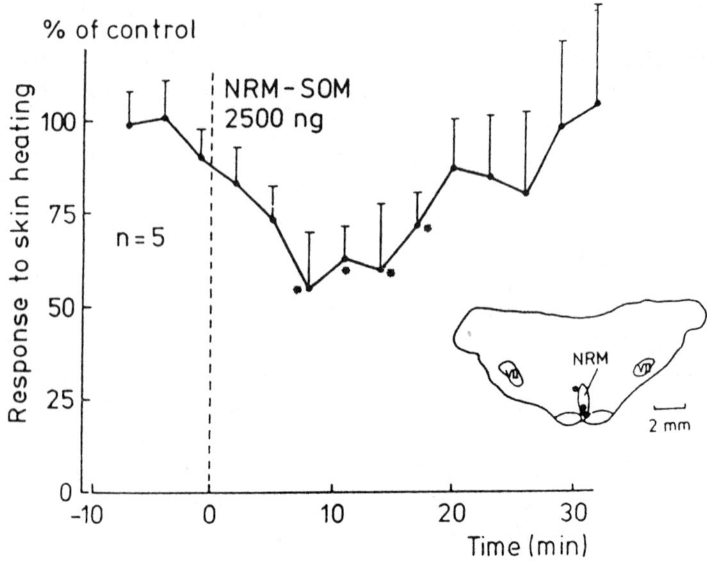

Figure 17.1 Inhibition of noxious heat-evoked responses by micro-injection of somatostatin (SOM) into the nucleus raphe magnus (NRM). Mean responses of five dorsal horn neurons (ordinate) plotted versus the time (abscissa) before and after the micro-injection of SOM (2.5 µg). Vertical dotted line indicates time of injection, vertical bars show SEM. *, $P < 0.02$. Effective micro-injection sites are shown on the coronal section through the medullary NRM, 8–8.5 mm caudal to the interauricular line (P 8.0–8.5). Reproduced from Helmchen *et al.* 1995, with permission.

mentally for other non-somatostatin peptides in animals (Gaumann *et al.* 1990). Studies on neuronal cells *in vitro* have shown somatostatin to have non-specific toxic effects on cells at concentrations in excess of 1 µM (Delfs and Dichter 1983). High concentrations of somatostatin, like other unrelated peptides such as substance P and vasoactive intestinal polypeptide, have also been shown to release histamine from mast cells in the human skin (Piotrowski and Foreman 1985). It would seem that somatostatin receptor agonists are needed which are not peptides and which will readily penetrate to potentially important brain or spinal receptors by more conventional routes of administration.

CLINICAL POTENTIAL

The clinical studies carried out to date have not demonstrated a robust analgesic effect of either somatostatin or octreotide. It remains to be determined why this is so. It could be that somatostatin is too readily metabolized (Gyr and Meier 1993). In the case of both somatostatin and octreotide, access to the site of action, particularly central, could be a major problem for such large peptides. In the absence of understanding about precise mechanisms and sites of action, the choice of dose could also be problematical. The knowledge that there are at least five different types of somatostatin receptor introduces another dimension, but one that offers promise in terms of drug discovery. Thus if analgesic mechanisms can be better defined and the receptor type or types involved identified, attempts to design appropriate selective agonists could be initiated. Thus it could be that although octreotide, unlike somatostatin, is metabolically stable, it does not have an optimal agonist profile. A non-peptide agonist will almost undoubtedly be essential for good pharmacokinetic characteristics. A further potential impediment to the development of a successful drug is receptor desensitization. It is evident that in many cases somatostatin receptors readily desensitize and if this is a feature of a target receptor it could prove an immutable problem (Sicuteri *et al.* 1984b, Feniuk *et al.* 1993). Nevertheless, not all somatostatin receptors desensitize, as exemplified by somatostatin's ability to inhibit growth hormone release in the pituitary or inhibit acid secretion in the gastric mucosa (Brazeau *et al.* 1973, Feniuk *et al.* 1994). Whether or not this relates to the fact that these two actions are important physiologically remains to be determined.

Acknowledgements

I am pleased to acknowledge the important contributions made by my colleagues within the Glaxo Institute of Applied Pharmacology and by our collaborators towards a better understanding of the pharmacology of somatostatin.

REFERENCES

Araujo, D.M., Lapchak, P.A., Collier, B. and Quirion, R. (1990) Evidence that somatostatin enhances endogenous acetylcholine release in the rat hippocampus. *Journal of Neurochemistry*, **55**, 1546.

Brazeau, P., Vale, W., Burgus, R., Ling, N., Butcher, M., Rivier, J. and Guillemin, R. (1973) Hypothalamic polypeptide that inhibits secretion on immunoreactive pituitary growth hormone. *Science*, **179**, 77–79.

Bruno, J.F., Xu, Y., Song, J. and Berelowitz, M. (1993) Tissue distribution of somatostatin receptor subtype messenger ribonucleic acid in the rat. *Endocrinology*, **133**, 2561.

Chapman, V. and Dickenson, A.H. (1992) The effects of sandostatin and somatostatin on nociceptive transmission in the dorsal horn of the rat spinal cord. *Neuropeptides*, **23**, 147–152.

Chesselet, M.-F. and Reisine, T.D. (1983) Somatostatin regulates dopamine release in rat striatal slices and cat caudate nuclei. *Journal Neuroscience*, **3**, 232–236.

Delfs, J.R. and Dichter, M.A. (1983) Effects of somatostatin on mammalian cortical neurons in culture: physiological actions and unusual dose response characteristics. *Journal of Neuroscience*, **3**, 1176–1188.

Dimech, J., Doyle, A.R., Latimer, R.D., Feniuk, W. and Humphrey, P.P.A. (1995) Somatostatin (SRIF)-induced contraction of human vascular smooth muscle. *Journal of Cardiovascular Pharmacology*, **26**, 721–728.

Dodd, J. and Kelly, J.S. (1978) Is somatostatin an excitatory transmitter in the hippocampus? *Nature*, **273**, 674–675.

Feniuk, W., Dimech, J. and Humphrey, P.P.A. (1993) Characterisation of somatostatin receptors in guinea-pig isolated ileum, vas deferens and right atrium. *British Journal Pharmacology*, **110**, 1156–1164.

Feniuk, W. and Humphrey, P.P.A. (1994) Somatostatin-induced inhibition of neurotransmission in the mouse isolated vas deferens is resistant to pertussis toxin. *European Journal of Pharmacology*, **261**, 333–337.

Feniuk, W., Jarvie, E. and Humphrey, P.P.A. (1994) Somatostatin (SRIF)-induced inhibition of gastric acid secretion in the rat isolated gastric mucosa. *British Journal of Pharmacology*, **113**, 43P.

Gaumann, D.M., Grabow, T.S., Yaksh, T.L., Casey, S.J. and Rodriguez, M. (1990) Intrathecal somatostatin, somatostatin analogs, substance P analog and dynorphin A cause comparable neurotoxicity in rats. *Neuroscience*, **39**, 761–774.

Gazelius, B, Brodin, E., Olgart, L. and Panopoulos, P. (1981) Evidence that substance P is a mediator of antidromic vasodilatation using somatostatin as a release inhibitor. *Acta Physiologica Scandinavica*, **113**, 155–159.

Gothert, M. (1980) Somatostatin selectivity inhibits noradrenaline release from hypothalamic neurones. *Nature*, **288**, 87–88.

Gullo, L. and Barbara, L. (1991) Treatment of pancreatic pseudocysts with octreotide. *Lancet*, **338**, 540–541.

Gyr, K.E., and Meier, R. (1993) Pharmacodynamic effects of sandostatin® in the gastrointestinal tract. *Digestion*, **54**, 14–19.

Helmchen, C., Fu, Q-G. and Sandkühler, J. (1995) Inhibition of spinal nociceptive neurons by microinjections of somatostatin into the nucleus raphe magnus and the midbrain periaqueductal gray of the anesthetized cat. *Neuroscience Letters*, **187**, 137–141.

Hoyer, D., Lubbert, H. and Bruns, C. (1994) Molecular pharmacology of somatostatin receptors. *Naunyn-Schmiedeberg's Archives of Pharmacology*, **350**, 441–453.

Hoyer, D., Bell, G.I., Berelowitz M., Epelbaum, J., Feniuk, W., Humphrey, P.P.A., O'Carroll, A-M, Patel, Y.C., Schonbrunn, A., Taylor, J.E. and Reisine, T. (1995) Classification and nomenclature of somatostatin receptors. *Trends in Pharmacological Sciences*, **16**, 86–88.

Humphrey, P.P.A. and Goadsby, P.J. (1994) The mode of action of sumatriptan is vascular? A debate. *Cephalalgia*, **14**, 401–410.

Lewin, M.J.M. (1992) The somatostatin receptor in the GI tract. *Annual Review of Physiology*, **54**, 455–468.

Long, J.B. (1988) Spinal subarachnoid injection of somatostatin causes neurological deficits and neuronal injury in rats. *European Journal of Pharmacology*, **149**, 287–296.

Long, J.B., Rigamonti, D.D., Dosaka, K., Kraimer, J.M. and Martinez-Arizala, A. (1992) Somatostatin causes vasoconstriction, reduces blood flow and increases vascular permeability in the rat central nervous system. *Journal of Pharmacology and Experimental Therapeutics*, **260**, 1425–1432.

Matsubara, T., Moskowitz, M.A. and Huang, Z. (1992) UK-14, 304, R(-)-α-methyl-histamine and SMS 201–995 block plasma protein leakage within dura mater by prejunctional mechanisms. *European Journal Pharmacology*, **224**, 145–150.

Meyer, D.K., Conzelmann, U. and Schultheiss, K. (1989) Effects of somatostatin-14 on the *in vitro* release of [^{3}H]GABA from slices of rat caudatoputamen. *Neuroscience*, **28**, 61–68.

Mollenholt, P., Post, C., Rawal, N., Freedman, J., Hokfelt, T. and Paulsson, I. (1988) Antinociceptive and 'neurotoxic' actions of somatostatin in rat spinal cord after intrathecal administration. *Pain*, **32**, 95–105.

Mollenholt, P., Post, C., Paulsson, I. and Rawal, N. (1990) Intrathecal and epidural somatostatin in rats: can antinociception, motor effects and neurotoxicity be separated? *Pain*, **43**, 363–370.

Mollenholt, P., Rawal, N., Gordh, T. and Olsson, Y. (1994) Intrathecal and epidural somatostatin for patients with cancer. *Anesthesiology*, **81**, 534–542.

Mollenholt, P., Post, C., Paulsson, I. and Rawal, N. (1992) Intrathecal somatostatin in the guinea pig: effects on spinal cord blood flow, histopathology and motor function. *Pain*, **51**, 343–347.

Murase, K., Nedeljkov, V. and Randic, M. (1982) The actions of neuropeptides on dorsal horn neurons in the rat spinal cord slice preparation: an intracellular study. *Brain Research*, **234**, 170–176.

O'Carroll, A.-M., Raynor, K., Lolait, S.J. and Reisine, T. (1994) Characterisation of cloned human somatostatin receptor SSTR5. *Molecular Pharmacology*, **46**, 291–298.

Panconesi, A., Luigi, Del Bianco, P., Franchi, G., Anselmi, B., and Andreini, R. (1987) Somatostatin: peripheral venoconstrictive activity and interaction with monoamines in man. *Regulatory Peptides*, **18**, 267–276.

Penn, R.D., Paice, J.A., and Kroin, J.S. (1992) Octreotide: a potent new non-opiate analgesic for intrathecal infusion. *Pain*, **49**, 13–19.

Piotrowski, W. and Foreman, J.C. (1985) On the actions of substance P, somatostatin, and vasoactive intestinal polypeptide on rat peritoneal mast cells and in human skin. *Naunyn-Schmiedeberg's Archives of Pharmacology*, **331**, 364–368.

Randic, M. and Miletic, V. (1978) Depressant actions of methionine-enkephalin and somatostatin in cat dorsal horn neurones activated by noxious stimuli. *Brain Research*, **152**, 196–202.

Sandkühler, J., Fu, Q.-G. and Helmchen, C. (1990) Spinal somatostatin superfusion *in vivo* affects activity of cat nociceptive dorsal horn neurons: comparison with spinal morphine. *Neuroscience*, **34**, 565–576.

Schmidt, K., Althoff, P.H., Harris, A.G., Prestele, H., Schumm-Draeger, P.M. and Usadel, K.H. (1993) Analgesic effects of the somatostatin analogue octreotide in two acromegalic patients: a double-blind study with long-term follow-up. *Pain*, **53**, 223–227.

Señaris, R.M., Schindler, M., Humphrey, P.P.A. and Emson, P.C. (1995) Expression of somatostatin receptor 3 mRNA in the motorneurons of the rat spinal cord and the sensory neurons of the spinal ganglia. *Molecular Brain Research*, **29**, 185–190.

Shirahase, H., Kanda, M., Shimaji, H., Usui, H., Rorstad, O.P. and Kurahashi, K. (1993) Somatostatin-induced contraction mediated by endothelial TXA$_2$ production in canine cerebral arteries. *Life Sciences*, **53**, 1539–1544.

Sicuteri, F., Geppetti, P., Marabini, S. and Lembeck, F. (1984a) Pain relief by somatostatin in attacks of cluster headache. *Pain*, **18**, 359–365.

Sicuteri, F., Panconesi, A., Del Bianco, P.L., Franchi, G. and Anselmi, B. (1984b) Venospastic activity of somatostatin *in vivo* in man: naloxone reversible tachyphylaxis. *International Journal of Clinical and Pharmaceutical Research*, **4**, 253–257.

Tanaka, S. and Tsujimoto, A. (1981) Somatostatin facilitates the serotonin release from rat cerebral cortex, hippocampus and hypothalamus slices. *Brain Research*, **208**, 219–222.

Taura, P., Planella, V., Balust, J., Beltran, J., Anglada, T., Carrero, E. and Burgues, S. (1994) Epidural somatostatin as an analgesic in upper abdominal surgery: a double-blind study. *Pain*, **59**, 135–140.

Tsujimoto, A. and Tanaka, S. (1981) Stimulatory effect of somatostatin on norepinephrine release from rat brain cortex slices. *Life Sciences*, **28**, 903–910.

DISCUSSION

Glover: Is analgesia the main function for somatostatin or are there many functions?

Humphrey: It has many. Physiologically somatostatin controls acid in our stomachs. It is a very powerful paracrine inhibitor in the gastric mucosa.

Fozard: Which receptor or combination of receptors is likely to be involved in the analgesic effect?

Humphrey: *In situ* hybridization studies suggest that it might be the somatostatin 3 receptor (sst_3), but we do not know. Most actions of somatostatin that we have studied, such as inhibition of acid secretion, seem to be mediated by somatostatin receptor 2 (sst_2). We have found a negative inotropic effect of somatostatin in the guinea-pig and a negative chronotropic effect in human atria that looks as though it might be mediated by the somatostatin receptor 5 (sst_5), but we've no evidence of a functional 1, 3 or 4 receptor subtype.

Sandler: What's the basis of the use of octreotide in certain endocrine syndromes?

Humphrey: It's used in the treatment of acromegaly and it's very good at turning off growth hormone release. In carcinoid it stops proliferation of enterochromaffin cells. We're working on how that happens because obviously that could potentially provide an anticancer mechanism. Most tumour cells appear to have somatostatin receptors on them, so that is an interesting avenue.

Diener: We looked at a large group of females who had hypophyseal tumours (May *et al.* 1994). It's well known that most of them have headaches, and that these do not depend on the size of the tumour. We treated a few patients who underwent successful operations with octreotide. They developed a migraine-like headache without autonomic symptoms. It started in the early morning, was pulsating and very intense, and it improved immediately after they took octreotide. Six of them developed a type of dependency. So we used the same protocol as for ergotamine and sumatriptan withdrawal, which is to stop it totally, and the headache went away. This indicates that octreotide may induce migraine-like headaches.

Humphrey: That's interesting. Whether vascular events are involved or not is not clear yet. Certainly acromegalic patients sometimes have profound headaches which octreotide treats effectively. Whether they then become dependent on octreotide is not clear from the clinical studies. This is why we need to understand the pharmacology, and to know which receptors are doing what. We need selective compounds.

Moskowitz: Octreotide is a peptide and probably enters the brain, but very poorly. But it would enter the pituitary: there is no blood–brain barrier there.

Goadsby: Is the inhibition of dorsal horn firing opiate sensitive?

Humphrey: Yes, opiates do the same thing as somatostatin: both can activate descending inhibitory pathways, probably by the same mechanism, turning off GABA release.

Goadsby: So does somatostatin mediate this effect through a distinct somatostatin receptor?

Humphrey: The somatostatin receptors, in terms of their structure and homology, are most closely related to the opioid receptors and octreotide in high doses has been shown to bind μ opioid receptors. So there is an overlap, but they are a completely distinct receptor family and there is no reason why you can't make highly selective compounds that will specifically and selectively only activate one somatostatin receptor type.

Fozard: Does the lack of vasoconstrictor response reflect a lack of an ongoing cyclase 'tone' in your model? Is the relevant somatostatin receptor linked negatively to adenylyl cyclase?

Humphrey: All five known recombinant receptors transfected into stable cell lines appear to couple negatively to adenylyl cyclase. But I don't think that's the normal coupling mechanism in the body. Everywhere one looks in whole tissues it is something else: linked to a potassium channel, or positively or negatively linked to a calcium channel, for example.

Peatfield: Earlier studies did not see the profound inhibition within the dorsal horn seen by Helmchen *et al.* (1995). What were the differences between the studies?

Humphrey: Somatostatin has been shown to cause hyperpolarization in an isolated spinal cord preparation (Murase *et al.* 1982). However, Helmchen *et al.* (1995) demonstrated *in vivo* a central excitatory effect leading to inhibition at the spinal level, something that others, for some reason, have missed. Thus, this could be an important site of action for centrally penetrating somatostatin receptor agonists.

Peatfield: Where is the receptor?

Humphrey: I suspect the receptors are both at the level of the periaqueductal grey and in the spinal cord itself. But we haven't done a study to confirm that. The fact that somatostatin can work intravenously is surprising, because I wouldn't expect it to have access to the relevant central sites. Obviously, further studies are required.

REFERENCES

Helmchen, C., Fu, Q-C. and Sandkühler, J. (1995) Inhibition of spinal nociceptive neurons by microinjections of somatostatin into the nucleus raphe magnus and the midbrain periaqueductal grey of the anesthetized cat. *Neuroscience Letters*, **187**, 137–141.

May, A., Lederbogen, S. and Diener, H.C. (1994) Octreotide dependency and headache: a case report. *Cephalalgia*, **14**, 303–304.

Murase, K., Nedeljkov, V. and Randic, M. (1982) The actions of neuropeptides on dorsal horn neurons in the rat spinal cord slice preparation: an intracellular study. *Brain Research*, **234**, 170–176.

18

Abnormal cortical information processing between migraine attacks

J. Schoenen

INTRODUCTION

Despite an impressive accumulation of scientific data over the past decade the pathogenesis of migraine is still unknown. Various theories have been proposed, but none can account for all available clinical and pathophysiological features. The pendulum has been swinging between vascular and neural mechanisms, between extra- and intracranial vessels, between platelets and the autonomic nervous system or between 5-hydroxytryptamine (5-HT, serotonin) and opioids (for review see Lance 1993).

In recent years much attention has been paid to the essence of the migraine phenotype, the migraine attack and the trigeminovascular system (Moskowitz and Cutrer 1993). We will not review the data indicating that the trigeminovascular system is activated during a migraine attack involving chemical (neurogenic inflammation) (Moskowitz 1991), vascular (vasodilation) (Friberg *et al.* 1991) and neural (nociception) (Goadsby *et al.* 1990) processes. Progress in this area was fostered by the development of animal models (Moskowitz 1993, Goadsby and Edvinsson 1993) and of novel effective drugs for acute migraine, such as the 5-HT$_{1D}$ agonist sumatriptan (Humphrey 1991) and led to a renewed interest in 5-HT mechanisms (Ferrari and Saxena 1993)

Migraine: Pharmacology and genetics
Edited by Merton Sandler, Michel Ferrari and Sara Harnett
Published in 1996 by Chapman & Hall
ISBN 1 86036 006 8

Table 18.1 Interictal pathophysiology of migraine

Data	Method	Author	Hypothesis
Decreased cerebral magnesium	NMR spectroscopy	Ramadan *et al.* 1989	Hypersensitivity of NMDA receptors favouring spreading depression
Increased excitatory amino acids in plasma and platelets	HPLC	Ferrari *et al.* 1990 D'Andrea *et al.* 1991	
Deranged energy metabolism in brain and muscle	NMR spectroscopy	Welch *et al.* 1989 Barbiroli *et al.* 1992 Montagna *et al.* 1994	Mitochondrial abnormality reducing energy reserve
Increased amplitude of visual evoked potentials Normalization by β-blockade	Neurophysiology	Kennard *et al.* 1978 Diener *et al.* 1989	Cortical hyperexcitability
Contingent negative variation: increased amplitude and decreased habituation Normalization by β-blockade	Neurophysiology	Schoenen *et al.* 1985 Kropp and Gerber 1993 Besken *et al.* 1993 Schoenen *et al.* 1986	Cortical hyperexcitability Deficient habituation in cognitive processing
Plasma noradrenaline and dopamine-β-hydroxylase increased or decreased	Biochemistry	Schoenen and Maertens de Noordhout (review, 1988)	Sympathetic instability, stress sensitivity
5-HT increased in platelets, decreased in plasma	Biochemistry	Anthony and Lance 1975 D'Andrea *et al.* 1989 Ferrari *et al.* 1989	Low 5-HT disposition; increased systemic turnover
Nitroglycerin induces headache in migraineurs	Clinical, blood flow studies	Olesen *et al.* 1993	Nitric oxide supersensitivity

NMR, nuclear magnetic resonance; HPLC, high-performance liquid chromatography; NMDA, *N*-methyl-D-aspartate; 5-HT, 5-hydroxytryptamine.

and to new concepts such as nitric oxide supersensitivity (Olesen *et al.* 1993).

The trigeminovascular system seems to be the major pain-signalling system of the visceral organ brain (Moskowitz 1991) and it can be activated by various triggers such as meningitis, subarachnoid haemorrhage, trauma, chemicals, acute hypertension, seizures or ischaemia (Edmeads 1992, Hardebo 1992, Moskowitz and Cutrer 1993). Some of these may have in common their ability to produce a cortical excitatory wave, similar to the one that initiates spreading depression (Leão 1944), which is able to depolarize trigeminovascular nerve fibres (Hardebo 1992). There is indirect evidence from clinical descriptions of the march of visual aura symptoms (Milner 1958) and from regional blood flow studies using single photon emission computerized tomography (SPECT) (Olesen *et al.* 1981, Lauritzen *et al.* 1983a,b) that cortical spreading depression occurs at the beginning of an attack in migraine with aura, and from blood flow studies using positron emission tomography (PET) (Woods *et al.* 1994) and magneto- (Barkley *et al.* 1990) and electroencephalography studies (Schoenen *et al.* 1987) that this may hold true for migraine without aura.

If spreading depression or a comparable physiological event is an aspecific reaction of the cerebral cortex to a variety of aggressions (ischaemia, ionic shifts, mechanical trauma etc.) able to trigger the major pain-signalling system of the cerebral parenchyma, it seems of no surprise that an exceptional migraine attack can occur in any human being (Blau 1987). The primary aetiopathogenetic mechanisms of migraine must therefore be related to factors that are capable of perpetuating migraine attacks and of explaining some interictal abnormalities, i.e. factors that cause the 'migraine disease'. These pathogenetically relevant factors, if they exist, should be detectable in the headache-free period and thus represent permanent dysfunctions in established migraine.

Many different biochemical and neurophysiological abnormalities have been described in migraine patients between attacks. Some are listed in Table 18.1. We shall focus on the neurophysiology and nuclear magnetic resonance (NMR) spectroscopy studies.

ABNORMAL INFORMATION PROCESSING: MIGRAINEURS 'OVERREACT'

Clinical neurophysiology is particularly suited for exploring functional disorders such as migraine. Various neurophysiological studies have been performed in migraine, especially between attacks (see review by Schoenen 1992). Taken together, they provide results favouring an increased cortical excitability or reagibility. For instance, visual evoked responses elicited by flash (Camp and Wolff 1961, Lehtonen 1974, Lehtonen *et al.* 1979, Connolly *et al.* 1982, Winter and Cooper 1985) or pattern-reversal stimulation (Kennard *et al.* 1978, Gawel *et al.* 1983, Diener *et al.* 1984) and studied by averaging a number of single responses have an increased amplitude in migraineurs between attacks. We have also reported exaggerated amplitude of an event-related potential, contingent negative variation (CNV), in migraine without aura (Schoenen *et al.* 1985, Maertens de Noordhout *et al.* 1986): habituation of CNV amplitude, as assessed in sequential blocks of averaged trials, was absent in 60% of patients. In a study analysing CNV habituation in more detail, Kropp and Gerber (1993) conclude that deficient habituation on trial repetition is the main CNV abnormality in migraine and is possibly sufficient to account for the increased amplitude of grand averages. The question therefore arises whether deficient habituation in cortical information processing might be a more general abnormality able to explain the high amplitude of other averaged evoked potentials. To provide an answer, we analysed the habituation phenomenon for various sensory modalities and cerebral potentials using repetitive stimulations at constant intensity (visual evoked potential), repetition of the same stimulus at increasing intensities (auditory evoked potential) and repetition of novel stimuli (passive 'oddball' auditory event-related potential).

As shown in Figure 18.1, in every study between attacks in migraine with or without aura a defect of habituation was found compared to healthy controls. During sequential averagings of 50 responses of pattern-reversal visual evoked potentials (VEP) at a 3 Hz stimulation rate, there was a clear-cut, though transient, decrement (i.e. habituation) of N1–P1 and P1–N2 amplitudes in healthy controls, but a transient increment (i.e. potentiation) exceeding 30% in migraine with and without aura (Schoenen *et al.* 1995) (Figure 18.1a). The N1–P2 component of the auditory evoked potential (AEP) was markedly increased at the 70 dB SL stimulation intensity compared to the 40 dB intensity in both types of migraine, while it underwent little change in controls. The intensity dependence of the AEP was thus strong in migraine (amplitude–stimulus function (ASF) slopes, 0.6 and 0.7 μV/10 dB), but weak in healthy controls (ASF slope, 0.07 μV/10 dB). Analysis

---

Figure 18.1 Histograms illustrating the amplitude change of: a) pattern-reversal visual evoked; b) cortical auditory (70 db SL) evoked; and c) passive 'oddball' auditory event-related potentials in successive blocks of averaged responses (a, 50; b and c, 40 responses per block). MO, migraine without aura; MA, migraine with aura.

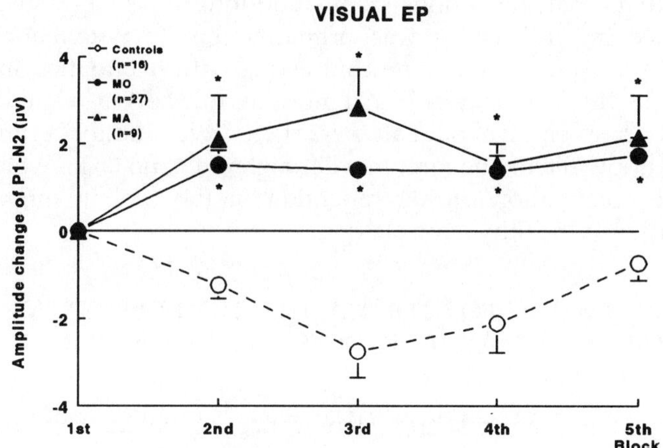
VISUAL EP
Controls (n=16)
MO (n=27)
MA (n=9)
Amplitude change of P1-N2 (μv)
4
2
0
-2
-4
1st
2nd
3rd
4th
5th Block
(a)

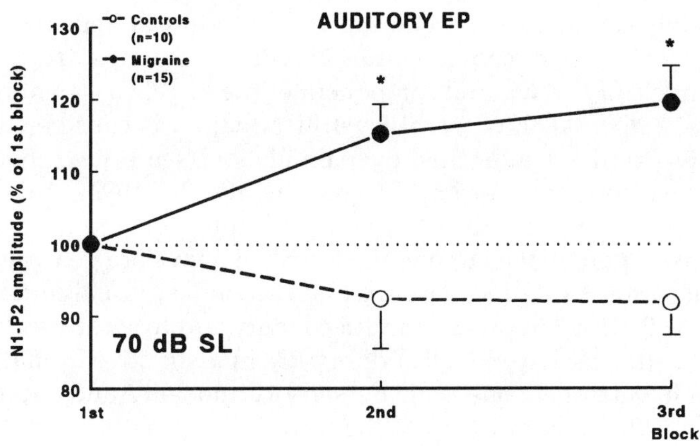
AUDITORY EP
Controls (n=10)
Migraine (n=15)
N1-P2 amplitude (% of 1st block)
130
120
110
100
90
80
70 dB SL
1st
2nd
3rd Block
(b)

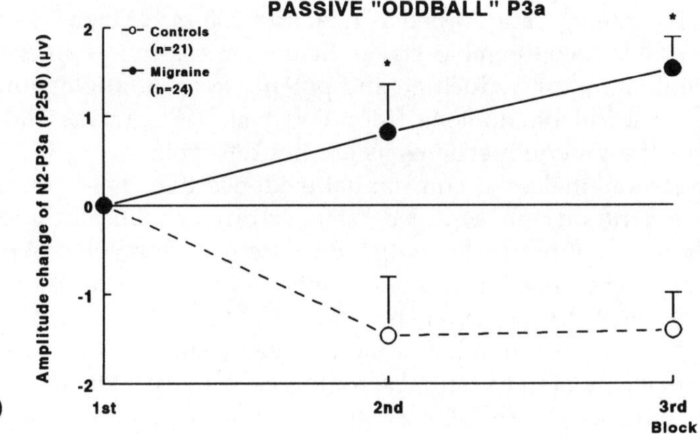
PASSIVE "ODDBALL" P3a
Controls (n=21)
Migraine (n=24)
Amplitude change of N2-P3a (P250) (μv)
2
1
0
-1
-2
1st
2nd
3rd Block
(c)

of habituation at the various stimulation intensities suggested that the difference in ASF slopes was primarily due to potentiation of the potential at 70 dB in migraine contrasting with habituation in controls (Figure 18.1b). The novelty P3a, a more complex event-related potential studied in a passive oddball paradigm (two auditory stimuli: one frequent, low pitch; one rare, 'novel', high pitch; no task involved), also showed potentiation during repetition of the trial in migraine, but habituation in healthy controls (Figure 18.1c).

POSSIBLE CAUSES FOR THE HABITUATION DEFICIT IN CENTRAL INFORMATION PROCESSING: THE 'CEILING' CONCEPT AND 5-HT

The exact mechanisms and significance of habituation are largely speculative and probably pleiomorphic. Habituation, as its counterpart potentiation (or sensitization), can be demonstrated in neuronal circuits of varying complexities, from the gill withdrawal reflex in Aplysia (Kandel *et al.* 1983) or spinal reflexes in rodents (Thompson *et al.* 1979) to autonomic and behavioural component of the so-called 'orienting reflex' (Sokolov 1963). At the cortical level, habituation is considered to be a protective mechanism against overstimulation (see below), but also an elementary form of learning (review by Kandel 1992) and a model phenomenon for the study of behaviour (Thompson and Spencer 1966). The evoked potential components described above are generated in the cerebral cortex: VEP P100 in primary and secondary visual cortices (areas 18,19); AEP N1–P2 in primary and secondary auditory cortices (Scherg *et al.* 1989); and passive oddball auditory P3a in associative frontal cortices. Although heterogeneous both by sensory modality and experimental paradigm (the total duration of the recording procedure is ± 4 min for AEPs, ± 3–5 min for passive oddball auditory P3a and ± 1 min for VEP), the three cerebral potentials have in common their occurrence within comparable latency ranges (between 80 and 250 msec), which suggests that they reflect comparable stages in the processing of information. Their habituation (or 'reducing') and potentiation (or 'augmenting') are doubtless cortical phenomena (Monnier *et al.* 1976, Lukas and Siegel 1977), but the precise mechanisms are not determined.

There is nonetheless circumstantial evidence that these phenomena are dependent on the so-called 'state-setting, chemically addressed connections' that originate in the brainstem and involve serotonin, dopamine, noradrenaline, acetylcholine or histamine as transmitters (Mesulam 1990). In particular, the intensity dependence of AEPs, and thus probably its potentiation at high intensity stimulations, is thought to be inversely related to central serotonergic activity (Hegerl and Juckel 1993). The increased AEP ASF slope in migraine would thus indicate a

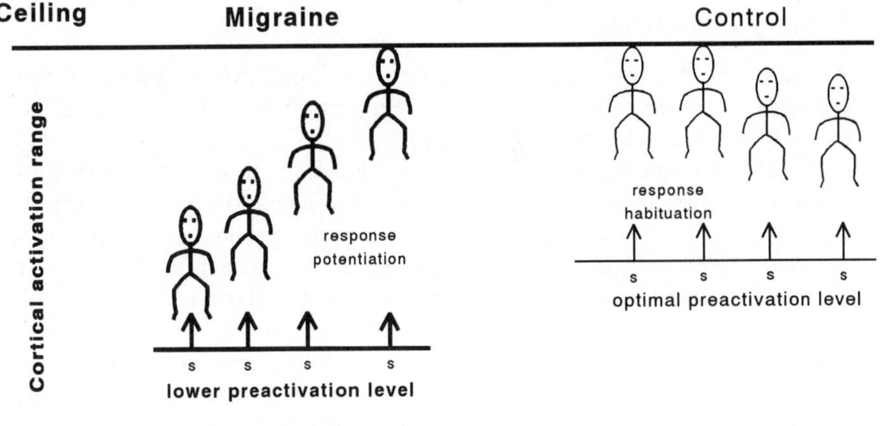

Figure 18.2 Illustration of the hypothesis of a low cortical preactivation level and the 'ceiling' concept.

low central 5-HT disposition, which is concordant with similar trends for 5-HT in the periphery (Ferrari 1992). The raphe serotonergic neurons are indeed ideally organized to modulate information processing in the cerebral cortex and 'to coordinate the activity of target structures (or set the tone) in conjunction with the organism's level of motor activity and behavioral arousal' (Jacobs and Azmitia 1992). Both their anatomical organization (i.e. widespread cortical innervation mainly of pyramidal cells and γ-aminobutyric acid (GABA) -ergic inhibitory interneurons in layer IV, the major site of thalamo-cortical input) and their physiological features (i.e. regular, tonic 'pacemaker' activity) would promote such a state-setting function. Low activity in these serotonergic pathways may be responsible for low cortical preactivation (Hegerl and Juckel 1993), which in models of competitive neuronal networks (Grossberg and Gutowski 1987) leads to high cortical reagibility with increased detection, but lowered tolerance thresholds. The latter can be explained by the 'ceiling' concept (Knott and Irwin 1973) (Figure 18.2), which postulates that the low cortical preactivation level in migraine offers a large range for suprathreshold activation up to the 'ceiling', explaining strong intensity dependence of responses (augmenting pattern) as well as the potentiation of the response after repetition of the same stimulus.

Whatever the causes for abnormal cortical information processing in migraine might be, the lack of habituation may have deleterious consequences on the metabolic homeostasis of the brain parenchyma.

ABNORMAL INFORMATION PROCESSING: A CORNERSTONE IN MIGRAINE PATHOGENESIS?

As mentioned above, habituation or 'reducing' in the 'augmenting/ reducing' concept (Buchsbaum and Silvermann 1968) is thought to protect the cerebral cortex against overload. PET (Fox *et al.* 1988, Phelps and Kuhl 1981) and NMR spectroscopy (Prichard *et al.* 1991) studies of the normal human cortex show that photic stimulation induces a rapid, though transient, excess of glycolysis over respiration accompanied by a significant rise in lactate. Using NMR spectroscopy, Sappey-Marinier *et al.* (1992) found that during pattern reversal stimulation cortical lactate levels begin to decrease only after amplitude of the visual evoked potential has diminished by more than 50%, suggesting that the response habituation, i.e. the diminished neuronal activity, is an adaptive mechanism decreasing lactate production.

In addition, ^{31}phosphorus NMR spectroscopy studies performed between attacks (Table 18.2) demonstrate a significant reduction of the mitochondrial energy reserve in occipital cortex, i.e. reduction of phosphocreatine (Welch *et al.* 1989) and phosphorylation potential, both in migraine with (Barbiroli *et al.* 1992) and without aura (Montagna *et al.* 1994). The mitochondrial dysfunction is thought to be of a sufficient severity to induce a significant rupture of metabolic homeostasis in the cerebral cortex of migraineurs under circumstances of overload and increased energy demands (Montagna *et al.* 1989). These data may provide some direct support for the 'oxygen theory' of migraine (Amery 1982), which postulates that an episode of cerebral hypoxia resulting from any imbalance between neuronal energy supply and energy consumption is at the core of the pathophysiology of a migraine attack. Although mitochondrial dysfunction can reduce the neuronal energy supply, this may not be sufficient to develop migraine, which is not

Table 18.2 Mitochondrial phosphorylation and energy reserve in occipital areas of migraine patients and control subjects[a]

	Phosphocreatine (μM)	*ADP concentration* (μM)	*Phosphorylation potential*
Migraine with aura			
($n = 18$)	3.73 ± 0.3	37 ± 6.5	55 ± 10.3*
Migraine without aura			
($n = 22$)	3.39 ± 0.3*	45 ± 6.5*	50 ± 8.2*
Healthy controls			
($n = 50$)	4.45 ± 0.2	29 ± 2.5	84 ± 7.0

[a] Barbiroli *et al.* 1992, Montagna *et al.* 1994
* $p < 0.001$

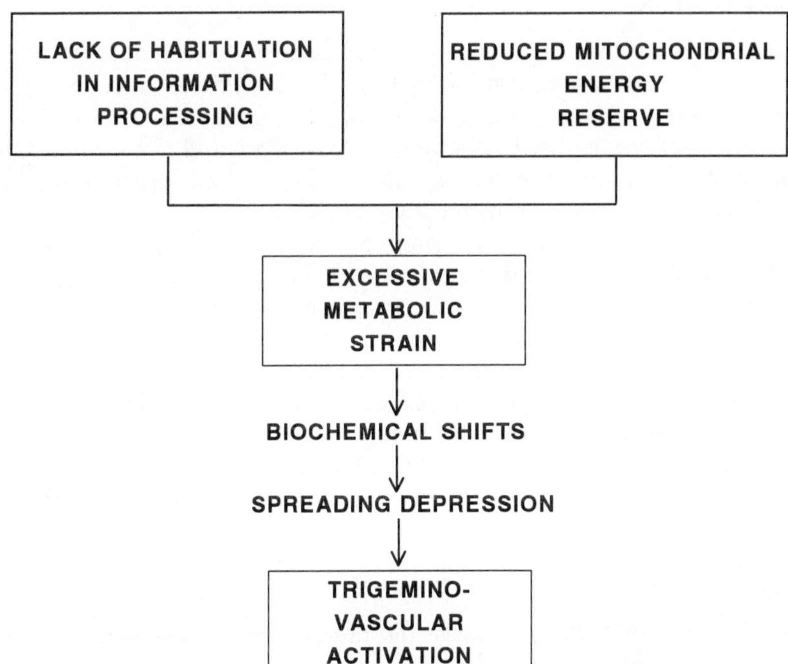

Figure 18.3 Model of migraine pathogenesis hypothesizing that coexistence of a habituation defect in sensory processing and a reduced mitochondrial energy reserve may lead to a rupture of brain metabolic homeostasis, triggering a migraine headache as a protective mechanism.

always associated with various known mitochondriopathies. Hence, a supplementary central nervous system dysfunction in migraine is likely.

Considering these biochemical data, one may hypothesize that the lack of habituation in information processing and the reduced mitochondrial phosphorylation potential can concur in migraine to favour metabolic shifts in the cerebral cortex. The deranged oxygen metabolism would accelerate and exaggerate the lactate and proton accumulation that occurs after physiological stimulation, since it is not compensated for by habituation of neuronal activity. This might lead to rupture of the metabolic homeostasis and trigger spreading depression under certain circumstances, especially in the visual cortex, where the neuron/glia ratio is high (Figure 18.3). The hypothesis that physiological stimuli cause glucose uptake and blood flow increase in excess of oxygen consumption as well as exaggerated lactate levels in the brain of migraine patients between attacks can be tested with PET and NMR spectroscopy.

CONCLUSIONS

Migraineurs are characterized between attacks by a deficient habituation in cortical information processing and by a reduced mitochondrial energy reserve. These abnormalities may be independent factors that (genetically?) predispose to migraine or may be related to each other. In concert they can favour metabolic shifts in the cerebral cortex, triggering an attack as a nociceptive, protective mechanism.

Moreover, the abnormal information processing and oxygen metabolism in the cerebral cortex of migraine patients may have behavioural correlates. It seems indeed reasonable to think that a lower ability to distract from novel or repeated stimuli in the environment can influence behaviour and cognition. Limited internal resources due to the low cortical activation or reduced energy reserve may also influence behavioural patterns, and in particular promote self-stimulating processes (Gerber and Schoenen 1995). The physiological abnormalities could thus be relevant for the biobehavioural concept of migraine (Welch 1986).

REFERENCES

Amery, W.K. (1982) Brain hypoxia: the turning-point in the genesis of the migraine attack? *Cephalalgia*, **2**, 83–109.

Anthony, M. and Lance, J.W. (1975) Serotonin in migraine. In: *Topics in migraine*, (ed. J.M.S. Pearce). London, Heinemann.

Barbiroli, B., Montagna, P., Cortelli, P., Funicello, R., Iotti, S., Monari, L., Pierangeli, G., Zaniol, P. and Lugaresi, E. (1992) Abnormal brain and muscle energy metabolism shown by ^{31}P magnetic resonance spectroscopy in patients affected by migraine with aura. *Neurology*, **42**, 1209–1214.

Barkley, G.L., Tepley, N., Simkins, R., Moran, J. and Welch, K.M.A. (1990) Neuromagnetic fields in migraine: preliminary findings. *Cephalalgia*, **10**, 171–176.

Besken, E., Pothmann, R. and Sartory, C. (1993) Contingent negative variation in childhood migraine. *Cephalalgia*, **13**, 42–43.

Blau, J.N. (1987) Adult migraine: the patient observed. In: *Migraine, Clinical, Therapeutic, Conceptual and Research Aspects*. (ed. J.N. Blau), pp. 3–30, Chapman & Hall, London.

Buchsbaum M.S. and Silverman J. (1968) Stimulus intensity control and the cortical evoked response. *Psychosomatic Medicine*, **30**, 12–22.

Camp W.A. and Wolff H.G. (1961) Studies on headache. Electroencephalographic abnormalities in patients with vascular headache of the migraine type. *Archives of Neurology*, **4**, 475–485.

Connolly, J.F., Gaxel, M. and Clifford Rose, F. (1982) Migraine patients exhibit abnormalities in the visual evoked potential. *Journal of Neurology Neurosurgery Psychiatry*, **45**, 464–467.

D'Andrea, G., Welch, K.M.A., Riddlle, J.M. and Grunfeld, S. (1989) Platelet serotonin metabolism and ultrastructure in migraine. *Archives of Neurology*, **46**, 1187–1189.

D'Andrea, G., Gananzi, A.R., Joseph, R. *et al.* (1991) Platelet glycine, glutamate and aspartate in primary headache. *Cephalalgia*, **11**, 197–200.

Diener, H.C., Ndosi N.K., Koletzki, E. and Langohr, H.D. (1984) Visual evoked potentials in migraine. In: *Updating Headache,* (eds V. Pfaffenrath, P.J. Lundberg and O. Sjaastad), pp. 439–465. Springer Verlag, Berlin

Diener, H.C., Scholz, E., Dichgans, J. and Gerber, W.D. (1989) Central effects of drugs used in migraine prophylaxis evaluated by visual evoked potentials. *Annals of Neurology*, **25**, 125–130.

Edmeads, J. (1992) Migraine: Disease or syndrome? *Pathologie Biologie*, **40**, 279–283.

Ferrari, M.D. (1992) Biochemistry of migraine. *Pathologie Biologie*, **40**, 284–292.

Ferrari, M.D., Odink, J., Tapparelli, C., Van Kempen, G.M.J., Pennings, E.J.M. and Bruyn, G.W. (1989) Serotonin metabolism in migraine. *Neurology*, **39**, 1239–1242.

Ferrari, M.D. and Saxena P.R. (1993) On serotonin and migraine: a clinical and pharmacological review. *Cephalalgia*, **13**, 151–165.

Ferrari, M.D., Odink, J., Bos, K.D., Malessy, M.J.A. and Bruyn, G.W. (1990) Neuroexcitatory plasma amino acids are elevated in migraine. *Neurology*, **40**, 1582–1586.

Fox, P.T., Raichle, M.E., Mintum, M.A. and Dence, C. (1988) Nonoxidative glucose consumption during focal physiological neural activity. *Science*, **241**, 462–464.

Friberg, L., Olesen, J., Iversen, H.K. and Sperling B. (1991) Migraine pain associated with middle cerebral artery dilation reversal by sumatriptan. *Lancet*, **338**, 13–17.

Gawel, M., Connolly, J.F. and Clifford Rose, F.C. (1983) Migraine patients exhibit abnormalities in the visual evoked potential. *Headache*, **23**, 49–52.

Gerber, W.D. and Schoenen, J. (1995) Migraine etiopathogenesis: new vistas. *Born to be wild*. 3rd Congress on Headache in Childhood and Adolescence. May 4–6, Budapest.

Goadsby, P.J., Edvinsson, L. and Ekman, R. (1990) Vasoactive peptide release in the extracerebral circulation of humans during migraine headache. *Annals of Neurology*, **28**, 183–187.

Goadsby, P.J. and Edvinsson, L. (1993) The trigeminovascular system and migraine: studies characterizing cerebrovascular and neuropeptide changes seen in humans and cats. *Annals of Neurology*, **33**, 48–56.

Grossberg, S. and Gutowski, W.E. (1987) Neural dynamics of decision making under risk: an effective balance and cognitive-emotional interactions. *Psychology Review*, **94**, 300–318.

Hardebo, J.E. (1992) A cortical excitatory wave may cause both the aura and the headache of migraine. *Cephalalgia*, **12**, 75–80.

Hegerl, U. and Juckel, G. (1993) Intensity dependence of auditory evoked potentials as an indicator of central serotonergic neurotransmission: a new hypothesis. *Biological Psychiatry*, **33**, 173–187.

Humphrey, P.P.A. (1991) 5-Hydroxytryptamine and the pathophysiology of migraine. *Journal of Neurology*, **238**, S38–S44.

Jacobs, B.L. and Azmitia, E.C. (1992) Structure and function of the brain serotonin system. *Physiology Review*, **72**, 165–229.

Kandel, E.R. (1992) Cellular mechanisms of learning and biological basis of individuality. In: *Principles of Neurological Science*, (eds E.R. Kandel, J.H. Schwartz and T.M. Jessell), pp. 1009–1031. Elsevier, New York.

Kandel, E.R., Abrams, T., Bernier, L., Carew, T.J., Hawkins, R.D. and Schwartz, J.H. (1983) Classical conditioning and sensitization show aspects of the same molecular cascade in Aplysia, *Cold Spring Harbor Symposia on Quantitative Biology*, **48**, 821–830.

Kennard, C., Gawel, M., Rudolf, N. and Clifford Rose, F. (1978) Visual evoked potentials in migraine subjects. *Research and Clinical Studies in Headache*, **61**, 73–80.

Knott, J.R. and Irwin, D.A. (1973) Anxiety, stress and contingent negative variation. *Archives of General Psychiatry*, **29**, 538–541.

Kropp, P. and Gerber, W.D. (1993) Is increased amplitude of contingent negative variation in migraine due to cortical hyperactivity or to reduced habituation? *Cephalalgia*, **13**, 37–41.

Lance, J.W. (1993) *Mechanisms and Management of Headache*, 5th edition. Butterworth & Heinemann, Oxford.

Lauritzen, M., Skyhøj Olsen, T., Lassen, N.A. and Paulson, O.B. (1983a) The changes of regional cerebral blood flow during the course of classical migraine attacks. *Annals of Neurology*, **13**, 633–641.

Lauritzen, M., Skyhøj Olsen, T., Lassen N.A. and Paulson, O.B. (1983b) Regulation of regional cerebral blood flow during and between migraine attacks. *Annals of Neurology*, **14**, 569–572.

Leão, A.A. (1944) Spreading depression of activity in cerebral cortex. *Journal of Neurophysiology*, **7**, 359–390.

Lehtonen, J.B. (1974) Visual evoked potentials for single flashes and flickering light in migraine. *Headache*, **14**, 1–12.

Lehtonen, J.B., Hyyppä, M.T., Kaihola, H.L., Kangasniemi, P. and Lang, A.H. (1979) Visual evoked potentials in menstrual migraine. *Headache*, **19**, 63–70.

Lukas, J.H. and Siegel, J. (1977) Cortical mechanisms that augment or reduce evoked potentials in cats. *Science*, **198**, 73–75.

Maertens de Noordhout, A., Timsit-Berthier, M., Timsit, M. and Schoenen, J. (1986) Contingent negative variation in headache. *Annals of Neurology*, **19**, 78–90.

Mesulam, M.M. (1990) Large-scale neurocognitive networks and distributed processing for attention language and memory. *Annals of Neurology*, **28**, 597–613.

Milner, P.M. (1958) Note on a possible correspondence between the scotomas of migraine and spreading depression of Leao. *Electroencephalography and Clinical Neurophysiology*, **10**, 705.

Monnier, M., Boehmer, A. and Scholer, A. (1976) Early habituation, dishabituation and generalization induced in the visual centers by colour stimuli. *Vision Research*, **16**, 1479–1504.

Montagna, P., Sayuegna, T., Cortelli, P. and Lugaresi, E. (1989) Migraine as a defect of brain oxidative metabolism: a hypothesis. *Journal of Neurology*, **236**, 124–125.

Montagna, P., Cortelli, P., Monari, L., Pierangeli, G., Parchi, P., Lodi, R., Iotti, S., Zaniol, P., Lugaresi, E. and Barbiroli, B. (1994) ^{31}P-Magnetic resonance spectroscopy in migraine without aura. *Neurology*, **44**, 666–668.

Moskowitz, M.A. (1991) The visceral organ brain: implications for the pathophysiology of vascular head pain. *Neurology*, **41**, 182–186.

Moskowitz, M.A. (1993) Neurovascular mechanisms in the pathogenesis and treatment of migraine. In: *Abstracts 7th World Congress on Pain, Seattle*, p. 253. IASP Publications.

Moskowitz, M.A. and Cutrer, F.M. (1993) Sumatriptan: a receptor-targeted treatment of migraine. *Annual Review of Medicine*, **44**, 145–154.

Olesen, J., Larsen, B. and Lauritzen, M. (1981) Focal hyperemia followed by spreading oligemia and impaired activation of rCBF in classic migraine. *Annals of Neurology*, **9**, 344–352.

Olesen, J., Friberg, L., Olsen, T.S., Andersen, A.R., Lassen, N.A., Hansen, P.E. and Karle, A. (1993) Ischaemia-induced (symptomatic) migraine attacks may be more frequent than migraine-induced ischaemic insults. *Brain*, **116**, 187–202.

Phelps, M.E. and Kuhl, D.E. (1981) Metabolic mapping of the brain's response to visual stimulation: studies in humans. *Science*, **211**, 1445–1448.

Prichard, J.W., Rothman, D.L., Novotny, E., Petroff, O.A.C., Kuwabara, T., Avison, M., Howseman, A., Hanstock, C.C. and Shulman, R.G. (1991) Lactate rise detected by ^{1}H NMR in human visual cortex during physiologic stimulation. *Proceedings of the National Academy of Sciences USA*, **88**, 5829–5831.

Ramadan, N.M., Halvorsen, H., Vande-Linde, A., Levine, S.R., Helpern, J.A. and Welch, K.M.A. (1989) Low brain magnesium in migraine. *Headache*, **29**, 590–593.

Sappey-Marinier, D., Galabrese, G., Fein, G., Hugg, J.W., Biggins, C. and Weiner, M.W. (1992) Effect of photic stimulation on human visual cortex lactate and phosphates using ^{1}H and ^{31}P magnetic resonance spectroscopy. *Journal of Cerebral Blood Flow and Metabolism*, **12**, 584–592.

Scherg, M., Vajsar, J. and Picton, T.W. (1989) A source analysis of the late human auditory evoked potentials. *Journal of Cognitive Neuroscience*, **1**, 336–355.

Schoenen, J. (1992) Clinical neurophysiology studies in headache: a review of data and pathophysiological hints. *Functional Neurology*, **7**, 191–204.

Schoenen, J. and Maertens de Noordhout, A. (1988) The role of the sympathetic nervous system in migraine and cluster headache. In: *Basic Mechanisms of Headache. Pain Research and Clinical Management*, Vol. 2, (eds J. Olesen and L. Edvinsson), pp. 393–410. Elsevier, Amsterdam.

Schoenen J., Maertens de Noordhout, A., Timsit-Berthier, M. and Timsit, M. (1985) Contingent negative variation (CNV) as a diagnostic and physiopathologic tool in headache patients. In: *Migraine: Clinical and Research Advances*, (ed. F. Clifford Rose), pp. 17–25. Karger, Basel.

Schoenen, J., Maertens de Noordhout, A., Timsit-Berthier, M. and Timsit, M. (1986) Contingent negative variation and efficacy of beta-blocking agents in migraine. *Cephalalgia*, **6**, 229–233.

Schoenen, J., Jamart, B. and Delwaide, P.J. (1987) Cartographie électroencéphalographique dans les migraines en périodes critique et intercritique. *Revue d'Electroencephographie et de Neurophysiologie Clinique*, **17**, 289–299.

Schoenen, J., Wang, W., Albert, A. and Delwaide, P.J. (1995) Potentiation instead of habituation characterizes visual evoked potentials in migraine patients between attacks. *European Journal of Neurology*, **2**, 115–122.

Sokolov, E.N. (ed.) (1963) *Perception and the Conditioned Reflex*. Pergamon, Oxford.

Thompson, R.F. and Spencer, W.A. (1966) Habituation: a model phenomenon for the study of neuronal substrates of behavior. *Psychology Review*, **7**, 16–43.

Thompson, R.F., Berry, S.D., Rinaldi, P.C. and Berger, T.W. (1979) Habituation and orienting reflex: the dural-process theory revised. In: *The Orienting Reflex in Humans*, (eds H.D. Kimmel, E.H. van Olst and J.F. Orlebeke) pp. 21–60. Laurence Erlbaum, Hillsdale, New Jersey.

Welch, K.M.A. (1986) Migraine: a biobehavioral disorder. *Cephalalgia*, **6** (Suppl. 4), 103–110.

Welch, K.M.A., Levine, S.R., D'Andrea, G., Schultz, L. and Helpern, J.A. (1989)

Preliminary observations on brain energy metabolism in migraine studied by in vivo [31]phosphorus NMR spectroscopy. *Neurology*, **39**, 538–541.

Winter, A.L. and Cooper, R. (1985) Neurophysiological measures of the visual system in classic migraine. In: *Migraine: Clinical and Research Advances*, (ed. F. Clifford Rose), pp. 11–16. Karger, Basel.

Woods, R.P., Iacoboni, M. and Mazziotta, J.C. (1994) Bilateral spreading cerebral hypoperfusion during spontaneous migraine headache. *New England Journal of Medicine*, **331**, 1689–1692.

DISCUSSION

Fozard: Do you see any gross difference between migraine patients receiving prophylactic therapy and those not on therapy?

Schoenen: Contingent negative variation (CNV) in patients receiving β-blockers tends to normalize (Schoenen *et al.* 1986) and the amplitude of the visual evoked potential also decreases (Diener *et al.* 1989). Now we are looking at possible pharmacological effects on other phenomena such as habituation.

Fozard: Were these β-blockers that penetrate the brain?

Schoenen: Yes. They were propranolol and metropolol.

Glover: How do your findings compare with what's been found with patients with different psychiatric disorders, such as anxiety or depression? Did you ensure that your migraine patients didn't have a history of such disorders?

Schoenen: This is a difficult question, to which I have only a partial response. CNV is a complex activity. Most anxiety patients seen by Martine Timsit-Berthier do not have a high CNV: they tend to have a low CNV and a high P3. Usually there is an inverse correlation: the higher the CNV, the lower the P3; and the higher the P3, the lower the CNV. In depressed patients, the CNV is usually also low, except in a subgroup of about 10% of her patients who have a high CNV resembling that in migraineurs. Habituation seemed to be normal in these depressed patients and they usually had a large post-imperative negative variation (PINV), which is considered to reflect psychopatho-logical changes.

In most published studies depressed patients have a low intensity dependence of the evoked potentials. They are reducers not aug-menters. That contrasts with our group of migraineurs. Personality traits have been related to some of these responses. For example, strong intensity dependence has been correlated with sensation-seeking behaviour. So we used the Zuckermann scale and found the opposite: migraineurs have a low propensity for sensation-seeking. So our impression is that in migraineurs there is some kind of disconnection of the usual correlations between electrophysiology and psychology or psychopathology. We do not find the expected correlation between some of these physiological patterns and the expected personality or behavioural patterns.

Diener: We took blood samples from all our families with migraine, and Professor Reichmann and his colleagues in Würzburg analysed mitochondrial RNA. They didn't find any deletions or repeats. This could differ for brain mitochondrial function, but in peripheral blood cells in a large sample of migraine patients we couldn't find anything.

Schoenen: Montagna *et al.* (1994) and Barbiroli *et al.* (1992) studied mitochondrial function rather than RNA.

Diener: In all known diseases with mitochondrial dysfunction there are genetic changes in RNA.

Schoenen: I'm not saying that migraine is a mitochondrial disease. I am not even certain that the mitochondrial dysfunction is primary. It could be secondary to some other change, for example, in transmitter activity. But the data about energy reserves between the attacks are quite convincing.

Tournier-Lasserve: Although Dr Diener found that RNA isolated from mitochondria were normal in migraine patients, most of the proteins which are functional in the mitochondria are encoded by the nuclear genome.

Ferrari: Dr Schoenen suggested that reduced mitochondrial function might lower the threshold for cortical spreading depression. Have experiments been done in animals to reduce mitochondrial function in an attempt to induce spreading depression?

Diener: In humans the stroke-like episodes in mitochondrial encephalopathy resemble migraine attacks with aura. A typical feature of this disorder is that patients have aura symptoms which spread faster than migraine symptoms, and they have the typical headache.

Schoenen: It is not possible to slightly reduce mitochondrial activity because mitochondrial poisons used in animal research are very toxic. In some mitochondriopathies patients have been ameliorated by receiving high doses of riboflavin (vitamin B_2) or nicotinamide (vitamin B_3), which are the only available nontoxic substances that are able to increase mitochondrial activity (Penn *et al.* 1992). We thought it would be interesting to try high dose riboflavin as a prophylactic treatment. The open study is encouraging: we had a responder rate of 65%. We are now doing a double-blind study against placebo.

Tournier-Lasserve: Some patients with MELAS (mitochondrial encephalopathy with lactic acidosis and strokes) present only as having migraine with aura for a long time: the only indication is that magnetic resonance imaging shows white matter lesions.

Moskowitz: The threshold for causing a spreading depression can be affected by whether the animals are fed or fasted. That might relate in some way to your metabolism arguments.

Tournier-Lasserve: It would be interesting to test with Dr Schoenen's model what is happening in families of migraineurs, specifically where the family tree gives the impression that migraine might be inherited with a mitochondrial pattern.

Schoenen: I agree. Martine Timsit looked at CNV in pairs of mothers and daughters with migraine and found that mothers and daughters have very similar CNV patterns. Dieter Gerber is now doing a larger family study, looking at CNV in relatives.

Goadsby: What happens to CNV with ageing, particularly in Alzheimer's disease and Parkinson's disease? We know noradrenergic activity is reduced in Alzheimer's disease and there is a reasonable model for reduction in dopaminergic activity in Parkinson's disease.

Schoenen: CNV is decreased in Parkinson's disease and the amplitude can be increased again by giving DOPA. CNV is also decreased in Alzheimer's disease.

Goadsby: Therefore, does this CNV abnormality in migraine patients imply that the noradrenergic activity must be increased, rather than reduced?

Schoenen: It's difficult to relate a physiological activity precisely to just one neurotransmitter. CNV is not only modulated by noradrenaline and there are some indirect arguments that it's the early component which is mostly modulated by noradrenaline and that the late component is mostly modulated by dopamine. But acetylcholine and GABA also play a role. Initially we thought, and it might still be true, that the increased CNV reflected hyperactivity in the catecholamine system. But it could be that it is a hyper-reactivity, let's say like receptor supersensitivity. The argument we were using was the effect of β-blockers on the CNV amplitude. But I think it is more complicated than that, because in Dieter Gerber's studies of CNV before the attack, the late component is mainly increased just before the attack. This would suggest dopaminergic hyperactivity just before the attack.

Goadsby: Signal-to-noise can be modulated favourably, at least by noradrenergic systems, when the systems act normally. So I was surprised that your hypothesis necessitates overactivity.

Schoenen: One hypothesis which correlates with what is known from neuronal networks and serotonin activity in the brain would be a low cortical activation due to a hypoactive serotonin innervation, at least for the intensity dependence and the potentiation instead of the habituation. But CNV is a much more complicated cerebral activity than the auditory evoked potential or the visual evoked potential, and therefore we are dealing with more actors.

Lance: I'm interested in the possible relationship between the failure of habituation and photophobia and phonophobia in migrainous patients. Many chronic daily headache patients also complain of these symptoms and it would be interesting to investigate them in the same way. Have you examined any patients during a headache when they have photophobia and phonophobia to see if this phenomenon is even more evident?

Schoenen: We have no data about the other evoked potentials during attacks, but Dieter Gerber has looked at CNV in patients before and during migraine attacks. He found some dynamic changes: CNV starts to increase the day before the attack, decreases just before the attack, and reaches a normal amplitude during the attack. With Martin Timsit we found that during an attack the CNV is normal: compared to the headache-free interval the amplitude is decreased and the habituation is normal. I think phono- and photophobia during the attack are not related to the hypersensitivity to, for example, visual stimuli in headache-free intervals. The latter could be a consequence of the lack of habituation, the former seems more to be related to the pain.

Moskowitz: In other neurological conditions in which photo- and phonophobia occur, there has usually been meningeal irritation, the most profound form being during meningitis. I wonder whether in migraine photo- and phonophobia occur as a consequence of abnormal irritation of the meninges, particularly in proximity to those areas that are subserving sound and light.

Lance: There is a hypersensitivity not only to light and sound, but also to smells. There is often hyperaesthesia of the skin. In migraine there is a general disinhibition of all afferent stimuli, including painful stimuli. Rather than irritation of dura or any particular part of the brain, I think there is a generalized disinhibition or failure to gate afferent impulses of all sorts, whether they be through the special senses, in the case of light, sound or smells, or whether they be tactile or pain pathways. Therefore I'd place the cause centrally as a part of a failure of the endogenous pain control system. I think Dr Schoenen's observations give us an important insight into failure of habituation. If habituation normally depends on the body's own gating mechanism, and it fails to work in migraine patients between headaches, this could be an indication of a central failure. The only point against this is the fact that habituation of the CNV returns to normal during the headache phase of migraine.

Schoenen: Several studies show that migraineurs between attacks are also more sensitive to light stimuli. Also, several studies show some permanent dysfunction in visual processing between attacks. For example, migraineurs are more susceptible to visual illusions, which suggests an imbalance between excitation and inhibition in the visual cortex, or at least in certain visual pathways. It is not likely that this hypersensitivity to sensory stimuli has a direct relation to the more pronounced and disabling one we see during the attack.

Moskowitz: There is a difference between the phenomenon of sensitivity and the presence of photophobia and phonophobia. Light perception, a light source and an intact trigeminal nerve are necessary to develop photophobia. During a migraine headache, the photophobia and phonophobia may be reflecting an abnormal brain plus hypersensitive trigeminovascular afferents innervating the meninges overlying occipital and temporal cortex, respectively.

Schoenen: That's my feeling also.

Lance: Drummond (1986) showed there are two components to photophobia in migraine. One is localized to the eye on the side of the migrainous headache and is clearly related to irritation or activation of the first division of the trigeminal nerve. The other is a general sensitivity to light, which is not dependent on the side of the headache and is a part of a generalized hyperacuity of special senses. So there are at least two components here. One is a sort of generalized failure to inhibit the visual stimuli, and the other is a unilateral irritative phenomenon related to the trigeminal nerve.

Moskowitz: However, light entering the opposite eye is going to affect function in the ipsilateral hemisphere. Shining light in the left eye affects the trigeminal nerve innervating the meninges in the right occipital lobe. So the fact that there is light sensitivity in both eyes is quite consistent with a strictly right hemispheric disturbance.

Lance: I'm talking about anterior visual pathways here, about activation of the first division of the trigeminal nerve causing hypersensitivity in that particular eye as a retinal phenomenon rather than a hemispheric phenomenon.

Moskowitz: You also described a disturbance in the left eye as well.

Lance: There is a generalized diffuse hypersensitivity to light, which is present irrespective of the side of the headache, but there is a localized sensitivity in the affected eye. One sees this in cluster headache as well.

Humphrey: Dr Schoenen, how do you envisage spreading depression activating the trigeminovascular system? I can't see how it can do that unless the depolarization and electrical activity penetrate to the level of the nucleus caudalis and possibly activate incoming primary afferents. I can't envisage that happening.

Schoenen: I may have put a questionmark on spreading depression. What I wanted to say is that if the trigeminovascular system is a protective defensive system any threat, biochemical or metabolic, to the cerebral cortex should be able to activate it.

Humphrey: I agree that it is an attractive concept. I'm just trying to think how you can link that up, from a knowledge of the neuroanatomy.

Moskowitz: We now know that it can occur, and that it's not a central 'down-the-neural-axis' kind of activation, because the sides don't match up. The ipsilateral trigeminal system can be activated by the brain. We've certainly shown this under intense pathological conditions, with blood flow, and we've seen it with c-*fos* with less intense activity.

Humphrey: I still don't understand. You need a central activation that's independent of blood flow and associated changes in order to link in with Dr Schoenen's hypothesis.

Moskowitz: I have no problem with that. The most important factor is that brain events occur in proximity to the meninges in the outer perimeter of the brain. Drainage and the removal of chemicals released into the brain tissue have access to the vessels that are innervated by the trigeminal nerve. For example, basal ganglia or deep structures would not qualify as a headache generator for a migraine attack. This need not be restricted to visual cortex or primary sensory cortex. The hypothalamus is a candidate because it is located in close proximity to the meninges.

Humphrey: That implies activation of the trigeminovascular system at the peripheral end rather than the central end, but it is integral to Dr Schoenen's hypothesis that it's the depolarization of brain neurons that activates the trigeminal.

Moskowitz: I'm not sure about the depolarization of central neurons. Clearly there is something going on in the cortex. The hypothesis is that there is build-up in the brain that is not cleared by blood vessels.

Humphrey: That makes sense. But it just means that spreading depression goes hand in hand with things that are going on at the level of the blood vessel wall. You are saying that spreading depression *per se* does not activate the trigeminovascular system.

Moskowitz: That's correct. There is nothing unique about spreading depression with respect to activating the trigeminal system. Post-ictal headache may develop from the same phenomenon. In epilepsy there is a flood of ions and chemicals entering the extracellular space. Patients waken from an epileptic attack with a terrible headache. That is an extreme example. I wouldn't say that migraine is like an epileptic attack, but both develop chemical activation of primary afferents innervating the meninges. There is nothing incompatible with what Dr Schoenen is saying.

Humphrey: Given that explanation, one wouldn't look for drugs that block spreading depression, because it's just another epiphenomenon of what's going wrong at the level of those metabolites or mediators that are activating brain neurons and, in particular, the trigeminal nerve.

Moskowitz: I hope we will know in the next decade. If there is a common mechanism for events within the central nervous system, that would become the therapeutic target. Right now the target is the perivascular afferent and that works quite nicely, but it doesn't address the issue of cause and that's why the recurrences happen.

Fozard: Is the build up of chemicals/mediators subsequent to spreading depression sufficient to activate trigeminal fibres?

Moskowitz: There is poor documentation that spreading depression occurs in the human brain. In lissencephalic brain it is very easy to elicit, but in primates it is much more difficult. Neurosurgeons have looked for spreading depressions in thousands of exposed human brains during epilepsy surgery, some with sophisticated techniques. They claim not to have seen it. Some spreading event appears to occur in human brain during classic migraine that is accompanied by spreading oligaemia. Does every spreading depression have an accompanying slow oligaemic phase? We don't know.

Peatfield: It has been suggested that the blood flow changes can occur without clinical symptoms.

Moskowitz: That's exactly the point. Our ability to detect what's going on in the nervous system based on clinical information alone seems to be limited.

Peatfield: The other issue is that only a minority of people are affected. There is obviously some idiosyncrasy within a proportion of humans which leaves them susceptible. Neurosurgeons may be operating on people with quite another neurological disease who haven't this biochemical propensity.

Moskowitz: But among thousands of people you'd expect a few with the propensity for developing migraine. In the epileptic population the epidemiologists tell us that there is a higher incidence. However, epileptic surgeons are not looking in the occipital cortex, which is the most susceptible region, because in migraine the visual aura is clearly predominant. You could argue that the correct regions of the brain are not being examined, or that anti-epileptic drugs obscure the effect. More data and better techniques are needed. To study neurons, techniques that evaluate neuronal function are required. Blood flow is a fingerprint that is not necessarily phase-linked to events occurring within the brain.

Fozard: Do you have thoughts on alternative mechanisms which could cause the build up of chemicals/mediators which could then activate the trigeminal fibres?

Moskowitz: I hope that the answers might come from geneticists, who may identify the genes and proteins. Then we can fit them into a cascade, and have a better understanding of what makes somebody susceptible to migraine.

REFERENCES

Barbiroli, B., Montagna, P., Cortelli, P., Funicello, R., Iotti, S., Monari, L., Pierangeli, G., Zaniol, P., and Lugaresi, E. (1992) Abnormal brain and muscle energy metabolism shown by ^{31}P-magnetic resonance spectroscopy in patients affected by migraine with aura. *Neurology*, **42**, 1209–1214.

Drummond, P.D. (1986) A quantitative assessment of photophobia in migraine and tension headache. *Headache*, **26**, 465–469.

Diener, H.C., Scholz, E., Dichgans, J. and Gerber, W.D. (1989) Central effects of drugs used in migraine prophylaxis evaluated by visual evoked potentials. *Annals of Neurology*, **25**, 1025–1030.

Montagna, P., Cortelli, P., Monari, L., Pierangeli, G., Parchi, P., Lodi, R., Iotti, S., Zaniol, P., Lugaresi, E. and Barbiroli, B. (1994) ^{31}P-magnetic resonance spectroscopy in migraine without aura. *Neurology*, **44**, 666–668.

Penn, A.M.W., Lee, J.W.K., Thuillier, P., Wagner, M., Maclure, K.M., Hennard, M.R., Hail, L.D. and Kennaway, N.G. (1992) MELAS syndrome with mitochondrial tRNA$^{Leu(VVR)}$ mutation: correlation of clinical state, nerve conduction and muscle ^{31}P magnetic resonance spectroscopy during treatment with nicotinamide and riboflavin. *Neurology*, **42**, 2147–2152.

Schoenen, J., Maertens de Noordhout, A., Timsit-Berthier, M. and Timsit, M. (1986) Contingent negative variation and efficacy of beta-blocking agents in migraine. *Cephalalgia*, **6**, 229–233.

19

Sources of genetic complexity of migraine

Kathleen Ries Merikangas

GENETIC STUDIES OF MIGRAINE

The rapid developments in molecular biology have introduced a new era in human genetics. Only a decade ago the identification of genes for human traits depended upon inferences from the expression of traits that were known to be a manifestation of genes, such as colour blindness. Methods are now available to inspect DNA directly in order to identify genes involved in human diseases. Since the exciting discovery of a DNA marker for Huntington's disease (Gusella *et al.* 1982), numerous other diseases have followed and the primary gene defect has been discovered for Duchenne's muscular dystrophy (Kunkel *et al.* 1986) and cystic fibrosis (Beaudet *et al.* 1986).

The most exciting implication of these developments is the use of a genetic study design called linkage studies to identify markers for human diseases *without* knowledge of an abnormal gene product involved in their aetiology. Genetic researchers use information on the distance between specific DNA segments, or markers, to quantify the association between these DNA markers and a particular disease within families. If a close association is found, molecular geneticists and clinical researchers can work together to identify candidate genes located nearby on that chromosome which may actually cause the disease.

For example, if migraine were found to be associated with a marker in close proximity to a gene involved in the function of the 5-

Migraine: Pharmacology and genetics
Edited by Merton Sandler, Michel Ferrari and Sara Harnett
Published in 1996 by Chapman & Hall
ISBN 1 86036 006 8

hydroxytryptamine (5-HT) system, the association between the DNA segment which codes for the particular 5-HT gene could be investigated directly in families of subjects with migraine. If this gene were present in the majority of family members with migraine, other families could be studied to test the role of this gene in migraine. The identification of a DNA marker for migraine, irrespective of its role in the aetiology, would have major implications for the classification, treatment and patho-physiology of migraine.

The power of this approach lies in its ability to bypass assessment of the complex pathways involved in the expression of a particular gene, such as measurement of 5-hydroxyindoleacetic acid (5-HIAA) in spinal fluid or urine to infer differences in the underlying metabolism of 5-HT. The lack of trait markers for migraine to date can be attributed at least in part to the complexity of the neurochemical systems purported to be involved in its manifestation. The ultimate output of a gene may be altered by literally thousands of factors, including the specific tissue in which it is expressed, characteristics of its receptor(s), or different levels of neurotransmitters, neuropeptides, hormones, or immunological factors that may influence its expression.

The recent discovery of a genetic locus on chromosome 19 for familial hemiplegic migraine (FHM) in several families has led to a resurgence of interest in the genetic basis of the more common forms of migraine (Joutel *et al.* 1993). However, the application of linkage and association techniques to complex diseases is controversial (Risch 1994). There are several critical differences between the disorders to which the molecular biologists' tools have been successfully applied and complex human disease. Linkage has been reported for diseases which are extremely rare (<0.01% population prevalence), exhibit simple patterns of inheritance, and are clearly diagnosed with extremely high specificity and sensitivity. In contrast, disorders such as migraine, the spectrum of psychiatric disorders, and cardiovascular disease are characterized by high popula-tion prevalence, a lack of clear distinction between affected and unaffected (with an arbitrary threshold for case definition) and failure to adhere to Mendelian patterns of transmission.

Although recent progress in identification of the human gene map through the Human Genome Project and development of statistical methods to assess complex models of transmission have enhanced the power of studies to identify the genetic basis of more complex diseases, such as insulin-dependent diabetes (Davies *et al.* 1994, Hashimota *et al.* 1994), breast cancer (Hall *et al.* 1990, Easton *et al.* 1993, Miki *et al.* 1994), and Alzheimer's disease (Clark and Goate 1993), linkage studies of common diseases with imprecise phenotypic definitions continue to be plagued by lack of replication and inconsistent findings. For example, initial reports of linkage between affective disorders and DNA markers

(Egeland *et al.* 1987) could not be replicated by several studies (Kelsoe *et al.* 1989, Baron *et al.* 1993). Despite a decade of intensive effort to identify the genetic basis of bipolar disorder, there is still not a single replicated linkage or association finding for this condition or any of the other major psychiatric disorders (Risch and Merikangas 1993, McGuffin and Merikangas 1995). The lack of success of association studies is illustrated by the series of studies of the dopamine D_2 receptor and alcoholism which was announced with great fanfare and yet could not be replicated in five subsequent studies (Holden 1994). The most likely explanations are genetic and phenotypic heterogeneity and the inability of current studies to detect genes when the disease results from the effects of multiple genes or gene–environment interactions.

Family studies

Since Tissot first suggested the importance of familial transmission of migraine in 1834, there have been nearly 40 family history studies based on patient report, 10–90 % of whom had at least one relative who suffered from migraine. However, it is quite astonishing that in the literature over the past 100 years the evidence on the genetic mechanisms in migraine is quite sparse. Aside from a few studies described below, there are almost no family studies of migraine that would meet modern methodological standards. This underscores the need for family studies meeting such standards, including systematic ascertainment of probands, controls comparable to the probands on relevant confounding variables, sufficient sample size for adequate statistical power, application of standardized diagnostic criteria for migraine and related subtypes of headache, and direct interviews of relatives and spouses with blindness of the interviews to the diagnostic status of the proband (Weissman *et al.* 1986). The importance of obtaining direct and blind interviews of the relatives in family studies of migraine was demonstrated by Ottman *et al.* (1993) who reported that less than half of the true cases of migraine are detected via patient report compared to direct interview. Moreover, the introduction of operational diagnostic criteria for headache syndromes by the International Headache Society (IHS; Headache Classification Committee 1988) necessitates a new series of studies to facilitate comparability of phenotypic definitions.

The six controlled studies of adult or child probands with migraine report an average six-fold increase in the risk of migraine among relatives of migraine patients compared to the risk among relatives of controls (Ely 1930, Lennox 1941, Ask-Upmark 1953, Childs and Sweetnam 1961, Bille 1962, Waters and O'Connor 1971, Couch *et al.* 1986). However, these studies all reported a positive family history based on the proportion of migraine patients with a positive family history rather than the actual recurrence risk of migraine among relatives. The first controlled family study of a non-clinical sample of migraine subjects with direct and blind assessment of relatives yielded a three-fold increased risk of migraine among the relatives compared to those of controls (Merikangas *et al.* 1988).

Factors related to increased familial aggregation of migraine include early age of onset (Barolin and Sperlich 1969, Steiner *et al.* 1980, Baier 1985, Devoto *et al.* 1986), parental concordance for migraine (Buchanan 1920, Allan 1928, Devoto *et al.* 1986, Baier 1985), and sex of the affected parent, with elevated rates of migraine reported on the maternal side of the family (Mobius 1894, Bille 1962, Dalsgaard-Nielsen 1964, Barolin and Sperlich 1969, Couch *et al.* 1986). However, data from studies of systematically selected samples of migraineurs using direct interviews of probands and relatives indicate that there is virtually no difference in the proportion of affected relatives by maternal and paternal lineage (Baier 1985, Merikangas *et al.* 1988, Mochi *et al.* 1993).

Despite the inclusion of migraine as an autosomal dominant disorder (#15730) in the catalogue of *Mendelian Inheritance in Man* (McKusick 1988), the aggregate evidence from segregation analyses is contradictory and fails to support any specific Mendelian pattern of transmission over another (e.g. Devoto *et al.* 1986, D'Amico *et al.* 1991). Segregation analyses of data from the only controlled family study rejected autosomal dominant and X-linked transmission and favoured an autosomal recessive model with reduced penetrance (Mochi *et al.* 1993). In addition, the results suggested greater heritability of migraine without aura than migraine with aura, but also some common genetic basis for both subtypes. In contrast, a family study using IHS criteria reported that migraine with aura was associated with a greater magnitude of familial aggregation than migraine without aura (Russell and Olesen 1993).

Twin studies

Several twin studies of migraine provide support for a strong genetic component in its aetiology. Data from clinical samples (Spaich and Ostertag 1936, Ebbing, 1956, Harvald and Hauge 1956, Ziegler 1975, Lucas 1977) and population registries of twins with migraine (Corey *et al.* 1991, Larsson 1993, Merikangas *et al.* 1994, Honkasalo *et al.* 1995) reveal consistently elevated migraine concordance rates among monozygotic (MZ) rather than dizygotic (DZ) twin pairs. These clinical studies yield estimates of the proportion of variance attributable to genes (i.e. heritability) that are highly variable, ranging from 0.24 to 0.90. However, methodological differences preclude derivation of aggregate rates across studies of twins ascertained in clinical settings.

Table 19.1 Twin studies of recurrent migraine: population-based samples

Population samples	Authors	Probandwise concordance rates		
		Monozygotic	Dizygotic	Heritability
USA	Corey *et al.* (1991)	0.35	0.17	0.36
Norway	"	0.32	0.18	0.28
Sweden	Larsson (1993)	0.52	0.34	0.36
Australia	Merikangas *et al.* (1994)	0.42	0.24	0.36
Finland	Honkasalo *et al.* (1995)	0.28	0.12	0.32

The results of five large-scale studies of population twin registries are presented in Table 19.1. The Swedish and Australian studies were the only ones that employed IHS criteria and the latter study was the only population-based study that used direct interviews of the twin sample. Probandwise concordance rates ranged from 0.28 to 0.52 for monozygotic twins and from 0.12 to 0.34 for dizygotic twins. Estimates of the heritability of migraine were strikingly similar: the results indicate that approximately one-third of the variance in the aetiology of migraine is attributable to genetic factors. Application of statistical models that accounted for the population prevalence and partitioned the variance into genetic and environmental components in the Swedish, Australian and Finnish studies revealed that about half of the variation of migraine could be attributed to an additive genetic component, with most of the remainder being due to the unshared rather than shared environment of twin pairs. Furthermore, there were no differences in the components of these models by sex.

Apart from the Australian Twin Study, which investigated the genetic relationship between migraine and tension-type headache as described below, the only twin study that examined the difference between headache subtypes among monozygotic and dizygotic twins revealed no difference in the heritability of classic (i.e. migraine with aura) versus common migraine (i.e. migraine without aura) (Lucas 1977). This study also revealed an association between twin concordance for migraine and the magnitude of familial aggregation of migraine in other relatives of the twins. Additional twin studies which investigate the genetic overlap between the headache subtypes defined by the IHS criteria are clearly necessary.

GENETIC EPIDEMIOLOGICAL STUDIES

The application of the methods of genetic epidemiology, the study of risk factors and aetiology of familial diseases, appears to be one of the most promising avenues to unravel the complex mechanisms through which genes may exert their influence. The research designs of genetic epidemiology attempt to hold environmental factors constant while allowing genetic factors to vary or the converse, employing paradigms such as comparisons between discordant monozygotic twins, and cross-fostering studies. These research paradigms are all based upon the lack of one-to-one correspondence between the genotype and phenotype. One basic approach of genetic epidemiology is the use of the within-family design to minimize the probability of heterogeneity, assuming that the aetiology of a disease is likely to be homotypic within families. This design reduces or eliminates the danger of genetic heterogeneity which is likely to characterize migraine.

Application of genetic epidemiological studies to define phenotype

Rather than for their usual purpose of identifying the patterns of genetic transmission of diseases, genetic epidemiological study designs may also be used to refine phenotypic definitions of disorders and to increase the homogeneity of diagnostic classes. Although the family study design has usually been employed to elucidate the degree and mode of transmission of most disorders, there are numerous other purposes for the application of such data, including validation of phenotypic definitions, identification of sources of heterogeneity and mechanisms for comorbidity, and detection of gene–environment interactions or epistasis.

The use of familial transmission data in disease classification was first suggested in the 16th century by Paracelsus (see Rosenthal 1970). Family studies can be used to study the validity of diagnostic categories by assessing the specificity of transmission of symptom patterns and disorders within as compared to between families (Tsuang 1994). Data from family studies may also provide evidence regarding aetiological or phenotypic heterogeneity. Phenotypic heterogeneity is suggested by variable expressivity of symptoms, whereas aetiological heterogeneity is demonstrated by homotypic expression of different aetiological factors between families. Genetic heterogeneity may also be identified in family study data. Different patterns of transmission in families or distinct patterns of clinical phenomenology that 'breed true' in families may be associated with different mutations at the same locus or different genetic loci underlying the expression of a particular disease. Moreover, the family study method permits assessment of mechanisms for associations between disorders by evaluation of specific patterns of co-segregation of two or more disorders within families.

Another source of evidence provided by family study data is the estimate of recurrence risk as a function of population prevalence (λ) (Risch 1990). Whereas λ tends to exceed 20 for most autosomal dominant diseases and those for which the genetic basis has been identified, the values of λ derived from family studies of migraine tend to range from 2 to 3. In general, there is an inverse relationship between the magnitude of the effect of a gene that contributes to disease susceptibility and the population prevalence because of selective disadvantage. Common diseases are far more likely to result from multiple genes or interactions between several predisposing loci (Risch 1994). In general, the power of linkage and association studies of disorders with λ values less than 10 is extremely low.

Decrement in risk according to the degree of genetic relatedness can be examined to detect interactions between several loci. If the risk to second and third degree relatives decreases by more than 50% this implies that more than one locus must contribute to disease risk, and no single locus can predominate. Such interactive effects among loci contributing to the risk for common familial disorders have been demonstrated for schizophrenia, cleft lip and palate, diabetes mellitus and multiple sclerosis (Risch 1994). The lack of information on second and third degree relatives of migraine probands precludes assessment of the relationship between recurrence risk and genetic relationship in family study data.

The aggregate data from the twin studies reviewed above does not suggest that multiple loci are involved in the aetiology of migraine. The genetic models consistently yield a significant additive component based on a decrement in risk between monozygotic and dizygotic twins of approximately 50%. However, these results are often sex-specific and highly dependent upon variable phenotypic definitions.

Although the traditional application of the twin design focuses on the estimation of the heritability of a trait, there are several other research questions for which twin studies may have value. Differences in concordance rates between monozygotic and dizygotic twins may be investigated at the level of symptoms, or symptom clusters, to study the validity of symptom complexes. Varying forms or degrees of expression of a particular disease or trait in monozygotic twins may be a source of evidence of the validity of the construct or disease entity. One of the most thoughtfully designed twin studies has found a significant degree of heritability for gastrointestinal symptoms, nature of the headache pain, neurological prodromata, a history of childhood vomiting, personal and family history of eczema and motion sickness, but **not** for the common–classic distinction, unilaterality, severity, duration or precipitants (Lucas 1977).

Australian twin study

Data from the Australian twin study were used to identify sources of heterogeneity in the expression of migraine. Specifically, the genetic

Table 19.2 Probandwise concordance rates for migraine and tension-type headache in the Australian twin study

Sex of co-twin	Headache subtype		Monozygotic		Dizygotic	
	Proband	Co-twin	N of pairs	Concordance rates (S.E.)	N of pairs	Concordance rates (S.E.)
Female	Tension-type	Tension-type	171	0.161* (0.037)	155	0.073* (0.026)
		Migraine	186	0.113 (0.023)	191	0.273 (0.036)
	Migraine	Tension-type	409	0.054 (0.011)	324	0.102 (0.018)
		Migraine	388	0.433** (0.031)	208	0.293** (0.033)
Male	Tension-type	Tension-type	97	0.165 (0.051)	110	0.124 (0.040)
		Migraine	107	0.082 (0.028)	108	0.029 (0.016)
	Migraine	Tension-type	82	0.108 (0.036)	179	0.085 (0.022)
		Migraine	74	0.324* (0.070)	187	0.170* (0.032)

*, $p < 0.01$; **, $p < 0.02$

overlap between the major subtypes of headache and the heritability of the individual symptoms of migraine were examined (Merikangas *et al.* 1994, Tierney *et al.* 1995). The sample of 5996 twins derived from a volunteer-based Australian National Health and Medical Research Council Twin Registry. This sample included 940 identical (MZ) female, 540 fraternal same-sex female, 400 identical male, 236 fraternal same-sex male and 604 opposite-sex complete twin pairs. The twins were interviewed directly regarding symptoms of migraine or recurrent headaches, and the diagnostic criteria of the IHS were used to classify recurrent headaches (Table 19.2).

A total of 2739 (45.73%) twins screened positive for recurrent headaches. The lifetime prevalence of migraine was 21.54% for females ($n = 3899$) and 7.89% for males ($n = 2090$). The probandwise concordance rates for migraine were significantly higher for MZ twins than for DZ twins (females, 0.433 vs 0.293, $p = 0.001$; males, 0.324 vs 0.170, $p = 0.02$), indicating a genetic influence. When migraineurs were further divided based on the presence of visual problems, significant differences in concordance rates remained only for migraine with visual problems. The best fitting model that resulted from application of structural equations models included an additive genetic model for migraine with visual problems with a narrow sense heritability estimate of 51.3% and no shared familial environment. These results also suggest that approximately half of the variance in the aetiology of migraine cannot be attributed to transmitted genes. The data did not suggest any genetic influence on tension-type headache, nor was there any evidence of an overlap in genetic factors between tension-type headache and migraine. These results provide evidence for the validity of the distinction between migraine and tension-type headache.

The twin study data were also examined to investigate the heritability of the symptoms of migraine. At the univariate level, the symptoms that provided the best discrimination between the monozygotic and dizygotic pairs were visual problems, and photophobia/phonophobia/osmophobia. However, multivariate analyses revealed that visual problems were the most important source of heritability of headache: after accounting for the increase in heritability associated with visual problems, no other symptoms were associated with a significant increase in the heritability of recurrent headache (Tierney *et al.* 1994). Analyses of the Finnish Twin Registry revealed highest levels of heritability for visual symptoms and/ or nausea (Honkasalo *et al.* 1995).

COMORBIDITY AND MIGRAINE: A SOURCE OF HETEROGENEITY

The term 'comorbidity', introduced by Feinstein, refers to the presence of any additional coexisting ailment in a patient with a particular index disease (Feinstein 1970). Failure to classify and analyse comorbid diseases can create misleading medical statistics and may cause spurious comparisons during the planning and evaluation of treatment for patients. Comorbidity can alter the clinical course of patients with the same diagnosis by affecting the time of detection, prognostic anticipations, therapeutic selection and post-therapeutic outcome of an index diagnosis (Kaplan and Feinstein 1974).

Non-random co-occurrence of two conditions may be attributable to several methodological artefacts, including: samples selected from clinical settings that are non-representative of persons with the index disease in the general population, i.e. 'Berkson's Paradox' (Berkson 1946); assessment bias, in which the co-occurrence of two conditions is an artefact of overlap in the diagnostic criteria or in the assessments used to ascertain the criteria; and the lack of an appropriate comparison group with which to control for factors which confound the association between the two conditions.

Aside from identification of bias, investigation of patterns of comorbidity is important for several reasons. First, identification of differential patterns of comorbidity may lead to the elucidation of subtypes of a particular index disorder for which the comorbid condition may indicate a different form or subtype, thereby enhancing the validity of their distinction in the classification system. Second, differential associations between particular pairs of diseases may yield clues regarding the pathogenesis of the index disease. If two conditions emanate from the same underlying aetiological factors, investigations of their aetiology can be targeted to risk factors that are common to both conditions. Finally, if the comorbid disorders are a consequence of the index disease, interventions can be developed to prevent the development of the secondary conditions.

Associations between migraine and a variety of somatic and psychiatric conditions have been reported in the literature since it was first described as a discrete syndrome. Because most of the early descriptions of such associations were based on clinical case series, empirical evidence was lacking. Several factors complicate the investigation of comorbidity of migraine and other conditions, including: discrimination from 'migraine equivalents' defined as alternative manifestations of migraine that occur in an 'attack-like' fashion, including abdominal pain, dizziness or vertigo, or visual symptoms; lack of specificity of symptom expression or constellations within individuals over time; and the involvement of several systems, including the cardiovascular, gastrointestinal and sensory organs, as well as both the peripheral and central nervous systems.

There is dramatic variability in the methodology of studies of comorbidity and migraine, which limits their conclusiveness. Studies of comorbidity require valid definitions and reliable ascertainment of each of the disorders under consideration. Most studies were conducted prior to the introduction of the IHS criteria and used idiosyncratic definitions of migraine ranging from recurrent headaches to classical migraine with neurological prodromes. Moreover, standardized definitions of both disorders were included in few of the clinical or epidemiological studies of comorbidity and migraine. In general, clinical series and case-control studies have used the most thorough clinical evaluations of the subjects. Epidemiological studies tended to apply less rigorous definitions because collection of extensive diagnostic information on both conditions was precluded by the sheer magnitude of the studies.

Epidemiological studies generally have sufficient statistical power to detect associations between migraine and rare diseases. However, the negative associations in the smaller sample sizes of the clinical and case-control studies are often the result of β-type errors rather than a true lack of association between migraine and other diseases.

Another methodological limitation of most studies of migraine comorbidity is the failure to incorporate confounding risk factors that could explain the association between several diseases and migraine. In addition, the interrelationships between the comorbid disorders themselves are often not accounted for in multivariate analyses, thereby yielding spurious associations. Finally, as noted above, the samples of both the clinical series and case-control studies may be biased with respect to the increased probability that persons with two or more conditions are represented in clinical samples (Berkson's paradox). Thus, the epidemiological studies are necessary to identify such biases in treatment samples.

Comorbidity of migraine and several other disorders has been reported in clinical series, case-control studies, and epidemiological surveys (Merikangas and Fenton 1994). The most widely implicated are disorders of the cardiovascular, allergies/asthma, epilepsy, psychiatric and gastrointestinal systems. In a large-scale epidemiological US study of the association between migraine and disorders which had been previously purported to be non-randomly associated with migraine, Merikangas and Fenton (1994) confirmed the associations between migraine and asthma, allergies, stroke, epilepsy and psychiatric disorders. However, in contrast to previous clinical studies, no association was found for migraine and hypertension after controlling for other well-known risk factors for hypertension.

Evidence for comorbidity of migraine and depression

There is now substantial evidence that corroborates early anecdotal clinical descriptions of the co-occurrence of migraine and depression. Clinicians have often described a set of characteristic features of migraineurs including anxiety, depression, and social fears. Wolff (1937) was so convinced of this constellation of attributes that he is often credited as being the initiator of the concept of the 'migraine personality'. However, careful inspection of his description reveals that the characteristics of 'extreme physical fatigue, apathy, and anxious anticipation' are more akin to psychiatric symptoms than personality traits. Earlier descriptions of these characteristics can be found throughout the clinical literature. The most common features of these descriptions are depression characterized by anergia and anxiety disorders, particularly panic disorder and phobia. The contemporary equivalent to these features is the 'atypical' subtype of depression.

Studies of the association between migraine, depression and anxiety in clinical samples which used standardized diagnostic criteria consistently revealed associations between the two disorders, irrespective of the index disorder for which the subjects sought treatment. The results of studies of community samples are summarized in Table 19.3. There is remarkable similarity in the magnitude of the association between depression and migraine across studies. The odds ratios in the

Table 19.3 Association of migraine with depression and anxiety: community studies

Author (year)	n	Anxiety (odds ratio)	Depression (odds ratio)
Merikangas *et al.* (1988)	115	–	2.9
Merikangas *et al.* (1990, 1993)	591	2.7	2.2
Stewart *et al.* (1989)	10169	5.3	–
Breslau *et al.* (1991)	1007	1.9	3.6

Odds ratio calculated by this author from rates given in Breslau *et al.* (1991)

latter three studies were nearly identical, despite the variation in the subjects' characteristics, geographic site, and specific assessments of migraine and depression. These findings exclude sampling as a source of bias in the co-occurrence of depression and migraine reported in previous clinical samples. The relationship between migraine and anxiety disorders has also been investigated because of the well-known association between depression and anxiety. When experienced without depression, anxiety disorders are also associated with migraine in both clinical and community studies (Harper and Roth 1962, Garvey *et al.* 1984; Stewart *et al.* 1989; Merikangas *et al.* 1990, 1993, Breslau *et al.* 1991). However, the simultaneous association between all of these disorders needs to be examined systematically.

Longitudinal studies may be used to identify sources of comorbidity by studying the stability of expression of an index disorder either with or without the comorbid disorders over the long-term course. The prospective design enables elucidation of the causal relationship between the index disorder and the comorbid disorder, and the risk factors and sequelae of each condition. Homogeneous subtypes of these conditions may also be identified according to their patterns of longitudinal course.

The course and order of onset of comorbid conditions with respect to migraine were investigated using data from a prospective longitudinal cohort study of young adults in Zurich, Switzerland. The prospective design of the study avoided the bias inherent in retrospective recall of the course and onset of such conditions. The findings revealed that the onset of anxiety disorders tended to precede that of migraine in about 80% of the cases of migraine with comorbid anxiety/depression, and that the onset of depression followed that of migraine in 75% of the comorbid cases (Merikangas *et al.* 1990). Retrospective data from a community survey in Detroit, Michigan produced strikingly similar findings (Breslau *et al.* 1991). The associations between migraine, anxiety

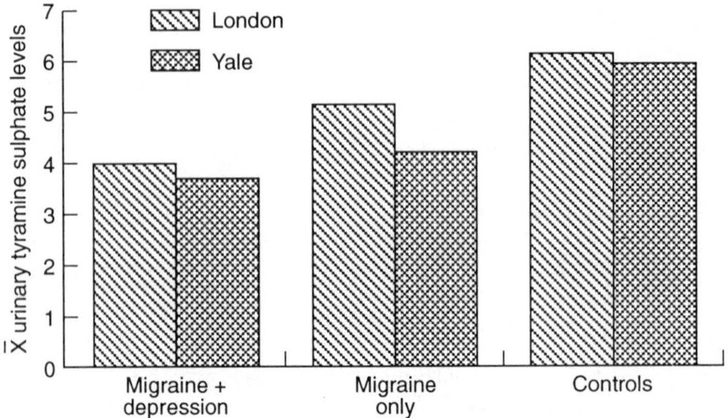

Figure 19.1 Tyramine sulphate levels in urine from subjects with migraine and depression. London, M. Sandler *et al.*; Yale, K.R. Merikangas *et al.*

and depression were not only of the same magnitude, but also the order of onset of the three conditions was the same, with anxiety in childhood and adolescence, followed by migraine and then depression (Merikangas *et al.* 1993).

The most likely explanation for these findings is that the combination of these disorders comprise a subtype of either migraine or depression/ anxiety in which symptoms of all three disorders are manifest at some point during the longitudinal course. Because disturbances in the same neurochemical systems have been implicated in migraine, depression and anxiety disorders, perturbation of a particular system or systems may produce symptoms of all three conditions, thereby producing one syndrome rather than three discrete entities. Support of this interpreta- tion derives from a large-scale epidemiological study in the USA in which persons with a history of migraine who no longer suffered from episodic attacks of headache continued to have significantly more depression than those without a history of migraine.

Comorbidity may be an important source of heterogeneity in studies of biochemical or psychophysiological parameters or treatment outcome as well. For example, in collaboration with Professor M. Sandler and Dr V. Glover, our research group has conducted studies of tyramine sulphate deficit after an oral tyramine load among subjects with migraine and tension-type headache stratified by major depression. As shown in Figure 19.1, we found that subjects with both migraine and depression had lower urinary excretion of tyramine sulphate than subjects with migraine alone or controls (Merikangas *et al.* 1995).

Yale family study

One major goal of the investigation of comorbidity is to elucidate the mechanisms for non-random associations between diseases. Documentation of the association is only the first step in this process. The two major classes of explanations for associations between disorders are: aetiological models, in which an index disease causes or precipitates the manifestation of the comorbid condition; and common underlying causes, in which shared risk factors lead to differential pathways of expression. In addition to elucidating the mode of disease transmission and genetic markers, family and genetic studies can be used to investigate the mechanisms for comorbidity as described below.

Specificity of transmission of the pure form of the comorbid condition in probands with the index disorder and the converse suggest shared underlying aetiological factors involved in the expression of two conditions. Alternatively, if the comorbid disorder is elevated among the relatives of probands with the 'pure' index disorder, but only when coupled with the index disorder, an aetiological model would be more likely to explain the association (Merikangas *et al.* 1988). Patterns of co-segregation of migraine and depression were investigated in two of our previous family studies, one with probands with depression (Merikangas *et al.* 1988) and the other with probands with migraine (Merikangas *et al.* 1993). The results of both studies indicated that migraine and depression share a syndromic relationship, representing manifestation of the same disease, as opposed to their representing distinct diseases resulting from the same underlying aetiological factors (Merikangas *et al.* 1988, 1993).

Our recent large-scale family study of probands with migraine, depression, anxiety disorders and controls using direct interviews of adult and child relatives and clinical assessments of both headache syndromes and psychopathology illustrates the application of family studies to investigate mechanisms for comorbidity. There were 219 probands, 42 with migraine, 98 with depression or anxiety disorders without migraine, and 60 controls from the general community. Complete pedigrees of first and second degree relatives and spouses were obtained on first degree relatives, including children over age 7, and spouses were assessed directly by clinically experienced interviewers, who were blind to the diagnostic status of the proband. Information on relatives who were deceased, refused to participate, or geographically distant was obtained blindly from multiple relatives and best estimate diagnostic assessments were made by clinicians based on all available information. Treatment records were requested for all probands and relatives who had received treatment for one of these conditions. Diagnoses were made according to the Diagnostic and Statistical Manual of the American Psychiatric Association (DSM-III-R,

Table 19.4 Yale family study: comorbidity of migraine and psychopathology

Psychiatric disorder	Odds ratio[a]
Affective disorders	
Bipolar	4.1***
Dysthymia	2.0**
Major depression	2.0**
Anxiety disorders	
Generalized anxiety disorder	2.8***
Panic disorder	3.4***
Agoraphobia	4.1***
Simple phobia	1.8*
Social phobia	1.8*
Substance abuse	
Alcoholism	0.7
Drug abuse	0.9
Antisocial personality	1.7

***, $p < 0.001$; **, $p < 0.01$; *, $p < 0.05$
[a] Adjusted for sex

American Psychiatric Association 1990) for affective and anxiety disorders and according to IHS criteria for migraine.

Associations between migraine and psychiatric disorders in the 1218 first degree relatives are presented in Table 19.4. As in previous epidemiological and clinical studies, migraine was strongly associated with both the affective and anxiety disorders, the greatest associations emerging for the bipolar subtype of depression and for the agoraphobia and panic subtypes of anxiety disorders. There was an inverse relationship with alcoholism and drug abuse, suggesting that migraine may be protective against the development of alcoholism.

The results of the co-segregation analyses of the transmission of migraine, depression and anxiety are presented in Table 19.5. The patterns of transmission of migraine with major depression and anxiety were consistent with a transmissible association between depression and migraine, and a non-transmissible association between anxiety and migraine. That is, probands with depression had an increased risk of migraine in their relatives, whereas probands with anxiety did not. Additional analyses revealed that the transmissible association between depression and migraine was most strongly attributable to the bipolar subtype of depression. This suggests that migraine and bipolar depression may have a partially shared underlying diathesis.

Table 19.5 Yale family study: co-transmission of migraine, anxiety and major depression

Factors in model	Migraine in relatives (risk ratio)[a]
Probands	
Migraine	2.6***
Anxiety	0.8
Depression	1.8*
Relatives	
Anxiety	1.9**
Depression	1.5*

[a] Adjusted for sex of proband and relative, interview status and age of relative
*, $p < 0.05$; **, $p < 0.01$; ***, $p < 0.001$.

However, migraine in probands was not associated with an increased risk of depression in relatives. The lack of symmetry of the transmissible association between migraine and depression suggests that migraine and depression are syndromic rather than equivalent expressions of the same underlying aetiological factors. Studies of treatment response, biological markers and longitudinal course comparing subjects with pure migraine and those with comorbid psychopathology could be used to examine whether the familial patterns truly indicate distinct pathways to migraine.

The association between migraine and depression/anxiety, particularly in the light of the findings from prospective data, warrants further study to determine whether depression can be used as an index of a discrete syndrome. Studies which differentiate pure migraine from migraine associated with affective and anxiety disorder on such domains as psychophysiology, neurobiology and treatment response are indicated. In fact, failure to discriminate between migraine with and without concomitant depression could obscure the results of studies across all domains of migraine research.

SUMMARY

Convergent evidence suggests that migraine is familial, and that genetic factors explain a significant degree of the variance in its aetiology. However, evidence regarding the specific mode of transmission and the specificity of transmission of the subtypes and the symptoms of headache is either inconsistent or absent. Moreover, the heritability of migraine is only moderate and suggests multifactorial aetiology of this syndrome and that gene–environment interactions may be important.

Based on the aggregate evidence from family and twin studies, migraine is a complex disorder, characterized by either genetic and/or phenotypic heterogeneity or the lack of single loci with effects of sufficient magnitude to allow detection with current methodology. The lack of conclusive evidence about the role of genes in the aetiology of migraine may result from either limitations in its definition, measurement and ascertainment or truly complex genetic mechanisms.

Genetic analysis of migraine is complicated by: 1) the high population prevalence; 2) the lack of valid definitions of the phenotype and subtypes thereof; 3) absence of diagnostic trait markers with high sensitivity and specificity; 4) lack of evidence regarding the mode(s) of transmission; 5) comorbidity of headache subtypes and other disorders; 6) variable age of onset; 7) sex differences in expression; 8) lack of specificity of symptom expression across episodes; and 9) high frequency of bilineal transmission of migraine.

Research on the genetics of migraine should profit from the knowledge gleaned from linkage studies of other complex disorders which rely solely upon clinical definitions of the phenotype. A reminder of the dangers of overeager acceptance of simple explanations of the transmission of complex phenotypes was provided by McGuffin and Huckle (1990) who reported that the results of complex segregation analyses were consistent with a single recessive gene for attending medical school! They concluded that the application of segregation or linkage analysis is not a panacea for the problems of complex phenotypes and that genetic studies must be developed in the context of information gleaned from the application of classical methods of genetic epidemiology, including family, twin and adoption studies.

The lack of replication and inconsistent findings which have plagued other complex diseases could be avoided through a cautious approach to study of the genetic basis of migraine. Family and twin study paradigms should be used to examine the specificity of transmission of the components of migraine, comorbid disorders, and putative markers before linkage analyses are applied to migraine. Moreover, application of the within-family design can minimize the heterogeneity that is likely to characterize samples of unrelated patients. This approach, which controls for both shared genetic and environmental factors within families, comprises an extremely powerful method with which to identify the underlying neurobiological mechanisms involved in the pathogenesis of migraine.

Large-scale controlled family studies of extended pedigrees of systematically selected probands should also be conducted using phenotypic definitions to clarify the modes of transmission of migraine. Simulation studies indicate that a very large number of families is necessary to detect Quantitative Trait Loci in the presence of oligogenic inheritance and to replicate linkage claims in order to avoid false positive findings (Suarez *et al.* 1994). The large number of families necessary to detect the underlying genetic mechanisms in the presence of genetic heterogeneity, gene–environment interactions, epistasis or polygenic inheritance would best be obtained through collaborative research with standardized methodology.

Although caution is warranted in the investigation of the aetiology of complex disorders, this does not imply that discovery of the role of genes is a phenomenon in the distant future. Recent developments in identifying the genetic basis of insulin-dependent diabetes (Davies *et al.* 1990, Hashimota *et al.* 1994) and some forms of breast cancer (Hall *et al.* 1990, Easton *et al.* 1993, Miki *et al.* 1994) demonstrate the importance of inheritance of genetic factors which, in the presence of particular environmental factors, lead to the development of disease. These studies illustrate the strength of the combined approach of genetic epidemiology and molecular genetics to gain understanding of the gene – environment interactions involved in the pathogenesis of complex diseases (Hall *et al.* 1990, Friend *et al.* 1986).

REFERENCES

Allan, W. (1928) The inheritance of migraine. *Archives of Internal Medicine*, **13**, 590–599.

American Psychiatric Association (1987) *Diagnostic and Statistical Manual of Mental Disorders*, 3rd Edn, Washington DC.

Ask-Upmark, E. (1953) Inverted nipples and migraine. *Acta Medica Scandinavica*, **167**, 191–197.

Baier, W.K. (1985) Genetics of migraine and migraine accompagnee: a study of eighty-one children and their families. *Neuropediatrics*, **16**, 84–91.

Barolin, G.S. and Sperlich, D. (1969) Migraine familien. *Fortschitte der Neurologie-Psychiatrie und ihrer Grenzgebiete*, **37**, 521–544.

Baron, M., Freimer, N.F., Risch, N., Lerer, B., Alexander, J.R., Straub, R.E., Asokan, S., Das, K., Peterson, A., Amos, J. *et al.* (1993) Diminished support for linkage between manic depressive illness and X-chromosome markers in three Israeli pedigrees. *Nature Genetics*, **3**(1), 49–55.

Beaudet, A., Bowcock, A., Buchwald, M. *et al.* (1986) Linkage of cystic fibrosis on two tightly linked DNA markers: joint report from a collaborative study. *American Journal of Human Genetics*, **39**, 681–693.

Berkson, J. (1946) Limitation of the application of the 4-fold table analysis to hospital data. *Biometrics*, **2**, 47–53.

Bille, B. (1962) Migraine in school children. *Acta Paediatrica Scandinavica*, **51** (Suppl. 136), 3–151.

Breslau, N., Davis, G.C. and Andreski, P. (1991) Migraine, psychiatric disorders, and suicide attempts: An epidemiologic study of young adults. *Psychiatry Research*, **37**, 11–23.

Buchanan, J.A. (1970) The mendelianism of migraine. *Medical Research*, **98**, 45–47.

Childs, A.K. and Sweetnam, M.T. (1961) A study of 104 cases of migraine. *British Journal of Industrial Medicine*, **18**, 234–236.

Clark, R.F. and Goate, A.M. (1993) Molecular genetics of Alzheimer's disease. *Archives of Neurology*, **50**, 1164–1172.

Corey, L.A., Berg, K., Nance, W.E., Solaas, M.K. and Delorenzo, R.J. (1991) Migraine headache in Virginian and Norwegian twins. *American Journal of Human Genetics*, (Abstract), H9, 40.

Couch, J.R., Bearss, C. and Verhulst, S. (1986) Importance of maternal heredity in the etiology of migraine. *Neurology*, **36**, Suppl 99.

D'Amico, D., Leone, M., Macciardi, F., Valentini, S. and Bussone, G. (1991) Genetic transmission of migraine without aura: a study of 68 families. *Italian Journal of Neurological Sciences*, **12**, 581–584.

Dalsgaard-Nielson, A.T. (1964) Migraene og epilepsi. *Ugeskrift Laeger*, **126**, 185–191.

Davies, J.L., Kawaguchi, Y., Bennet, S.T., Copeman, J.B., Cordell, J.H., Pritchard, L.E., Reed, P.W. *et al.* (1994) A genome-wide search for human type I diabetes susceptibility genes. *Nature*, **371**, 130–136.

Devoto, M., Lozito, A., Staffa, G., D'Allessandro, R., Sacquengna, T. and Romeo, G. (1986) Segregation analysis of migraine in 128 families. *Cephalalgia*, **6**, 101–105.

Easton, D.F., Bishop, D.T., Ford, D. and Crockford, G.P. (1993) Breast Cancer Linkage Consortium. Genetic linkage analysis in familial breast and ovarian cancer: results from 214 families. *American Journal of Human Genetics*, **52**, 678–701.

Ebbing, H.C. (1956) Migraine bei zwillingen vorlaufige mitteilung. *Acta Geneticae Medicae (Roma)*, **5**, 371–382.

Egeland, J.A., Gerhard, D.S., Pauls, D.L., Sussex, J.N., Kidd, K.K., Allen, C.R., Hostetter, A.M. and Housman, D. (1987) Bipolar affective disorders linked to DNA markers on chromosome 11. *Nature*, **325**, 783.

Ely, F.A. (1930) The migraine–epilepsy syndrome. *Archives of Neurology and Psychiatry*, **24**, 943.

Feinstein, A.R. (1970) The pre-therapeutic classification of co-morbidity in chronic disease. *Journal of Chronic Diseases*, **23**, 455–468.

Friend, S.H., Bernard, R., Rogeli, S. *et al.* (1986) A human DNA segment with properties of the gene that predisposes to retinoblastoma and osteosarcoma. *Nature*, **323**, 643–646.

Garvey, M.J., Tollefson, G.D. and Schaffer, C.B. (1984) Migraine headaches and depression. *American Journal of Psychiatry*, **141**, 986–988.

Gusella, J.F., Wexler, N.S., Conneally, P.M. *et al.* (1982) A polymorphic DNA marker genetically linked to Huntington's disease. *Nature*, **306**, 234–238.

Hall, J.M., Lee, M.K., Morrow, J., Newman, B., Anderson, L., Huey, B. and King, M.C. (1990) Linkage analysis of early onset familial breast cancer to chromosome 17q21. *Science*, **250**, 1684–1689.

Harvald, B. and Hauge, M. (1956) A catamnestic investigation of Danish twins. *Danish Medical Bulletin*, **3**, 150–158.

Harper, M. and Roth, M. (1962) Temporal lobe epilepsy and the phobic anxiety-depersonalization syndrome. Part I. A comparative study. *Comprehensive Psychiatry*, **3**(3), 129–151.

Hashimota, L., Habita, C., Beressi, J.P., Delepine, M., Besse, C., Cambon-Thomsen, A., Deschamps, I. *et al.* (1994) Genetic mapping of a susceptibility locus for insulin-dependent diabetes mellitus on chromosome 11q. *Nature*, **371**, 161–164.

Headache Classification Committee of the International Headache Society.

(1988) Classification and diagnostic criteria for headache disorders, cranial neuralgias, and facial pain. *Cephalalgia*, **8** (Suppl. 7), 1–96.

Holden, C. (1994) A cautionary genetic tale: the sobering story of D_2. *Science*, **264** (17), 1696–1697.

Honkasalo, M.L., Kaprio, J., Winter, T., Heikkilä, K., Sillanpää, M. and Koskenvuo, M. (1995) Migraine and concomitant symptoms among 8167 adult twin pairs. *Headache*, **35**, 70–78.

Joutel, A., Bousser, M., Biousse, V., Labauge, P., Chabriat, H., Nibbio, A., Maciazek, J., Meyer, B., Bach, M., Weissenbach, J., Lathrop, G.M. and Tournier-Lasserve, E.T. (1993) A gene for familial hemiplegic migraine maps to chromosome 19. *Nature Genetics*, **5**, 40–45, 1993.

Kaplan, M.H. and Feinstein, A.R. (1974) The importance of classifying initial co-morbidity in evaluating the outcome of diabetes mellitus. *Journal of Chronic Disease*, **27**, 387–404.

Kelsoe, J.R., Ginns, E.E., Egeland, J.A., Gerhard, D.S., Goldstein, A.M., Bale, S.J., Pauls, D.L., Long, R.T., Kidd, K.K., Conte, G., Housman, D.E. and Paul, S. (1989) Re-evaluation of the linkage relationship between chromosome 11p loci and the gene for bipolar affective disorder in the Old Order Amish. *Nature*, **16**, 238.

Kunkel, L.M. *et al.* (1986) Analysis of deletions in DNA from patients with Becker and Duchenne muscular dystrophy. *Nature*, **322**, 3.

Larsson, B. (1993) The genetic influence in headache: A Swedish twin study. *Cephalalgia*, **13** (Suppl. 13), 22.

Lennox, W.G. (1941) *Science and seizures: new light on epilepsy and migraine.* Harper, New York.

Lucas, R.N. (1977) Migraine in twins. *Journal of Psychosomatic Research*, **20**, 147–156.

McGuffin, P. and Huckle, P. (1990) Simulation of mendelism revisited: the recessive gene for attending medical school. *American Journal of Human Genetics*, **46**, 994.

McGuffin, P. and Merikangas, K.R. (1995) Definition of the phenotype in psychiatry. *Genetics of Human Behavior*, Cold Spring Harbor Laboratory, March 5–8, Long Island, New York.

McKusick, V. (1988) *Mendelian inheritance in man.* Eighth Edition. Baltimore: The Johns Hopkins University Press.

Merikangas, K.R. (1990) Genetic epidemiology of migraine. In: *Migraine: a Spectrum of Ideas*, (eds M. Sandler and G. Collins), pp. 40–49. Oxford University Press.

Merikangas, K.R., Risch, N.J., Merikangas, J.R., Weissman, M.M. and Kidd, K.K. (1988) Migraine and depression: association and familial transmission. *Journal of Psychiatric Research*, **22**, 119–129.

Merikangas, K.R., Angst, J. and Isler, H. (1990) Migraine and psychopathology: results of the Zurich cohort study of young adults. *Archives of General Psychiatry*, **47**, 849–853.

Merikangas, K.R. and Angst, J. (1993) Headache syndromes and psychiatric disorders: association and familial transmission. *Journal of Psychiatric Research*, **27**, 197–210.

Merikangas, K.R., Risch, N.J. and Weissman, M.M. (1994) Comorbidity and co-transmission of alcoholism, anxiety, and depression. *Psychological Medicine*, **24**, 69–80.

Merikangas, K.R. and Fenton, B. (1994) Comorbidity of migraine and somatic disorders. In: *Headache Classification and Epidemiology*, (eds J. Olesen *et al.*). Raven Press, New York.

Merikangas, K.R., Tierney, C., Martin, N.G. and Heath, A.C. (1994) The genetics of migraine in the Australian Twin Registry. In: *New Advances in Headache Research*, (ed. F. Clifford Rose), p. 27. Smith Gordon & Co., London.

Merikangas, K.R., Stevens, D.E., Merikangas, J.R., Katz, C.B.S., Glover, V., Cooper, M.A. and Sandler, M. (1995) Tyramine conjugation deficit in migraine, tension-type headache and depression. *Biological Psychiatry*, **38**, 730–736.

Miki, Y., Swensen, J., Shattuck-Eidens, D., Futreal, P.A., Harshman, K., Tavtigian, S., Liu, Q., *et al.* (1994) A strong candidate for the breast and ovarian cancer susceptibility gene BRCA1. *Science*, **266**, 66–71.

Möbius, P.J. (1894) *Die migraine*. pp. 14–17. Holder, Vienna.

Mochi, M., Sangiorgi, S., Cortelli, P., Carelli, V., Scapoli, C., Crisci, M., Monari, L., Pierangeli, G. and Montagna, P. (1993) Testing models for genetic determination in migraine. *Cephalalgia*, **13**(6), 389–394.

Ottman, R., Hong, S. and Lipton, R. (1993) Validity of family history data on severe headache and migraine. *Neurology*, **43**, 1954–1960.

Risch, N. (1990) Linkage strategies for genetically complex traits. I. Multilocus models. *American Journal of Human Genetics*, **46**, 222–228.

Risch, N. (1994) Mapping genes for psychiatric disorders. In: *Genetic Approaches to Mental Disorders*. (eds E.S. Gershon and C.R. Cloninger), pp. 47–61. American Psychiatric Press, Washington, D.C.

Risch, N. and Merikangas, K.R. (1993) Linkage studies for psychiatric disorders. *European Archives of Psychiatry and Clinical Neuroscience*, **243**, 143–149.

Rosenthal, D. (1970) *Genetic theory and abnormal behavior*. McGrawHill, New York.

Russell, M.B. and Olesen, J. (1993) The genetics of migraine without aura and migraine with aura. *Cephalalgia*, **13**, 245–248.

Spaich, D., Ostertag, M. (1936) Untersuchungen Über allergische Erkrankungen bei Zwillingen. *Zeitschrift fuer Menschliche Vererbungs und Konstitutions Lehre*, **19**, 730.

Steiner, T.J., Guha, P., Capildeo, R., Rose, F.C. (1980) Migraine in patients attending a migraine clinic: an analysis by computer of age, sex and family history. *Headache*, **20**, 190–195.

Stewart, W., Linet, M., Celantano, D. (1989) Migraine headaches and panic attacks. *Psychosomatic Medicine*, **51**, 559–569.

Suarez, B.K., Hampe, C.L., Eerdewegh, P.V. (1994) Problems of replicating linkage claims in psychiatry. In *Genetic Approaches to Mental Disorders*. (ed. E.S. Gershon and C.R. Cloninger), pp. 23–46. American Psychiatric Press, Washington, D.C.

Tierney, C., Merikangas, K.R., Martin, N.G., Heath, A.C. (1995) The genetics of headache symptoms in the Australian twin registry. *American Journal of Human Genetics*, **55**, 158.

Tsuang, M.T. (1994) Identification of clinical phenotypes for genetic research on mental disorders. In: *Genetic Approaches to Mental Disorders*, (eds E.S. Gershon and C.R. Cloninger). American Psychopathological Association, Washington D.C.

Waters, W.E., O'Connor, P.J. (1971) Prevalence of migraine. *Journal of Neurosurgery and Psychiatry*, **38**, 613–616.

Weissman, M.M., Merikangas, K.R., John, K., Wickramaratne, P., Prusoff, B.A., Kidd, K.K. (1986) Family-genetic studies of psychiatric disorders: developing technologies. *Archives of General Psychiatry*, **43**, 1104–1116.

Wolff, H.G. (1937) Personality features and reactions of subjects with migraine. *Archives of Neurology and Psychiatry*, **37**, 895–921.
Ziegler, D.K., Hassanein, R., Harris, D., Stewart, R. (1975) Headache in a non-clinic twin population. *Headache*, **14**, 213–218.

DISCUSSION

Haan: Although there are some methodological problems, the study of Russell *et al.* (1993) is the only family study so far to use the International Headache Society (IHS) criteria (Headache Classification Committee 1988) and to look at migraine with aura and without aura separately.

Merikangas: In my summary of family studies I only included controlled studies of migraine in which relatives of probands with migraine were compared to relatives of controls in order to calculate odds ratios or estimates of the relative risk. However, you are right that the study by Russell and Olesen (1993) is the first to investigate the familial aggregation of migraine with and without aura.

Connor: Is there any evidence for anticipation in migraine patients? With subsequent generations do we see an earlier age of onset and a more severe disease?

Peatfield: It would be extremely difficult to demonstrate that because a mother may bring her daughter to the clinic because her daughter has similar attacks of headache, whereas a patient without a family history may turn for clinical help later. A clinician would almost certainly find the phenomenon but it would be spurious. You'd need a population epidemiologist to look at the situation systematically. If it was linked with a trinucleotide repeat we'd have a much cleaner, dominant inheritance pattern, wouldn't we?

Haan: We've tried to study anticipation in families with familial hemiplegic migraine (FHM). Even in well-defined families this is difficult because there is a great variety of age of onset and severity of attacks. Clarke, who in 1910 was one of the first describers of FHM, is the only researcher who reported anticipation in FHM families: all descriptions after that don't mention it. We don't think it occurs.

Bruyn: Anticipation has been proven in two neurological diseases, Curschmann Steinert's myotonic dystrophy and Huntington's chorea. Anticipation is directly correlated with increasing length of CGT or CAG: the longer the repeat the earlier the onset, even to the age of one or two.

Tournier-Lasserve: We looked in 61 families with migraine with aura. The mean age of onset of migraine was 14 and the mean age of probands was 36. The accuracy of memory about the age of onset depends on the persons' age. We did not observe anticipation. It is easier to do for migraine with aura, because an aura would be reported by a child: migraine without aura is even more difficult to analyse for anticipation.

Ferrari: What would you call the age of onset? How do you define a migraineur? Is somebody who has had two attacks a migraineur?

Merikangas: After someone meets the criteria for migraine (i.e. five attacks or more), I would date the age of onset to the first attack. I would classify relatives with fewer than five attacks as 'probable-migraine' and analyse the risk of probable, and of definite, migraine in relatives.

Ferrari: Would you change liability classes according to the number of attacks?

Merikangas: No, only if I had *a priori* evidence of different liability classes based on the age at onset and/or the number of attacks.

Tournier-Lasserve: I'm concerned about the use of liability classes. I wonder if it's not better to quote as 'unknown' somebody whose status is not known. We should first use the IHS criteria, although they don't suffice, and then do subgrouping when possible. There is, for example, a subgroup of non-FHM with migraine with aura who appear more likely to have autosomal dominant inheritance. These families generally have a more complex rather than visual aura.

Merikangas: For linkage studies, counting persons who do not clearly meet threshold or subthreshold criteria for migraine as 'unknown' is the most conservative approach.

Ferrari: Does the increased risk for depression in migraine patients relate more to migraine with aura than migraine without aura?

Merikangas: In some of our work, we found that both those with or without aura had an elevated risk of depression, but the Zurich cohort study findings (Merikangas *et al.* 1990) suggested a stronger association between migraine with aura and depression than for migraine without aura. This was also found by Breslau *et al.* (1991).

Glover: I was particularly interested in your finding of greatest association with the bipolar II subtype, because what's emerging all the time with migraine is a link with a predisposition to instability. The migraine attack itself is often associated with an early agitation and a later depression, like a brief bipolar episode. What about links with brief recurrent depression?

Merikangas: We did not look at that in our family study. In our study it's the atypical variety of depression that is associated with hypomania. In the Zurich study, recurrent brief depression was not associated with migraine.

Peatfield: Are those the patients who often complain of pain, the depressive equivalents who have a pain syndrome rather than reporting themselves to be miserable?

Merikangas: These are not people who complain of chronic misery. They appear to be doing better than most people most of the time. Their episodes of depression tend to be rather short-lived.

Peatfield: Do they respond better to monoamine oxidase inhibitors (MAOIs) than to tricyclics?

Merikangas: Yes, this was reported by Anthony and Lance (1969). MAOIs are the most effective drugs for those with the atypical variety of depression. These patients tend to be hypersomnic, retain interest in their usual activities, and are hyperphagic during their episodes. It's the opposite to what we think of as 'depression'. We have recently replicated that work (Merikangas and Merikangas 1995).

Schoenen: For which of the psychiatric disorders is the link the strongest?

Merikangas: I believe that depression is the disorder most strongly associated with migraine. However, when one considers comorbidity of depression and anxiety disorders, the association with migraine is even stronger. Recent evidence from genetic, biochemical, clinical, and treatment studies suggest that anxiety and depression have shared underlying causes.

Glover: Breslau and Davis (1993) found that panic disorder had the highest odds ratio.

Merikangas: Yes, but again it's a rare disorder, affecting only 1.5% of the population. One should be careful because, as with bipolar disorder, the rarity means there is going to be a higher odds ratio. One must examine the confidence intervals as well.

Peatfield: What is known about the genetic markers of bipolar psychiatric illness now?

Merikangas: There is still not a single linkage study of a major psychiatric disorder that's been replicated.

Peatfield: So although there is a strong familial effect in bipolar illness, still nobody has found a marker?

Merikangas: Not as yet. And most of us would have bet on bipolar disorder! It has a 1% population prevalence and is believed to have a strong genetic basis.

Tournier-Lasserve: Although it is true that the linkage study for bipolar disorder has not been replicated, this arose for the Amish pedigree linked to chromosome 11 after another branch of the family was added to the first branch. Geneticists working in psychiatry are feeling defensive about the lack of replication but there are many explanations for it.

Merikangas: That is right, but it is totally unjustified to blame solely the clinicians; errors have been made in the laboratory and in the application of the statistical models as well.

Tournier-Lasserve: I do not think we shall see this in migraine, but in bipolar disorders there appears to be an attraction between people suffering from the same disorder. In a comparison of alleles for a particular candidate gene Jacque Mallet in Paris found that the frequency of a particular allele was much higher in affected subjects than in unrelated controls. However, in spouses, there was an intermediate level of the allele, which may be interpreted, among other hypotheses, as a 'non-random' choice of spouse by individuals with bipolar disorder. We should be extremely careful in the analysis of clinical data.

Merikangas: The most important thing is to be honest about our assumptions and the limitations of our methods and cautious in the claims we make for our work.

Frants: Could you expand on the reliability and meaning of a possible familial pattern of drug response? It sounds attractive but could be dangerous.

Merikangas: For example, there appears to be specificity of drug response in families with bipolar disorder. There is a suggestion that some families respond to lithium, whereas other families do not. The anti-epileptic drugs, particularly depakote, are now widely used in the treatment of bipolar disorder. If we found that there was a correlation in treatment response within families, this could be used as a potentially homogeneous subgroup which could be discriminated from families with preferential response to other agents. We do not usually ask migraine patients what drugs family members responded to, and sumatriptan wasn't available to previous generations. But in psychiatry where the same drugs have been available for two or three generations, one could use this to distinguish families.

Tournier-Lasserve: It's an interesting idea, but there are so many reasons why a treatment might not be effective, metabolism of the medicine etc. On the other hand, once genes are identified this might help enormously to sort out which medicine may be more efficient.

Diener: This is an important issue. Nobody has studied patients who claim to be non-responders to some drugs whereas other drugs are effective. In cases where this remains constant, for example non-response to sumatriptan, this would perhaps argue for a genetically induced change in receptor sensitivity.

Haan: Do the studies of Ottman and Lipton (1994) shed light on the relationship between epilepsy and migraine? They showed comorbidity of migraine and epilepsy in probands and a higher occurrence of migraine in families of probands with epilepsy.

Merikangas: They did not propose to focus on migraine, so they didn't conduct detailed interviews of people with both conditions. I believe that their work suggested that migraine and epilepsy are transmitted independently in families. An association between epilepsy and migraine has been suggested for a long time. There is certainly some evidence for comorbidity.

Ferrari: A 100 years ago Gowers said that the only relationship between migraine and epilepsy is the wrong diagnosis!

Merikangas: It is very difficult to make such clinical distinctions in population studies. That could be an important issue. This is why one must consider the aggregate evidence in drawing conclusions about such associations.

Moskowitz: Virtually any mammal, including humans, can develop a seizure. We know this from the Korean War Studies. Among American soldiers on leave who binged for 36 hours and then withdrew from alcohol and drugs, many had seizures and did not suffer one subsequently. Built into the organization of the nervous system is the potential for developing a seizure. I would say that the same principle applies for migraine. If an individual is sufficiently stressed with appropriate precipitants, a headache and probably migraine would occur. But there is a range of susceptibility. What we're trying to distinguish is what makes one person more susceptible than another.

Ferrari: In kindling research, at the end of a provoked seizure spreading depression is seen. Could that be a relationship between migraine and epilepsy?

Diener: I know of one young female patient for whom a migraine always led to an epileptic fit, or a fit led to aura and headache. That would be a strong argument that it could be both ways.

Haan: In migraine we are searching for susceptibility genes and not for disease genes. There might be a similar situation to that in Alzheimer's disease where the different alleles of the apolipoprotein E gene on chromosome 19 determine the susceptibility to the disease.

Schoenen: That relates to the earlier question about the number of attacks needed for someone to be designated a migraineur.

Ferrari: Yes, it's a threshold gene we're looking for, rather than a pathophysiological gene.

Glover: In terms of environment, apart from genes, is there any evidence about neurodevelopment or obstetric complications? These are emerging as risk factors for certain psychiatric diseases.

Merikangas: The environment here is completely confounded with random error of measurement in our models and is part of the residual error terms. Thus, we can only infer the degree to which environmental factors are involved by the lack of concordance among monozygotic relative to dizygotic twins.

Peatfield: Waters (1973) found in an epidemiological study in South Wales, that 92% of young women had had a headache in the previous year, and yet we found (Tannock *et al.* 1993) in a study of alcoholic subjects that many had never had a headache in their lives. I am unhappy about the sophisticated mathematical analysis of data collected using imprecise diagnostic criteria in imprecise patients.

Merikangas: That's a good point, but in a general population about 30 to 40% of people say they never have a headache, although there are far more men without headaches than women.

Peatfield: Could there be a familial element to that? Is there a protective gene which might be easier to look for than the positive causative genes, which are clearly multiple? You might go to an alcoholism treatment centre and find people who have not had a headache, probably, in my experience, liver failure patients, and then study whether there is a family history of lack of headaches. You may find genetic markers there.

Merikangas: We have data on that in our families of alcoholics, but I haven't looked at it that way.

REFERENCES

Anthony, M. and Lance, J.W. (1969) Monoamine oxidase inhibition in the treatment of migraine. *Archives of Neurology*, **21**, 263–268.

Breslau N. and Davis, G. (1993) Migraine, physical health and psychiatric disorder: a prospective epidemiogenetic study in young adults. *Journal of Psychiatric Research*, **27**, 211–222.

Breslau, N., Davies, G.C. and Andreski, P. (1991) Migraine, psychiatric disorders and suicide attempts: an epidemiological study of young adults. *Psychiatry Research*, **37**, 11–23.

Clarke, J.M. (1910) On recurrent motor paralysis in migraine, with report of a family in which recurrent hemiplegia accompanied the attacks. *British Medical Journal*, **1**, 1534–1541.

Headache Classification Committee of the International Headache Society (J. Olesen *et al.*) (1988) Classification and diagnostic criteria for headache disorders, cranial neuralgias, and facial pain. *Cephalalgia*, **8**(Suppl. 7), 1–96.

Merikangas, K.R., Angst, J. and Isler, H. (1990) Migraine and psychopathology: results of the Zurich cohort study of young adults. *Archives of General Psychiatry*, **47**, 849–853.

Merikangas, K.R. and Merikangas, J.R. (1995) Combination monoamine oxidase inhibitor and beta blocker, treatment of migraine, with anxiety and depression. *Biological Psychiatry*, **38**, 603–610.

Ottman, R. and Lipton, R.B. (1994) Comorbidity of migraine and epilepsy. *Neurology*, **44**, 2105–2110.

Russell, H.B. and Olesen, J. (1993) The genetics of migraine without aura and migraine with aura. *Cephalalgia*, **13**, 245–248.

Russell, M.B., Hilden, J., Sorensen, S.A. *et al.* (1993) Familial occurrence of migraine without aura and migraine with aura. *Neurology*, **43**, 1369–1373.

Tannock, C., Bullock, R. and Peatfield, R.C. (1993) Problem drinkers do not get headache. *Cephalalgia*, **13**, 365.

Waters, W.E. (1973) The epidemiological enigma of migraine. *International Journal of Epidemiology*, **2**, 189–194.

20

Genetics of familial hemiplegic migraine

E. Tournier-Lasserve

INTRODUCTION

Migraine is a common neurological, sometimes incapacitating, condition affecting about 10% of the general population (Lance 1982). Its mechanisms are still poorly understood. Familial hemiplegic migraine (FHM) is an autosomal dominant subtype of migraine with aura (International Headache Society (IHS) criteria, Headache Classification Committee 1988) characterized by the occurrence of hemiplegia or hemiparesis during the aura (Clarke 1910, Whitty 1953). FHM may be considered a good model to investigate the mechanisms of migraine for several reasons. The aura in hemiplegic migraine attacks very often includes visual as well as sensory symptoms similar to those observed in other subtypes of migraine with aura. In addition, patients suffering from hemiplegic migraine attacks also suffer from migraine without aura attacks as well as migraine with non-hemiplegic aura. Migraine is often a familial condition although, despite the numerous studies conducted in the past few years, it still remains difficult to establish its modes of inheritance. FHM is clearly an autosomal dominant condition and this feature eases considerably the search for mutated genes involved in its pathophysiology. Once those FHM genes are identified, it will be possible to screen for their implication in other types of migraine.

Migraine: Pharmacology and genetics
Edited by Merton Sandler, Michel Ferrari and Sara Harnett
Published in 1996 by Chapman & Hall
ISBN 1 86036 006 8

MAPPING OF A GENE FOR FHM TO CHROMOSOME 19

During the clinical investigation of CADASIL, an autosomal dominant vascular condition causing recurrent cerebral small deep infarcts and subcortical dementia, we noticed that the frequency of migraine with aura was unusually high in CADASIL patients (Tournier-Lasserve *et al.* 1991). This led us to hypothesize that the CADASIL gene, which we had previously mapped on chromosome 19, might also be responsible for FHM, although the clinical and neuroimaging features of these two conditions differ quite markedly (Tournier-Lasserve *et al.* 1993, Joutel *et al.* 1993).

We selected two large pedigrees fulfilling IHS criteria for FHM. Genetic linkage analysis was conducted in 54 members, using a panel of four markers spanning the CADASIL locus, namely D19S216, D19S221, D19S226 and D19S215 (Figure 20.1). The maximum lod score, greater than 8, was obtained with two markers strongly linked to CADASIL, establishing genetic mapping of the FHM gene in these two families to

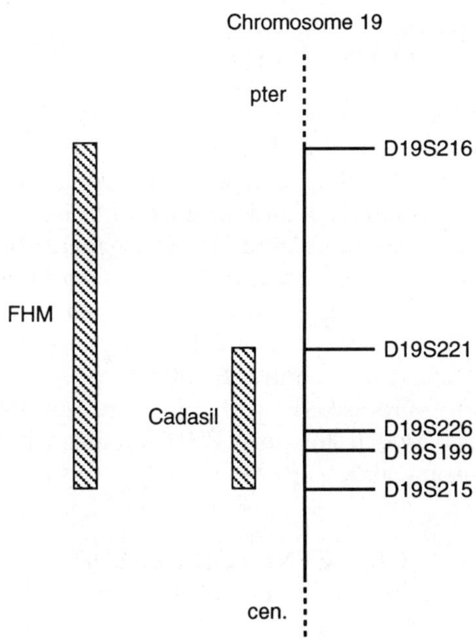

Figure 20.1 Chromosomal mapping of a gene responsible for familial hemiplegic migraine (FHM) on chromosome 19. Genetic linkage analysis conducted on two large FHM families with several chromosome 19 markers established genetic mapping of a gene for FHM on the short arm of chromosome 19.

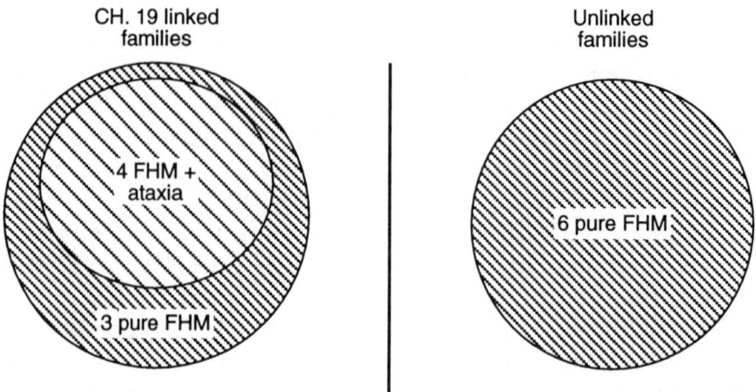

Figure 20.2 Genetic heterogeneity of familial hemiplegic migraine.

chromosome 19. Multipoint linkage analysis suggested that this FHM gene resides within a 30 cM interval, D19S216–D19S215, encompassing the CADASIL locus on chromosome 19.

GENETIC HETEROGENEITY OF FHM

We conducted linkage analysis on seven additional FHM families, using a set of seven markers spanning the D19S216–D19S215 interval. Two-point as well as multipoint lod score analysis provided strong evidence of linkage within two families, and absence of linkage in four families (Joutel *et al.* 1994). The same findings were made by other groups (Ophoff *et al.* 1994) and were further confirmed on additional families by our group (unpublished results). Interestingly, all families in which a cerebellar ataxia was associated with FHM were linked to chromosome 19 (Figure 20.2). On the contrary, of the 'pure' FHM families, approximately half were linked to 19. We were not able to show any clinical differences between the 'pure' FHM families whether or not they were linked to chromosome 19.

GENETIC MAPPING OF A GENE FOR HEREDITARY
PAROXYSMAL CEREBELLAR ATAXIA TO CHROMOSOME 19

Hereditary paroxysmal cerebellar ataxia (HPCA) is an autosomal dominant episodic ataxia highly responsive to acetazolamide. This condition, starting most often during childhood, is characterized by the recurrence of attacks of major unsteadiness, limb incoordination and dysarthria. The attacks generally last from a few minutes to a few days. Between attacks, neurological examination shows a gaze-evoked nystagmus and a mild permanent gait ataxia. The underlying mechanisms of this condition are poorly understood. Episodic ataxias are clinically heterogeneous conditions. In some of them, paroxysmal ataxia may be associated with other symptoms or signs such as kinesigenic movement disorders or neuromyotonia.

FHM and HPCA share several features such as the intermittent nature of their symptoms as well as the presence of a permanent cerebellar ataxia in 20% of the FHM families and most of the HPCA patients after several years of evolution. Based on these observations, we raised the hypothesis that these two conditions may be allelic disorders. We conducted a genetic linkage analysis with chromosome 19 markers on a large HPCA family and demonstrated that the most likely location of the affected gene was the same interval of 30 cM, D19S216–D19S215, encompassing the FHM locus as well as the CADASIL locus (Vahedi *et al.* 1995).

These results suggest that either these three conditions are allelic disorders, or that they are due to the alteration of distinct but closely linked genes belonging to a common gene family or metabolic pathway. Interestingly, the gene responsible for familial episodic ataxia with interictal myokimia has been shown to be a potassium channel gene located on chromosome 12, suggesting that ion channels may be excellent candidate genes for these conditions. Gene identification is the only way to solve this fascinating question. This or these genes will also be checked for their involvement in non-hemiplegic migraine with or without aura. To do that, we are now studying 200 families affected with migraine.

Acknowledgements

This work has been supported by INSERM, the Association Française contre les Myopathies, the Fondation de France. These data are the result of the intensive work of a number of scientists and physicians, including particularly Professor M.G. Bousser and Drs A. Joutel, A. Ducros, K. Vahedi, H. Chabriat and S. Alamowitch.

REFERENCES

Clarke, J.M. (1910) On recurrent motor paralysis in migraine. *British Medical Journal*, **1** 1534–1538.
Headache Classification Committee of the International Headache Society, (J. Olesen *et al.*) (1988) Classification and diagnostic criteria for headache disorders, cranial neuralgias and facial pain. *Cephalalgia*, **8** (Suppl. 7), 19–28.
Joutel, A., Bousser, M.G., Biousse, V., Labauge, P., Chabriat, H. *et al.* (1993) A

gene for familial hemiplegic migraine maps to chromosome 19. *Nature Genetics*, **5**, 40–45.
Joutel, A., Ducros, A., Vahedi, K., Labauge, P., Decrieu, O. *et al.* (1994) Genetic heterogeneity of familial hemiplegic migraine. *American Journal of Human Genetics*, **55**, 1166–1172.
Lance, J.W. (1982) *Mechanism and Management of Headache.* (4th edn) Butterworth Scientific, London.
Ophoff, R.A., Vaneisk, R., Sandkuijl, L.A., Terwindt, G.M., Grubben, C.P.M. *et al.* (1994) Genetic heterogenity of familial hemiplegic migraine. *Genomics*, **22**, 21–26.
Tournier-Lasserve, E., Iba-Zizen, M.T., Romero, N. and Bousser, M.G. (1991) Autosomal dominant syndrome with stroke-like episodes and leukoencephalo-pathy. *Stroke*, **22**, 1297–1302.
Tournier-Lasserve, E., Joutel, A., Melki, J., Weissenbach, J., Lathrop, G.M. *et al.* (1993) Cerebral autosomal dominant arteriopathy with subcortical infarcts and leukoencephalopathy maps to chromosome 19q12. *Nature Genetics*, **3**, 256–259.
Vahedi, K., Joutel, A., van Bogaert, P., Ducros, A., Maciazck, J. *et al.* (1995). A gene for hereditary paroxysmal cerebellar ataxia maps to chromosome 19p. *Annals of Neurology*, **37**, 289–293.
Whitty, C.W.M. (1953) Familial hemiplegic migraine. *Journal of Neurology Neurosurgery and Psychiatry*, **16**, 172–177.

DISCUSSION

Haan: You have FHM families with a maternal mitochondrial-like inheritance pattern. Are these linked to chromosome 19?

Tournier-Lasserve: In some families, the observed mode of inheritance could be consistent with a mitochondrial inheritance. Either this is due to the small size of the family, which decreases the chance of the father transmitting the disorder, or in these families migraine could be due to mitochondrial abnormalities.

Haan: Are you looking at both a mitochondrial gene and an ion channel gene on chromosome 19?

Tournier-Lasserve: We have not yet looked in these families at mito-chondrial genes encoded by the mitochondrial genome.

Merikangas: You said there were no candidate genes in the region. What about homologous areas in animal studies of chromosome 19?

Tournier-Lasserve: We were not able to find any in mouse syntechnic regions.

Merikangas: What about karyotyping?

Tournier-Lasserve: For two years, Dr M. Prieur at the Necker Hospital in Paris has used karyotyping on every index of every family and has not found any abnormality. We are now looking for very small chromo-somal rearrangements using probes located within the region of interest.

Lance: Forty percent of the patients carrying the CADASIL gene develop migraine in their 20s, although they may not develop CADASIL until they are in their 40s. How many have the magnetic resonance imaging (MRI) changes in their 20s and continue throughout life without developing CADASIL?

Tournier-Lasserve: This happens to very few people. In our series, there are three patients like that. One 82 year old woman has only migraine but her 60 year old daughter is already sick. So the phenotype can vary within a family, but some families are much more 'migraine-type' than others.

Bruyn: You have collected a large number of families of patients with migraine with aura only within the family. However, many patients suffer some attacks with aura and other attacks without aura.

Tournier-Lasserve: The probands fulfil the criteria of migraine with aura but in most cases they have migraine attacks with aura and also without aura.

Bruyn: From the clinician's point of view that is important. If the presumed gene has a size of 2000 nucleotide pairs, did you ever envisage the concept that FHM and CADASIL or the type with ataxia might be expressions of the same gene with allelic heterogeneity?

Tournier-Lasserve: There were at least two possibilities: either it would be the same gene for the three disorders with many different mutations within it; or it would be different genes which might have something in common.

Haan: Do you have a second FHM locus?

Tournier-Lasserve: These are preliminary data. We may have a second locus but we want to test new markers in our very large family and also to analyse the families unlinked to chromosome 19 with this particular marker.

Haan: St Clair *et al.* (1995) reported a CADASIL family not linked to chromosome 19. Do you think that was CADASIL?

Tournier-Lasserve: That Scottish pedigree is interesting. All 16 large CADASIL families that we analysed were linked to chromosome 19. There may be some families with CADASIL which are not linked, but we are waiting to check the other families for this. St Clair *et al.* (1995) published a pedigree for 87 people with what seems to be a CADASIL disorder. However, a significant number of the individuals who were studied genetically in this pedigree did not undergo MRI. MRI is crucial to establish the status for linkage analysis. In CADASIL families approximately half the people have the lesions but are not sick yet. All these individuals would be quoted as recombinants if MRI is not performed. Therefore, there is a high risk that the absence of linkage observed in the Scottish pedigree is due to a misclassification of the individuals.

Bruyn: If your findings are consistent with the fact that patients from CADASIL families may go through life with only migraine with aura, and you can prove it by means of MRI, would that imply that every patient suffering from migraine with aura with an onset from the age of 20 or above should be subjected to an MRI study to exclude the eventual presence of CADASIL?

Tournier-Lasserve: We are often asked this. I would not recommend MRI for every migraine patient because health systems could not cope. There are two criteria that may indicate that MRI should be used. One is the age of onset: this type of migraine with aura starts later than is normally observed. Secondly, it is simple to look at the family tree. If there is vascular dementia, if somebody has been diagnosed as having multiple sclerosis (a common misdiagnosis of this disorder), or if somebody has a mood disorder or manic episodes, I would recommend MRI.

Peatfield: To what use should a clinician put this information? It's a terrifying diagnosis to offer and I'm not sure what its value would be in the clinical management of the patient.

Tournier-Lasserve: That is a completely different question. We hope that once the gene is identified we may have a better understanding of the condition and thereby a better therapeutic approach. Paroxysmal ataxia has an effective treatment: it is sensitive to acetazolamide. This may suggest that acetazolamide could be effective in FHM but this has to be checked in a vigorous trial.

Glover: Has lithium been tried in CADASIL as it often has a bipolar link?

Tournier-Lasserve: As far as I know, Professor M. G. Bousser has not tried lithium.

Haan: You mentioned multiple sclerosis as a misdiagnosis. Several CADASIL patients have been described with oligoclonal bands in CSF, and you have described CADASIL patients with monoclonal gammopathies in the serum. Does that point to an immunological cause of CADASIL, and did you look for that kind of immunological abnormality in FHM also?

Tournier-Lasserve: In the first large CADASIL families that we reported with Professor Bousser there were three brothers and sisters with monoclonal gammopathy, and two of them died from a myeloma. This is extremely unusual. One offspring of one of these affected individuals had antiDNA antibodies. But we didn't find that in other families.

Haan: It is interesting that we have a CADASIL family in which one patient also had a monoclonal gammopathy in the serum. Perhaps he comes from France and is a member of your family!

Tournier-Lasserve: That would be interesting because I have not seen any others from France.

Merikangas: The manic depression link is interesting, particularly because association has been found between depression and migraine both with and without aura.

Tournier-Lasserve: I don't know what the relationship is between the manic episodes and this disorder. But these people have lacunar infarcts and lesions in the basal ganglia. My feeling would be that the manic episodes and mood disorders may be linked to these basal ganglia lesions. I would not advise a similar approach of looking for the chromosome 19 gene with manic episodes.

Merikangas: Have you looked in the region of the HLA system, on the grounds that some part of this is an immunological disorder? In diabetes, linkage was found at another site, and when they found linkage at that site, the secondary site was the HLA system. It required both genes. That model might be very interesting here.

Tournier-Lasserve: For CADASIL we did it because it was one of the very polymorphic sites, and we could exclude linkage to the HLA complex (on 20 cM on both sides).

Schoenen: Is it known which potassium channel is abnormal in paroxysmal ataxia?

Tournier-Lasserve: The one in the paroxysmal ataxia linked to chromosome 12 is known to be KCNA1.

Schoenen: Potassium channels, especially those acting at the late repolarization and the after-hyperpolarization, are very important for the discharge frequency of neurons and we know that the raphe serotonergic neurons have a very regular 'pacemaker-like' discharge, which might potentially be changed by changes in after-hyperpolarization.

Tournier-Lasserve: Ion channels are certainly excellent candidate genes, but there are so many that finding the right one in migraine would be a matter of chance.

Frants: There are channel genes on chromosome 19 but so far they are in the wrong place.

Tournier-Lasserve: There is a sodium channel on chromosome 19 on the long arm.

Haan: It is important that the episodic familial ataxia linked to chromosome 12 has myokymia, because all ion channel disorders have muscle symptoms.

Tournier-Lasserve: I agree. The story is not finished. I expect other diseases to be linked to ion channels. Epilepsy may be an excellent candidate disease.

Haan: All ion channel diseases are episodic diseases and all have environmental triggers that cause attacks.

Moskowitz: In animals it is possible to stop spreading depression by making the animals significantly hypercapnic and acidolic. If you put the same amount of potassium on the cortex you won't get the spread.

Peatfield: Familial periodic ataxia outgrows acetazolamide after a while, which suggests the metabolic adjustment of intracellular pH loses efficacy.

Bruyn: Acetazolamide inhibits carbonic anhydrase. Has carbonic anhydrase been pinpointed on the genome? Wouldn't that be, in view of the effect of acetazolamide on this disorder, an indication of where to look further?

Tournier-Lasserve: There are several genes and several pseudogenes.

Ferrari: Do you think the action of acetazolamide is specific to the enzyme or is it just altering the ionic conductance via changing the pH?

Tournier-Lasserve: We don't really understand how it works in other episodic neurological disorders. It can work in sodium channel disease, in potassium channel disease and also in other types of non-episodic disease like glaucoma.

Goadsby: Given current interest in magnesium, which has even been suggested as a therapy for migraine, it would be interesting to map the magnesium modulatory site on the NMDA receptor and see if it relates to these migraine families that you are studying.

REFERENCE

St Clair, D., Bolt, J., Morris, S. and Doyle, D. (1995) Hereditary multi-infarct dementia unlinked to chromosome 19_q12 in a large Scottish pedigree: evidence of probable locus heterogeneity. *Journal of Medical Genetics*, **32**, 57–60.

21

Chromosome 19 in migraine with and without aura

Rune R. Frants, Roel A. Ophoff, Gisela M. Terwindt, Christine Urban, Ronald van Eijk, Joost Haan, H. Christoph Diener, Dick Lindhout, Arne May, Lodewijk A. Sandkuijl, Michel D. Ferrari

INTRODUCTION

Migraine is a common paroxysmal neurological disorder affecting up to 8% of males and 25% of females in the general population (Rasmussen *et al.* 1991). There are two main types of migraine, migraine without aura, occurring in 85% of patients, and migraine with aura, occurring in 15% of patients (Headache Classification Committee 1988).

Attacks of migraine without aura are typically characterized by severe, unilateral, pulsating headache, associated with nausea, vomiting and photo- and phonophobia. In migraine with aura, attacks are preceded or accompanied by transient focal neurological, usually visual, symptoms.

Migraine frequently runs in families, suggesting that hereditary factors are involved (Ad hoc Committee on Classification of Headache 1962). Family and twin studies have yielded conflicting results with respect to the mode of inheritance of migraine (Allan 1928, Goodell *et al.* 1954, Dalsgaard-Nielsen 1965, Barolin and Sperlich 1969, Baier 1985, Devoto *et al.* 1986, D'Amico *et al.* 1991, Russell *et al.* 1993, Mochi *et al.* 1993, Lucas 1977, Ziegler *et al.* 1975). Methodological differences and

Migraine: Pharmacology and genetics
Edited by Merton Sandler, Michel Ferrari and Sara Harnett
Published in 1996 by Chapman & Hall
ISBN 1 86036 006 8

shortcomings may partly explain this confusion (Russell *et al.* 1993, Haan *et al.* 1994).

Familial hemiplegic migraine (FHM) is a rare subtype of migraine with aura characterized by hemiparesis in addition to other aura symptoms (for review see Haan *et al.* 1994). FHM shows a clear autosomal dominant mode of inheritance (Headache Classification Committee 1988). Studying the genetics of FHM may therefore help to unravel the genetics of the common migraine disease. A gene for FHM has been mapped to chromosome 19 (Joutel *et al.* 1993). We confirmed the localization of a gene for FHM on chromosome 19p13 in three families, while at least two other families provided evidence for locus hetero-geneity (Ophoff *et al.* 1994). In this study we investigate the involvement of the putative FHM gene on 19p13 in the common forms of migraine in 28 families with migraine with or without aura.

MATERIALS AND METHODS

Subjects

Index patients were ascertained from the headache outpatient clinic at the Essen University Hospital or from respondents to an article in a local Essen newspaper. Only individuals with migraine in at least two generations were asked to participate in the family study. Probandi ($n = 28$) and all available family members ($n = 170$) were asked to fill in a questionnaire and were subsequently interviewed personally by one of the authors (C.U. or A.M.). Information for eight persons was obtained through their relatives. Information on the occurrence of migraine in the previous generations was also obtained through family members.

Patients were diagnosed with migraine with or without aura according to the International Headache Society (IHS) classification criteria (Headache Classification Committee 1988).

Genetic analysis

Genomic DNA was isolated from 198 individuals according to Miller *et al.* (1988). The analysis of the highly informative microsatellite marker D19S394 (*UT705*) (Figure 21.1) was performed as described by Ophoff *et al.* (1994). The number and frequencies of alleles were estimated from the spouses in the 28 migraine families. The heterozygosity was estimated to be 0.89.

Statistical analysis

Affected sib-pairs analysis was done by comparing parental marker alleles found in one of the sibs of a given sib-pair with those of the other

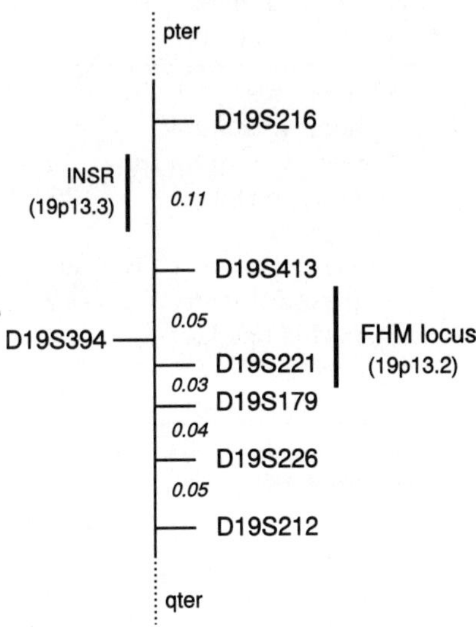

Figure 21.1 Genetic map of chromosome 19p region based on data from Genome Data Base. Distances are given in morgans.

sib. Alleles from homozygous parents were not scored; whenever parents had not been tested for the marker, their genotype probabilities were calculated and scores were computed as described by Sandkuijl (1989). Correction for multiple sib-pairs in a single sibship was according to Suarez and Hodge (1979).

In a separate analysis, pairs of affected sibs with only one affected parent were included. Only the allele inherited from the affected parent was scored. Significance levels were obtained through a one-sided test against a normal distribution.

In addition to sib-pair analysis, linkage analysis was carried out with the Linkage program package (Lathrop *et al.* 1985), version 5.04, applying the genetic model generated in our previous analysis of FHM (Ophoff *et al.* 1994). The liability classes are given in Table 21.1.

RESULTS

Description of families

Twenty-five of the 28 participating families were from Nordrhein-Westfalen. One family originated from Hessen, Germany. The remaining two families were from Afghanistan and the Netherlands. No apparent consanguinity was detected between the families. Out of 198 individuals, 23 (11.6%) had migraine with aura and 93 (47.0%) migraine

Table 21.1 Genetic model for the linkage analysis

Liability classes[a]	
Migraine with aura	8:1
Migraine without aura	2:1
Migraine, history	2:1
No migraine	1:4
<18 yrs:	2:3
Unaffected, history	3:8
Unspecific headache	1:1
Gene frequency	0.01

[a] Ratio indicates the odds of being gene carrier

Table 21.2 The distribution over the diagnostic categories for 28 families

Diagnostic groups	*Males* (n = 84)		*Females* (n = 114)		*Total* (n = 198)	
Healthy	52	(61.9%)	20	(17.5%)	72	(36.4%)
Healthy, but <18 yrs of age	3	(3.6%)	2	(1.8%)	5	(2.5%)
Atypical headache	2	(2.4%)	3	(2.6%)	5	(2.5%)
Migraine with aura	4	(4.8%)	19	(16.7%)	23	(11.6%)
Migraine without aura	23	(27.3%)	70	(61.4%)	93	(47.0%)

without aura (Table 21.2). Five family members had headache attacks not fulfilling the IHS criteria for migraine. The male: female ratio was 1:3.5 for migraine with aura and 1:2.2 for migraine without aura. As the preponderance of females among the migraineurs might suggest an X-linked dominant inheritance, we scored the parental transmission of migraine in the families. Observed male-to-male transmission argues against X-linked dominant as well as a mitochondrial inheritance. It should be noted that genetic heterogeneity could compromise this interpretation.

Genetic analysis

Affected sib-pair analysis was performed using the highly informative marker D19S394 which was previously shown to be closely linked to the FHM locus. We observed that affected sibs shared the same marker allele more frequently than expected (Table 21.3): 38.6 shared versus

Table 21.3 Numbers of shared and non-shared alleles within affected sibships[a]

	Shared alleles	*Non-shared alleles*	p *value*[b]
Alleles of both parents	38.6	27.2	≈0.08
Alleles of affected parents only	18.4	9.2	≈0.04

[a] Corrected for multiple sib-pairs occurring in a single family
[b] One-sided

27.2 non-shared alleles ($p = 0.08$). Taking into account only the alleles of the affected parents, the distribution of the marker alleles changed significantly: 18.4 alleles shared versus 9.2 non-shared alleles ($p = 0.04$). Family 25 contributed disproportionably to this result. In this family, five alleles were scored as shared in the main sibship after correction for multiple sib-pairs as mentioned before. Nevertheless, sharing was still increased in the remaining families, but not significantly. The results of the sib-pair analysis suggest that the putative 19p13 gene plays a role in 33% of the sib-pairs. This value drops to 18.6% if family 25 is excluded from the analysis.

Lod score calculations also support the involvement of this locus. When we applied a conservative model previously used for linkage analysis of FHM families (Ophoff *et al.* 1994) the overall lod score of marker D19S394 was 1.38 without recombination. A major contribution came from family 25 with a maximum lod score of 1.29.

DISCUSSION

So far it has been difficult to define the inheritance pattern of migraine. Phenomena such as reduced penetrance, variable expression and genetic heterogeneity, together with diagnostic and methodological problems, have prevented firm conclusions. Accordingly, various statistical methods must be applied to estimate the contribution of genetic factors. Affected sib-pair analysis is relatively insensitive to lack of specific inheritance models. However, since the method is not very powerful, large numbers of patients are required to detect genetic contributions. In our analysis of marker alleles transmitted by affected parents only, we detected increased sharing with borderline statistical significance. The ratio of shared versus non-shared alleles was 18.4:9.2, compared with the expected 1:1 ratio. Although an important contribution to this result came from one large family (family 25: five alleles scored as shared in the main sibship after correction for multiple sib-pairs), sharing is still increased in the remaining families, although not significantly.

For the lod score analysis, we chose to apply a very conservative model, identical to the one we used previously for the linkage analysis of families with hemiplegic migraine (see Ophoff *et al.* 1994). This model assumes that migraine is a common disorder, with population frequencies of 10.2% for all types of migraine, and 2.8% for migraine with aura. As an allowance is made for a large contribution of non-genetic factors in disease aetiology, only 5.4% of all migraine patients will carry a genetic predisposition to migraine under this model. Furthermore, the relative risk for gene carriers when compared to non-gene carriers to develop any type of migraine was calculated to be 2.82 under this model. A Finnish study excluded the involvement of the 19p FHM locus in four migraine families (Hovatta *et al.* 1994). Their estimate of the relative risk for gene carriers to develop migraine was ten times higher than ours, 84% of migraine patients being carriers. Accordingly, the two studies are difficult to compare.

Under our very conservative model, many families were almost completely uninformative. A major contribution to the overall positive lod score of 1.38 came, again, from family 25 (maximum lod score 1.29). A statistical test for genetic heterogeneity among the families yielded no evidence for such heterogeneity (data not shown), which was to be expected given the relatively small contributions coming from most families.

In regular gene mapping studies, a lod score of 1.38 is not regarded as definitive evidence for a gene localization, although the corresponding likelihood ratio of 24 to 1 is definitely significant ($p = 0.006$, one-sided) according to conventional statistical criteria. In random mapping studies stronger statistical evidence is required because no *a priori* knowledge exists about which of the 22 autosomes may carry a disease gene. This study, however, was initiated based on the earlier localization of a gene for hemiplegic migraine on 19p13. Therefore, regular statistical criteria can be applied in the interpretation of the lod score.

We conclude that our findings provide evidence for the involvement of a gene on 19p13 in the aetiology of migraine. It remains to be elucidated whether this genetic contribution constitutes a mild risk factor for migraine in the general population, or a major risk factor in only a small proportion of migraine families. Such questions can only be answered when the gene on 19p13 responsible for hemiplegic migraine has been cloned and characterized.

Acknowledgements

This work has been supported by the Phoenix Foundation (for R.A.O.) and the Netherlands Organization for Scientific Research (NWO) (number 950-10-615 for G.M.T.). The primers for marker D19S394 were synthesized by Isogen Bioscience Amsterdam.

REFERENCES

Ad hoc Committee on Classification of Headache (1962) Classification of headache. *Journal of the American Medical Association*, **179**, 717–718.

Allan, W. (1928) The inheritance of migraine. *Archives of Internal Medicine*, **13**, 590–599.

Baier, W.K. (1985) Genetics of migraine and migraine accompagneé: a study of eighty-one children and their families. *Neuropediatrics*, **16** 84–91.

Barolin, G.S. and Sperlich, D. (1969) Migränefamilien. Beitrag zum genetischen Aspekt des Migräneleidens. *Fortschritte der Neurologie Psychiatrie*, **37**, 521–544.

Dalsgaard-Nielsen, T. (1965) Migraine and heredity. *Acta Neurologica Scandinavica*, **411**, 287–300.

D'Amico, D., Leone, M., Macciardi, F., Valentini, S. and Bussone, G. (1991) Genetic transmission of migraine without aura: a study of 68 families. *Italian Journal of Neurological Sciences*, **12**, 581–584.

Devoto, M., Lozito, A., Staffa, G., D'Alessandro, R., Sacquegna, T. and Romeo, G. (1986) Segregation analysis of migraine in 128 families. *Cephalalgia*, **6**, 101–105.

Goodell, H., Lewontin, R. and Wolff H.G. (1954) Familial occurrence of migraine headache. A study of heredity. *American Medical Association Archives of Neurology and Psychiatry*, **72**, 325–334.

Haan, J., Terwindt, G.M., Bos, P.L.J.M., Ophoff, R.A., Frants, R.R. and Ferrari, M.D. (1994) Familial hemiplegic migraine in the Netherlands. *Clinical Neurology and Neurosurgery*, **96**, 244–249.

Headache Classification Committee of the International Headache Society (J. Olesen *et al.*) (1988) Classification and diagnostic criteria for headache disorders, cranial neuralgias and facial pain. *Cephalalgia*, **8** (Suppl. 7), 1–97.

Hovatta, I., Kallela, M., Färkkilä, M, and Peltonen, L. (1994) Familial migraine: exclusion of the susceptibility gene from the reported locus of familial hemiplegic migraine on 19p. *Genomics*, **23**, 707–709.

Joutel, A., Bousser, M.G., Biousse, V., Labauge, P., Chabriat, H., Nibbio, A., Maciazek, J., Meyer, B., Bach, M.A., Weissenbach, J., Lathrop, G.M., and Tournier-Lasserve, E. (1993) A gene for familial hemiplegic migraine maps to chromosome 19. *Nature Genetics*, **5**, 40–45.

Lathrop, G.M., Lalouel, J.M., Julier, C., and Ott, J. (1985) Multilocus linkage analysis in humans: detections of linkage and estimation of recombination. *American Journal of Human Genetics*, **5** 40–45.

Lucas, R.N. (1977) Migraine in twins. *Journal of Psychiatric Research*, **20**, 147–156.

Miller, S.A., Dykes, D.D. and Polesky, H.F. (1988) A simple salting out procedure for extracting DNA from nucleated cells. *Nucleic Acid Research*, **16**, 1215.

Mochi, M., Sangiorgi, S., Cortelli, P., Carelli, V., Scapoli, C., Crisci, M., Monari, L., Pierangeli, G., and Montagna, P. (1993) Testing models for genetic determination in migraine. *Cephalalgia*, **13**, 389–394.

Ophoff, R.A., Eijk van, R., Sandkuijl, L.A., Terwindt, G.M., Grubben, C.P.M., Haan, J., Lindhout, D., Ferrari, M.D. and Frants, R.R. (1994) Genetic heterogeneity of familial hemiplegic migraine. *Genomics*, **22**, 21–26.

Rasmussen, B.K., Jensen, R., Schroll, M., and Olesen, J. (1991) Epidemiology of headache in a general population: a prevalence study. *Journal of Clinical Epidemiology*, **44**, 1147–1157.

Russell, M.B., Hilden, J., Sorensen, S.A., and Olesen, J. (1993) Familial occurrence of migraine without aura and migraine with aura. *Neurology*, **43**, 1369–1373.

Sandkuijl, L.A. (1989) Analysis of affected sib pairs using information from extended families. In: *Multipoint Mapping and Linkage based upon Affected Pedigree Members. Genetic Analysis Workshop 6*, (eds R.C. Elston, M.A. Spence, S.E. Hodge and J.W. MacCluer) pp. 117–122. Alan R. Liss, New York.

Suarez, B.K. and Hodge, S.E. (1979) A simple method for detecting linkage for rare recessive diseases: an application to juvenile diabetes. *Clinical Genetics*, **15**, 126–136.

Ziegler, D.K., Hassanein, R.S., Harris, D. and Stewart, R. (1975) Headache in a non-clinic twin population. *Headache*, **4**, 213–218.

DISCUSSION

Peatfield: What is the result of excluding family 25 from the study?

Frants: In the linkage analysis we no longer have significant results, mainly because we used a very conservative model. In the sib-pair study we retain borderline significance.

Peatfield: That it is still borderline suggests that there is some linkage to chromosome 19 in many of Dr Diener's families, rather than just the one. Presumably the study needs to be extended to be confident of that.

Frants: Our results suggest that approximately a quarter of the families could be linked to chromosome 19.

Haan: But one 'normal' migraine family linked with chromosome 19 is very important because that would be the first 'normal' migraine family linked to a chromosome.

Goadsby: Is it still possible that chromosome 19 has nothing to do with migraine without aura? From Dr Tournier Lasserve's work (this volume) I was happy with the idea that chromosome 19 was important to some patients with familial hemiplegic migraine (FHM).

Frants: Our working hypothesis is that migraine is genetically heterogeneous, forming a distribution with mild, moderate and severe forms. There are several examples of other genes where mutations in different areas give different disorders and also different severity of disease.

Goadsby: I accept that, but how tightly do you think these data fit for a connection between chromosome 19 and migraine without aura?

Frants: According to the statistics, it's a weak effect, but the study has to be extended.

Lasserve: How many individuals, affected and healthy, were analysed within family 25? And was the lod score of 1.29 due to lack of information because the family was not large enough, or was it because of recombinants? If there are recombinants, how do they fit with your estimation of where the locus is in FHM?

Frants: The family has 12 affected sibs. We have looked only at the marker D19S394 and we also used the liability classes from FHM. That's why we have such a limited lod score even with such a large family. But we are extending this family. We have also some candidate genes for mutation screening. If we find mutations in these families then the circle is closed.

Peatfield: To what extent do you screen the rest of the genome in this project? Is your technique likely to turn up chromosomes elsewhere in the genome, or have we got to think of a candidate gene first?

Frants: To perform a genome screen for this disorder will be quite difficult. We are trying to collect more families and hope that we are lucky enough to find a few large families. We put great emphasis also on studying the spouses. Then we can also increase our threshold for the liability classes, because the probability of having other disorders, phenocopies, etc. in the specific families is very low. We are also looking for other loci and have already found one in other FHM families. The last approach is the sib-pairs technique, but we hope we don't need to use it, because even in a very simple model there are three genes involved in normal migraine. You need more than 200 sib-pairs for a feasible study, so it would be a major undertaking.

REFERENCE

Tournier-Lasserve, E. (1996) Genetics of familial hemiplegic migraine. In: *Migraine: Pharmacology and Genetics*, (eds M. Sandler, M.D. Ferrari and S. Harnett), pp. 282–290. Chapman & Hall, London.

22

Summing up

James W. Lance

INTRODUCTION

Our aim is to discover the cause of migraine and how to prevent it. To do this we must look first at the whole person, the family history, the emotional background and the factors that precipitate headache (Bruyn, this volume). Then we can dissect the hereditary pattern, the anatomical pathways and the pathophysiology responsible for headache. If we plunge deeper we examine the neurotransmitters and molecular biology involved, hoping to find some link in the chain that we can attack by pharmacological or other means. We must never lose sight of the fact that we are dealing with human beings and the hypotheses that we erect must be compatible with the symptoms described by our patients. The relevance of the experimental model to the human condition must be clearly demonstrable.

THE INHERITANCE OF MIGRAINE

The strongest case for a genetic basis for migraine is in familial hemiplegic migraine (FHM) in which 50% of the families have a gene limited to chromosome 19 (Tournier-Lasserve, this volume). Two other familial disorders have also been traced to this chromosome, dominantly inherited paroxysmal cerebellar ataxia (responsive to acetazolamide) and CADASIL (cerebral autosomal dominant arteriopathy with subcortical infarcts and leukoencephalopathy). In 20% of patients with hemiplegic migraine there are residual signs of cerebellar disturbance. Migraine

Migraine: Pharmacology and genetics
Edited by Merton Sandler, Michel Ferrari and Sara Harnett
Published in 1996 by Chapman & Hall
ISBN 1 86036 006 8

with aura occurs in 40% of patients with CADASIL, which is characterized by subcortical ischaemic strokes and cerebral white matter lesions on magnetic resonance imaging (MRI). Migraine with aura starts in the twenties but the mean age at which CADASIL patients present is 40. Nevertheless, the MRI changes may appear before that age and some may even persist through life without the patients developing dementia, stroke or other features of CADASIL. If the onset of migraine with aura is later than usual and there is a family history of dementia or cyclical mood disorder, an MRI investigation may be justifiable.

Genetic heterogeneity is present even within FHM and will certainly prove to be present in migraine with and without aura. Chromosome 19 may make a contribution to other forms of migraine in 25% of families (Frants *et al.*, this volume).

The risk of the close relatives of a migrainous patient developing migraine is two to three times that of control subjects (Merikangas, this volume). The Australian twin study included 5996 pairs with a lifetime prevalence of migraine of 21.5% for females and 7.9% for males. The concordance rates for monozygotic twins was significantly higher than for dizygotic twins. The results of the study indicate that about half of the variance in the aetiology of migraine is of genetic origin and the other half is due to environmental influences (Merikangas, this volume). There is a significant link between migraine, anxiety and depression.

ANATOMICAL PATHWAYS AND THEIR ASSOCIATED NEUROTRANSMITTERS

Pathways responsible for the perception of headache have been outlined by Goadsby (this volume). The importance of dural and vascular innervation to the genesis of headache was established by the pioneering studies of Harold G. Wolff. The trigeminal innervation of large basal cerebral blood vessels contains 5-hydroxytryptamine (5-HT), substance P, calcitonin gene-related peptide (CGRP) and neurokinin A (Edvinsson, this volume). The first order synapse is in the trigeminal nucleus caudalis, extending down to the second cervical segment of the spinal cord. Second order neurons are activated in these areas by stimulation of various cerebral vessels, demonstrated by c-*fos* immuno-reactivity or 2-deoxyglucose measurements of metabolism in rats, cats and monkeys (see Goadsby, this volume). Second order neurons terminate in the shell area of the ventroposteromedial thalamus. We must not forget the importance of the thalamus since some patients complain of pain extending from the head to the neck, shoulder and upper limb. Occasionally the pain extends down the whole of the affected side of the body, including the lower limb. A trigeminal syndrome can therefore extend to become a thalamic syndrome.

The other aspect of innervation concerns control of the cerebral blood vessels which participate in the migrainous process. The sympathetic nervous system contains noradrenaline (NA) and neuropeptide Y (NPY) and causes or modulates vasoconstriction. The parasympathetic outflow contains acetylcholine and vasoactive intestinal polypeptide (VIP) as well as peptide histidine isoleucine and pituitary adenylate cyclase-activating peptide (PCAP). This system is responsible for vasodilatation of intracerebral and extracerebral vessels.

Some years ago, Peter Goadsby and other members of our team demonstrated in monkeys that stimulation of the locus coeruleus at low frequencies reduced cerebral blood flow and, at high frequencies, increased extracranial blood flow through the parasympathetic nervous system. Stimulation of nucleus raphe dorsalis increased cerebral and extracranial blood flow through the same pathway (Lance *et al.* 1983). Vascular changes could therefore be secondary to activation of these brainstem centres.

Stimulation of the trigeminal ganglion in the cat (and in humans during thermocoagulation for the treatment of tic douloureux) releases CGRP and substance P into the external jugular vein (Edvinsson, Goadsby, this volume). The CGRP level in jugular venous blood increases in migraine and cluster headache, returning to normal after treatment with sumatriptan. The VIP level was also found to be increased in cluster headache and in two migrainous patients with autonomic symptoms.

CGRP is not released by experimental spreading depression (Edvinsson, this volume). The distribution of CGRP and SP-containing neurons is sparse on the cortical surface although dense on the proximal parts of the arteries. Trigeminally lesioned animals show a prolonged reaction to any vasoconstrictor substances other than NPY. The infusion of CGRP into patients with subarachnoid haemorrhage relieved vascular spasm but had no effect on normal vessels. It is possible that the release of CGRP is a mechanism to protect against vasospasm. CGRP and substance P produce vasodilatation but not pain in human subjects.

FACTORS TO BE CONSIDERED IN THE PATHOPHYSIOLOGY OF HEADACHE

Neurotrophins

Neurotropic factors probably remain active throughout life, mediating selective destruction and regeneration. They also have pharmacological actions when injected into animals or humans, causing muscle pain and hyperalgesia (Sandler, this volume).

Nerve growth factor and brain-derived neurotrophic factor are increased in rat cerebral cortex after experimental spreading depression or induced convulsions, possibly indicative of a neuroprotective effect. Overproduction of neurotrophins could conceivably be a mechanism for producing pain in migrainous patients. Basic fibroblast growth factor dilates rat pial arterioles and thus joins the long list of known vasodilators.

Depressive illness is common in migrainous patients and may be associated with neurotrophin deficiency. The time taken for induction of neurotrophins rules out their participation in the early phase of migraine headache but they could well play a part in the continuation of pain for hours or days.

5-Hydroxytryptamine

Seven 5-HT receptor families have now been identified, many with subtypes, five in the case of the 5-HT_1 group (Connor and Beattie, this volume). The most important in mediating contraction of cerebral and coronary vessels appears to be $5\text{-HT}_{1D\beta}$, the most abundant of all 5-HT_1 receptors, for which sumatriptan has a high affinity. There are important species differences in various vessels (Branchek *et al.*, this volume).

The subtype of 5-HT_{1D} receptors varies in different cerebral areas and vascular beds in humans. The alpha subtype is more common than beta in the trigeminal ganglion, whereas pial vessels are innervated predominantly by beta receptors (Bouchelet *et al.*, this volume). There are scanty alpha receptors on intracerebral vessels. One human coronary artery studied had predominantly beta receptors.

The 5-HT_{1D} receptor antagonist GR127935 is more potent in blocking the effects of sumatriptan than of 5-HT (Bax, this volume). In human coronary artery segments, ergotamine and dihydroergotamine (DHE) are more potent constrictors than sumatriptan although there is individual variability. The degree of the contractile response to sumatriptan is possibly related to the production of thromboxane A_2.

5-HT_1 receptors are present in the trigeminal innervation of the cerebral blood vessels, in the blood vessels themselves and within the central nervous system. Evidence from plasma protein extravasation (PPE) experiments (Moskowitz, this volume) indicates that sumatriptan acts at a neuronal prejunctional site as well as constricting arterial walls. Moskowitz speculates that substances acting on the $5\text{-HT}_{1D\alpha}$ receptor could be more effective than agonists of the $5\text{-HT}_{1D\beta}$ receptor in preventing PPE. A new agent CP-122, 288 is 2000 times more potent than sumatriptan in inhibiting PPE, but does so through an unknown mechanism. It will be of interest to see if this substance is effective in relieving migraine headache in doses that do not cause vasoconstriction.

Central 5-HT receptors are thought to play a role in pain control. Dihydroergotamine (a 5-HT_{1D} agonist) binds to neurons in the periaqueductal grey matter, the rostral part of the endogenous pain control system, as well as blocking the action of second order neurons. Sumatriptan exerts the latter effect if the blood–brain barrier is broken down experimentally (Goadsby, this volume). Since sumatriptan does not prevent headache if given during the aura but does stop the headache once it starts, its action may rely on penetration of the blood–brain barrier which may break down in the headache phase of migraine. This concept gains support from the observation of Goltman (1935/36) that a skull defect bulged during migraine headache, also reported by one of my patients, and by computed tomographic scans showing cerebral oedema in some patients.

Migraine attacks can be triggered by the 5-HT$_{2B/2C}$ receptor *m*-chlorophenyl piperazine (*m*-CPP), a breakdown product of trazodone, which dilates vessels by an endothelium-dependent mechanism (Fozard, this volume). Since migraine headache can be prevented by 5-HT$_{2B}$ antagonists such as methysergide and pizotifen, this receptor may play a part in pathophysiology.

Nitric oxide

Nitric oxide (NO) has a biological function mediating endothelium-dependent vasodilatation and the release of CGRP as well as modulating central neurotransmission (Thomsen and Olesen, this volume). The induction of headache by glyceryl trinitrate (NO donor) and histamine (NO liberator) relies on the release of NO. The duration of headache induced by glyceryl trinitrate correlated with dilatation of the middle cerebral artery, demonstrated by transcranial Doppler studies. As Thomsen and Olesen (this volume) point out, the moderate degree of intracranial vasodilatation is unlikely to cause headache unless vascular sensitivity is increased. Because NO is an unstable free radical with a half-life measured in seconds, it presumably initiates intermediary events that result in headache. NO itself produces pain when NO in solution is injected subcutaneously into forearm skin (Fozard, this volume).

Wines, commonly red wines in the United Kingdom, cause migraine headache (Peatfield *et al.*, this volume). The mechanism must involve a cascade of events in view of the latent period, possibly initiated by flavonoid pigments which might release NO.

Gamma aminobutyric acid

Valproate 10 mg/kg increases the amount of gamma aminobutyric acid (GABA) in the central nervous system. It blocks PPE whether it is induced by electrical or chemical stimulation by the application of capsaicin or substance P, unlike sumatriptan or ergotamine which block the former but not the latter. The action of valproate is negated by the $GABA_A$ antagonist bicuculline but not by $GABA_B$ antagonists. Since bicuculline methiodide does not cross the blood–brain barrier this indicates that the valproate effect is exerted on peripheral receptors, probably those of parasympathetic neurons (Moskowitz, this volume). Progesterone metabolites also appear to block PPE through $GABA_A$ receptors.

Somatostatin

Somatostatin is a peptide with 14 amino acids and five receptor subtypes which blocks the release of growth hormone and gastric secretion. Somatostatin and octreotide are also known to have analgesic actions (Humphrey, this volume). Possible mechanisms of analgesia that have been considered include: a) vasoconstriction, as somatostatin constricts human saphenous and hand veins, possibly by releasing noradrenaline; b) inhibition of hormone or enzyme release, although there is evidence that somatostatin actually releases 5-HT and NA; c) neuronal inhibition, although it has an excitatory action in some sites; d) release of neurotransmitters such as encephalins; and e) promoting neural degeneration.

Activity in rat dorsal horn neurons is inhibited when somatostatin is given intravenously or directly into the periaqueductal grey matter (PAG) or nucleus raphe magnus, possibly by turning off GABA inhibition in the pain control pathway. The somatostatin receptor is related to opioid (mu) receptors. Somatostatin has already been reported as useful in ameliorating cluster headache. Will it prove helpful for migraine?

CLINICAL STUDIES

Neurophysiology

What determines the recurrence of headaches in the susceptible 10% or so of the population? A number of differences between the normal and migrainous brain can be demonstrated by neurophysiological techniques. The contingent negative variation (CNV) is exaggerated in migrainous patients and does not habituate in the normal manner but does normalize during migraine headache (Schoenen, this volume). In the migrainous subject visual evoked responses do not habituate like those of normal controls. Auditory evoked responses at 70 db stimulation actually augment during repetition rather than habituating as in normal controls. When a random auditory signal was introduced, the initial amplitude of the response was lower but it potentiated with higher intensities of stimulation. Habituation of evoked responses could be regarded as a protective mechanism to prevent undue accumulation of lactate in the cerebral cortex should oxygen consumption exceed supply. Spreading depression could conceivably perform a similar protective task.

The contribution of positron emission tomography

Diener and May (this volume) studied by PET scanning nine patients, first examined within six hours of the onset of right-sided migraine without aura. There was a transient increase in regional cerebral blood flow (rCBF) in the cingulate cortex and the auditory and visual association cortex during headache, but these cortical changes disappeared after the headache was relieved by sumatriptan. Of greater interest were the higher rCBF values found in the medial brainstem, slightly contralateral to the headache side (covering the areas of the periaqueductal grey matter, locus coeruleus, dorsal raphe nucleus and midbrain reticular formation), which persisted after sumatriptan had provided relief from headache but were not present in headache-free intervals three days to four months later. These findings are of particular interest in view of the role of these structures in determining cerebral and extracranial blood flow in the monkey model (Lance *et al.* 1983).

Window on the brain

Fenfluramine releases 5-HT from the human hypothalamus, resulting in elevation of prolactin levels. This response is diminished in depression and increased in panic disorders. When fenfluramine (60 mg) was given to migrainous patients, the prolactin level rose significantly, suggesting hypersensitivity of 5-HT receptors (Glover *et al.*, this volume). Whether dietary factors will operate through a similar mechanism remains to be seen.

Recurrence of headache after sumatriptan

Migraine headache recurs after successful treatment with sumatriptan after 10 hours in about half of the patients given 6 mg subcutaneously and after 16 hours in about one third of patients receiving 100 mg orally (Ferrari and Visser, this volume). This applies to other agents such as ergotamine and analgesics as well. Ergotamine tartrate has a short half-life in the plasma resembling that of sumatriptan but recurrence takes place in 30% of cases after a mean of 23 hours. The tendency to recurrence is probably related to the natural history of the attacks, which may persist for 48 to 72 hours if untreated. Some patients report multiple episodes of recurrence within this time-frame, including the reappearance of an aura.

Plasma concentrations of sumatriptan are probably an unreliable measure of its potential effectiveness if it has to break through some hypothetical barrier to produce its clinical effect. Persistence of the drug effect appears to be determined by diffusion out of the receptor biophase rather than slow dissociation of the drug–receptor complex (Martin and Martin, this volume). This accounts for the longer time to recurrence of headache after the use of ergot alkaloids. The ideal drug for the treatment of migraine would appear to be a selective $5\text{-HT}_{1D\beta}$ agonist combining the slow diffusion properties of the ergots with an ability to access the site of action unimpaired by any biological barrier.

SUMMARY

What have we learned from this compilation of research and discussion? In the light of present knowledge, we can no longer argue whether migraine is a neurological or vascular disease because clearly both elements are involved. Prodromal symptoms of hypothalamic origin (elation, drowsiness or a craving to eat sweet foods) are experienced by some 25% of patients. The triggers for migraine are most often neurological: stress, excessive exposure to light, sounds or smells and so on. Other attacks arise at regular intervals set by some internal clock, the most obvious example being menstrual migraine.

The migrainous brain shows evidence of disturbance of 5-HT, NA and peptide transmitters, as well as magnesium ion content, excitatory amino acids and opioid receptors that have not been discussed in this volume. The discovery on PET scanning that the midbrain in the region of the periaqueductal grey matter, locus coeruleus and dorsal raphe nucleus becomes active during migraine headache and for some time thereafter reinforces the message from earlier animal experimental studies showing the potential significance of these areas in controlling the cerebral and extracranial circulations as well as playing a part in pain control.

Where will our new advances in pharmacology come from? Agents that block cranial vasodilatation and plasma protein extravasation, such as agonists for $5\text{-HT}_{1D\beta}$ receptors with a longer half-life and for GABA_A receptors, are obviously high on the list. Further study of hypothalamic and brainstem nuclei may disclose a means of selective blockade of the migrainous process. New agents like somatostatin may find a place in routine treatment. There are still many unanswered questions but the information provided in this volume forms a good starting point in the quest for more effective remedies in the prevention of migraine.

REFERENCES

Goltman, A.M. (1935/36) The mechanism of migraine. *Journal of Allergy*, **7**, 351–355.

Lance, J.W., Lambert, G.A., Goadsby, P.J. and Duckworth, J.W. (1983) Brain stem influences on the cephalic circulation: experimental data from cat and monkey of relevance to the mechanism of migraine. *Headache*, **23**, 258–265.

Index

Page numbers in **bold** type refer to figures and page numbers in *italics* refer to tables.

Acetazolamide, action in HPCA 284, 288, 290
Acetylcholine (ACh)
 transmitter 200, 202
 and NO release 155, **156**
Acetylsalicylic acid, *see* Aspirin
Ach, *see* Acetylcholine
Adenylyl cyclase, and somatostatin, discussion 231
AEP (auditory evoked potential), in migraineurs 234, 236, **237**, 238
Age of onset
 in CADASIL 285, 287, 301
 in familial migraine 257, 270
 in migraine 275–6
Alcoholic drinks
 effects of 127, 129–30
 and headache, discussion 135–6
 see also Red wine
Alcoholism
 and headache, discussion 136
 and migraine, inverse relationship 268
Altitude, and headache 159
Alzheimer's disease
 and neurotrophic factors, discussion 196, 197
 and pain 186
Amino acids
 in receptor protein 33–4, **35**, 37
 release of in SD 12
Amitriptyline, for headache, discussion 134

Amplitude–stimulus function (ASF), in migraineurs 236–9
Analgesia
 and blockade of *c-fos* expression 147
 somatostatin in 222–7, 305
 discussion 230–32
Angina pectoris 49
Antidepressant drug therapy 187, 188
Antimigraine drugs
 dependency on 94
 discussion 90–91
 effects of 43–50
 discussion 52–4
 and headache recurrence 82–3
 prophylactic agents (methysergide, pizotifen, propranolol) 98, 168, 171
 side-effects of 43
 discussion 78–9
 site of action 68–70
 see also Aspirin; Dihydro-ergotamine; Ergotamine; Methysergide; Pizotifen; Sumatriptan
Antimigraine drugs under development
 311C90 18, 19, 22, 32
 efficacy of, discussion 79
 and headache recurrence 82
 and nausea control 73, 74
 and plasma protein extravasation 22–3